Precision Medi
A Multidisciplinary
Approach

Editorial Advisor

JOEL J. HEIDELBAUGH

ELSEVIER

1600 John F. Kennedy Boulevard • Suite 1800 • Philadelphia, Pennsylvania, 19103-2899

http://www.theclinics.com

CLINICS COLLECTIONS
ISSN 2352-7986, ISBN-13: 978-0-323-78947-9

Editor: John Vassallo (j.vassallo@elsevier.com)

Clinics Collections (ISSN 2352-7986) is published by Elsevier Inc., 360 Park Avenue South, New York, NY 10010-1710. Business and editorial offices: 1600 John F. Kennedy Boulevard, Suite 1800, Philadelphia, PA 19103-2899. **POSTMASTER:** Send address changes to *Clinics Collections*, Elsevier Health Sciences Division, Subscription Customer Service, 3251 Riverport Lane, Maryland Heights, MO 63043. **Customer Service: Telephone: 1-800-654-2452** (U.S. and Canada); **1-314-447-8871** (outside U.S. and Canada). **Fax: 314-447-8029. E-mail: journalscustomerserviceusa@elsevier.com** (for print support); **journalsonlinesupport-usa@elsevier.com** (for online support).

Reprints. For copies of 100 or more of articles in this publication, please contact the Commercial Reprints Department, Elsevier Inc., 360 Park Avenue South, New York, NY 10010-1710. Tel.: 212-633-3874; Fax: 212-633-3820; E-mail: reprints@elsevier.com.

Contributors

EDITOR

JOEL J. HEIDELBAUGH, MD, FAAFP, FACG
Clinical Professor, Departments of Family Medicine and Urology, University of Michigan Medical School, Ann Arbor, Michigan, USA

AUTHORS

KIMBERLY ADERHOLD, DO
Thomas Jefferson University Hospital–Sidney Kimmel Cancer Center, Philadelphia, Pennsylvania, USA

THOMAS J. BALKIN, PhD
Behavioral Biology Branch, Walter Reed Army Institute of Research, Silver Spring, Maryland, USA

DEBASREE BANERJEE, MD, MS
Division of Pulmonary, Critical Care, and Sleep Medicine, Assistant Professor, The Warren Alpert School of Medicine at Brown University, Division of Pulmonary, Critical Care, and Sleep Medicine, Rhode Island Hospital, Providence, Rhode Island, USA

ANNE BARTON, FRCP, PhD
Professor, Division of Musculoskeletal and Dermal Sciences, Arthritis Research UK Centre for Genetics and Genomics, Centre for Musculoskeletal Research, Manchester Academic Health Science Centre, The University of Manchester, NIHR Manchester Musculoskeletal Biomedical Research Unit, Central Manchester NHS Foundation Trust, Manchester Academic Health Science Centre, Manchester, United Kingdom

IVOR J. BENJAMIN, MD, FAHA, FACC
Director, Cardiovascular Center, Department of Medicine, Division of Cardiology, Medical College of Wisconsin, Milwaukee, Wisconsin, USA

JOSEPH BENNETT, MD, FACS
Department of Surgery, Christiana Care Health System, Newark, Delaware, USA

ROBIN L. BENNETT, MS, CGC
Clinical Professor, Division of Medical Genetics, Department of Medicine, University of Washington, University of Washington Medical Center, Seattle, Washington, USA

ADAM C. BERGER, MD, FACS
Professor of Surgery and Chief of Melanoma and Soft Tissue Oncology, Rutgers Cancer Institute of New Jersey, New Brunswick, New Jersey, USA

PHILLIP J. BERON, MD
Associate Professor, Department of Radiation Oncology, Ronald Reagan University of California, Los Angeles Medical Center, Los Angeles, California, USA

JAMES BLUETT, MBBS, PhD
Division of Musculoskeletal and Dermal Sciences, Arthritis Research UK Centre for
Genetics and Genomics, Centre for Musculoskeletal Research, Manchester
Academic Health Science Centre, The University of Manchester, Manchester, United
Kingdom

ELISA BOGOSSIAN, MD
Fellow, Department of Intensive Care, Erasme University Hospital, Brussels,
Belgium

DON A. BUKSTEIN, MD
Allergy, Asthma & Sinus Center, Madison, Wisconsin, USA; Allergy, Asthma & Sinus
Center, Milwaukee, Wisconsin, USA

BRITTANY N. BURTON, MHS
Medical Student, School of Medicine, University of California, San Diego, La Jolla,
California, USA

MARCO CARBONE, MD, PhD
Division of Gastroenterology and Hepatology, Department of Medicine and Surgery,
University of Milan Bicocca, Milan, Italy; Academic Department of Medical Genetics,
University of Cambridge, Cambridge, United Kingdom

LOGAN COREY, MD
Resident, Department of Obstetrics and Gynecology, Ochsner Clinic Foundation, New
Orleans, Louisiana, USA

LAURA CRISTOFERI, MD
Division of Gastroenterology and Hepatology, Department of Medicine and Surgery,
University of Milan Bicocca, Milan, Italy

SHIBANDRI DAS, MD
Surgical Resident, University Hospitals Cleveland Medical Center, MetroHealth Hospitals,
Louis Stokes Veterans Administration Hospital, Case Western Reserve University,
Cleveland, Ohio, USA

ELIZABETH H. DIBBLE, MD
Department of Diagnostic Imaging, The Warren Alpert Medical School of Brown
University, Rhode Island Hospital, Providence, Rhode Island, USA

SHERIFF N. DODOO, MD
Department of Internal Medicine, Meharry Medical College, Nashville, Tennessee,
USA

HENRY MARK DUNNENBERGER, PharmD
Director, Pharmacogenomics, Mark R. Neaman Center for Personalized Medicine,
NorthShore University HealthSystem, Evanston, Illinois, USA

LAURA EISENMENGER, MD
Department of Radiology and Biomedical Imaging, University of California San Francisco,
San Francisco, California, USA

RODNEY A. GABRIEL, MD, MAS
Chief, Division of Regional Anesthesia and Acute Pain, Assistant Clinical Professor,
Departments of Anesthesiology and Medicine, Division of Biomedical Informatics,
University of California, San Diego, La Jolla, California, USA

IAN GREENWALT, MD
Chief Surgical Resident, University Hospitals Cleveland Medical Center, MetroHealth Hospitals, Louis Stokes Veterans Administration Hospital, Case Western Reserve University, Cleveland, Ohio, USA

COLIN HILL, MSc, PhD, DSc
School of Microbiology, APC Microbiome Ireland, University College Cork, Cork, Ireland

THOMAS A. HOPE, MD
Department of Radiology and Biomedical Imaging, University of California San Francisco, Department of Radiology, San Francisco VA Health Care System, San Francisco, California, USA

PETER J. HULICK, MD, MMSc, FACMG
Division Head, Center for Medical Genetics, Medical Director, Mark R. Neaman Center for Personalized Medicine, NorthShore University HealthSystem, Clinical Assistant Professor, University of Chicago, Pritzker School of Medicine, Evanston, Illinois, USA

EUGENE HUO, MD
Department of Radiology and Biomedical Imaging, University of California San Francisco, San Francisco, California, USA

STEVEN HURSH, PhD
Institutes for Behavior Resources, Inc, Baltimore, Maryland, USA

NADIM ILBAWI, MD
Department of Family Medicine, NorthShore University HealthSystem, Lincolnwood, Illinois, USA; Clinician Educator, University of Chicago, Pritzker School of Medicine, Chicago, Illinois, USA

PIETRO INVERNIZZI, MD, PhD
Division of Gastroenterology and Hepatology, Department of Medicine and Surgery, University of Milan Bicocca, Milan, Italy

PRASHANT NATARAJAN IYER, BE (Chem), MTPC, SCPM
Product Director, Healthcare Solutions, Oracle Corporation, Pleasanton, California, USA

ANDREW D. KRYSTAL, MD, MS
Ray and Dagmar Dolby Distinguished Professor, Director, Clinical and Translational Sleep Research Program Director, Dolby Family Center for Mood Disorders Director, Interventional Psychiatry Program, Vice-Chair, Research, Department of Psychiatry, University of California San Francisco, San Francisco, California, USA; Emeritus Professor, Psychiatry and Behavioral Sciences, Duke University School of Medicine, Durham, North Carolina, USA

AONGHUS LAVELLE, MB, PhD
Department of Medicine, APC Microbiome Ireland, University College Cork, Cork, Ireland

JISOO LEE, MD
Division of Pulmonary, Critical Care, and Sleep Medicine, Fellow, The Warren Alpert School of Medicine at Brown University, Division of Pulmonary, Critical Care, and Sleep Medicine, Rhode Island Hospital, Providence, Rhode Island, USA

SHOSHANA LEVI, MD
Department of Surgery, Christiana Care Health System, Newark, Delaware, USA

BENJAMIN D. LI, MD, MBA, FACS
MetroHealth Cancer Center Director, MetroHealth System, Edward Mansour Professor of Surgical Oncology, Case Western Reserve University, Cancer Care Pavilion, Cleveland, Ohio, USA

ALLAN T. LUSKIN, MD
Healthy Airways, Madison, Wisconsin, USA

GREGORY A. MASTERS, MD, FACP, FASCO
Attending Physician, Helen F. Graham Cancer Center and Research Institute, Newark, Delaware, USA; Associate Professor, Thomas Jefferson University Medical School, Philadelphia, Pennsylvania, USA

GEORGE MELLS, MRCP, PhD
Academic Department of Medical Genetics, University of Cambridge, Cambridge, United Kingdom

MARCO MENOZZI, MD
Fellow, Department of Intensive Care, Erasme University Hospital, Brussels, Belgium

ALESSANDRA NARDI, PhD
Department of Mathematics, Tor Vergata University of Rome, Rome, Italy

D. WILLIAMS PARSONS, MD, PhD
Section of Hematology/Oncology, Department of Pediatrics, Baylor College of Medicine, Texas Children's Hospital, Houston, Texas, USA

LUIS E. PICHARD, MHS, PhD
Division of Pulmonary and Critical Care Medicine, Department of Medicine, The Johns Hopkins University School of Medicine, Baltimore, Maryland, USA

ARIC A. PRATHER, PhD
Associate Professor, Director, Behavioral Sleep Medicine Program, Department of Psychiatry, University of California San Francisco, San Francisco, California, USA

LINDSAY SCHWARTZ, PhD
Institutes for Behavior Resources, Inc, Baltimore, Maryland, USA

NITA L. SEIBEL, MD
Division of Cancer Treatment and Diagnosis, Clinical Investigations Branch, National Cancer Institute, Rockville, Maryland, USA

DHAVAL R. SHAH, MBBS, MD
Attending Physician, Helen F. Graham Cancer Center and Research Institute, Newark, Delaware, USA

GUIDO SIMONELLI, MD
Behavioral Biology Branch, Walter Reed Army Institute of Research, Silver Spring, Maryland, USA

OSCAR E. STREETER Jr, MD
Medical Director, The Center for Thermal Oncology, Santa Monica, California, USA

RICHARD D. URMAN, MD, MBA, CPE, FASA
Associate Professor, Department of Anesthesiology, Perioperative and Pain Medicine, Center for Perioperative Research, Brigham and Women's Hospital, Harvard Medical School, Boston, Massachusetts, USA

ANA VALENTE, MD
Resident, Department of Obstetrics and Gynecology, Ochsner Clinic Foundation, New Orleans, Louisiana, USA

JEAN-LOUIS VINCENT, MD, PhD
Professor of Intensive Care Medicine, Université libre de Bruxelles, Consultant, Department of Intensive Care, Erasme University Hospital, Brussels, Belgium

KIEUHOA T. VO, MD, MAS
Department of Pediatrics, University of California San Francisco School of Medicine, Benioff Children's Hospital, San Francisco, California, USA

KATRINA WADE, MD
Gynecologic Oncologist, Department of Gynecologic Oncology, Ochsner Clinic Foundation, New Orleans, Louisiana, USA

DYSON T. WAKE, PharmD
Senior Clinical Specialist, Pharmacogenomics, Mark R. Neaman Center for Personalized Medicine, NorthShore University HealthSystem, Evanston, Illinois, USA

RUTH S. WATERMAN, MD, MSc
Chair, Associate Clinical Professor, Department of Anesthesiology, University of California, San Diego, San Diego, California, USA

DAVID M. WILSON, MD
Department of Radiology and Biomedical Imaging, University of California San Francisco, San Francisco, California, USA

MELISSA WILSON, MD, PhD
Associate Professor, Sidney Kimmel Medical College, Philadelphia, Pennsylvania, USA

DON C. YOO, MD
Associate Professor of Diagnostic Imaging (Clinical), Department of Diagnostic Imaging, The Warren Alpert Medical School of Brown University, Rhode Island Hospital, Providence, Rhode Island, USA

NORAH ZAZA, BA
Medical Student, Case Western Reserve University, Cleveland, Ohio, USA

Contents

with PET/MR imaging can change the diagnosis. This article discusses specific areas in which precision imaging with nontargeted and targeted diagnostic agents can change the diagnosis and treatment.

Genomic insights and analyses of Mendelian hypertension (HTN) syndromes and Genome-Wide Association study (GWAS) on essential hypertension have contributed to the depth of understanding of the genetics origins of hypertension. Mendelian syndromes are important for the field, since such knowledge leads to specific insights about disease pathogenesis and the potential for precision medicine. The clinical impact of findings of GWAS on essential hypertension is continuously evolving, and the insights accrued will refine efforts to combat the societal impact of hypertension. Comprehensive identification of all genomic variants of hypertension, along with their individual associated mechanisms, is paving the way forward in the era of personalized medicine. The overriding challenge for care providers is to reduce health inequities through improved compliance and, perhaps, new paradigms for implementation science that incorporate genomic medicine.

PET/computed tomography (CT) can evaluate the metabolic and anatomic involvement of a variety of inflammatory, infectious, and malignant cardiovascular disorders. PET/CT is useful in evaluating coronary vasculature, hibernating myocardium, cardiac sarcoidosis, cardiac amyloidosis, cerebrovascular disease, acute aortic syndromes, cardiac and vascular neoplasms, cardiac and vascular infections, and vasculitis. Novel targeted radiopharmaceutical agents and novel use of established techniques show promise in diagnosing and monitoring cardiovascular diseases.

The gut microbiome is fundamental to human health and development. Altered microbiomes have been associated with many diseases. However, variation between individuals, environmental effects, and a lack of standardization across studies makes differentiation between health and disease challenging. Large-scale population cohorts in different countries will be required to match disease subjects with healthy controls, whereas standardized, reproducible pipelines for analysis are required to compare findings between studies. Despite this, several conditions have already demonstrated great promise for developing microbiome-based biomarkers as well as providing a gateway into integrated personalized medicine.

> Metabolomics is an emerging field of research interest in sepsis. Metabolomics provides new ways of exploring the diagnosis, mechanism, and prognosis of sepsis. Advancements in technologies have enabled significant improvements in identifying novel biomarkers associated with the disease progress of sepsis. The use of metabolomics in the critically ill may provide new approaches to enable precision medicine. Furthermore, the dynamic interactions of the host and its microbiome can lead to further progression of sepsis. Understanding these interactions and the changes in the host's genomics and the microbiome can provide novel preventive and therapeutic strategies against sepsis.

> Improvements in outcome have been seen in children and adolescents with cancer. Nevertheless, challenges remain in trying to improve the outcomes for all children diagnosed with cancer, particularly in patients with metastatic disease or with cancers that are resistant or recur after standard treatment. Precision medicine trials using individualized tumor molecular profiling for selection of targeted therapies are ongoing in adult malignancies. Similar approaches are being applied to children and adolescents with cancer. This article describes how precision medicine is being applied to pediatric oncology and the unique challenges being faced with these efforts.

> Precision medicine and targeted therapies have a long history in the treatment of breast cancer and continue to show promise for further specialized and individualized care for this disease. From the discovery of endocrine and HER2 targeted therapies, to multigene arrays in chemotherapy for more specific patient selection, to radiomics and genetic subtyping, targeted therapies and precision medicine continue to push the management of breast cancer toward more individualized care. This article describes the foundation and future of targeted therapy and precision medicine in breast cancer.

> Lung cancer remains second most common cancer in men and women in the United States. More than 50% of patients are diagnosed in the advanced stage. Traditionally, chemotherapy has been the backbone of management of stage IV lung cancer. A better understanding of the molecular pathogenesis has led to rapid development of targeted therapy and immunotherapy. This has led to significant improvement in survival of patients with lung cancer stages III to IV. These drugs are being studied in early stage lung cancer. Several trials are ongoing to improve the survival and quality of life of our patients.

insufficiency in hopes for personalizing medical approach to improve patient outcomes. Following a discussion on causes and consequences of sleep loss, this article discusses tools for assessing sleep sufficiency, mitigating strategies to sleep loss, and sleep loss in the context of fatigue management.

Pharmacogenetics is the branch of personalized medicine concerned with the variability in drug response occurring because of heredity. Advances in genetics research, and decreasing costs of gene sequencing, are promoting tremendous growth in pharmacogenetics in all areas of medicine, including sleep medicine. This article reviews the body of research indicating that there are genetic variations that affect the therapeutic actions and adverse effects of agents used for the treatment of sleep disorders to show the potential of pharmacogenetics to improve the clinical practice of sleep medicine.

Pharmacogenomics (PGx) is the study of how individuals' personal genotypes may affect their responses to various pharmacologic agents. The application of PGx principles in perioperative medicine is fairly novel. Challenges in executing PGx programs into health care systems include physician buy-in and integration into usual clinical workflow, including the electronic health record. This article discusses the current evidence highlighting the potential of PGx with various drug categories (including opioids, nonopioid analgesics, sedatives, b-blockers, antiemetics, and anticoagulants) used in the perioperative process and the challenges of integrating PGx into a health care system and relevant workflows.

Preface

Clinics Review Articles have been a part of the physicians', nurses', and residents' library for nearly 100 years. This trusted resource covers more than 50 medical disciplines every year, producing thousands of articles focused on the most current concepts and techniques in medicine. This collection of articles, devoted to precision medicine, draws from this *Clinics* database to provide multidisciplinary teams with practical clinical advice on uses and management of this burgeoning field.

A multidisciplinary perspective is key to effective team-based management. Featured articles from the *Medical Clinics*, *Critical Care Clinics*, *Cardiology Clinics*, *PET Clinics*, *Clinics in Liver Disease*, and *Surgical Oncology Clinics* reflect the wide range of clinicians who manage patients using precision medicine.

I encourage you to share this issue with your colleagues in hopes that it may promote more collaboration, new perspectives, and informed, effective care for your patients.

Joel J. Heidelbaugh, MD, FAAFP, FACG
Departments of Family Medicine and Urology
University of Michigan Medical School
Ann Arbor, MI 48103, USA

Ypsilanti Health Center
200 Arnet, Suite 200
Ypsilanti, MI 48198, USA

E-mail address:
jheidel@umich.edu

https://doi.org/10.1016/j.ccol.2020.07.025
2352-7986/20/© 2020 Published by Elsevier Inc.

Individualizing Care
Management Beyond Medical Therapy

Laura Cristoferi, MD[a], Alessandra Nardi, PhD[b],
Pietro Invernizzi, MD, PhD[a], George Mells, MRCP, PhD[c],
Marco Carbone, MD, PhD[a,d,*]

KEYWORDS

- Primary biliary cholangitis • Precision medicine • Risk-stratification
- Autoimmune liver disease • Individualized care • Novel therapies • Omics

KEY POINTS

- The forthcoming availability of several novel drugs in primary biliary cholangitis (PBC) coupled with the rise of high-throughput omics technologies prompt changing the paradigm of the management of the disease.
- Precision medicine (PM), through the application of omics-based approaches, should enable identifying disease variants, stratifying patients according to disease trajectory, risk of disease progression, and likelihood of response to different therapeutic options in PBC.
- The development of PM needs specific interventions, such as sequencing more genomes, creating bigger biobanks, and linking biological information to health data in electronic medical record.
- The authors envisage that a diagnostic work-up of PBC patients will include information on genetic variants and molecular signature that may define a particular subtype of disease and provide an estimate of treatment response and survival.

Primary biliary cholangitis (PBC) is a chronic, autoimmune liver disease characterized by nonsuppurative granulomatous cholangitis, causing progressive duct destruction and portal fibrosis that progresses slowly to biliary cirrhosis. A substantial proportion of cases eventually develops cirrhosis with attendant complications, such as portal hypertension, chronic liver failure, or hepatocellular cancer (HCC). PBC, therefore, remains a leading indication for liver transplantation (LT).

This article originally appeared in *Clinics in Liver Disease*, Volume 22, Issue 3, August 2018. The authors have nothing to disclose.

[a] Division of Gastroenterology and Hepatology, Department of Medicine and Surgery, University of Milan Bicocca, Piazza dell'Ateneo Nuovo, 1, 20126 Milan, Italy; [b] Department of Mathematics, Tor Vergata University of Rome, Via della Ricerca Scientifica 1, Rome, Italy; [c] Academic Department of Medical Genetics, University of Cambridge, Hills Road 1, Cambridge, UK; [d] Academic Department of Medical Genetics, University of Cambridge, Cambridge, UK
* Corresponding author. Division of Gastroenterology and Hepatology, Department of Medicine and Surgery, University of Milan Bicocca, Piazza dell'Ateneo Nuovo, 1, 20126 Milan, Italy.
E-mail address: marco.carbone@unimib.it

https://doi.org/10.1016/j.ccol.2020.07.001
2352-7986/20/© 2020 Elsevier Inc. All rights reserved.

Advances over the past several years have improved the ability to individualize care in PBC. This is prescient: individualizing care is the aim of precision medicine (PM), described as "an emerging approach for disease treatment and prevention that takes into account individual variability in genes, environment, and lifestyle for each person."[1] The aim of PM is to enable health care workers and biomedical researchers to more accurately predict which treatment and prevention strategies for a particular disease will work in which groups of patients. It contrasts with a 1-size-fits-all approach, in which disease treatment and prevention strategies are developed for the average patient, with less consideration for interindividual variation.[1]

PM relies on biomarkers (or panels of biomarkers) that accurately predict key outcomes, such as treatment response or disease progression (**Fig. 1**). Biomarkers may be measurements in blood, urine, saliva, or other biofluids—but the concept also encompasses features on imaging and histology. Omics-based approaches, coupled with computational and bioinformatics methods, provide an unprecedented opportunity to accelerate biomarker discovery. Such approaches include genetic analysis (genome-wide genotyping of common to rare variants, exome sequencing, and whole-genome sequencing) and a plethora of approaches for profiling the epigenome, transcriptome, proteome, and metabolome (**Fig. 2**). PM is applicable to PBC, as it is to other chronic inflammatory conditions, especially now with the current and forthcoming availability of more efficacious medications.

The clinical features and investigations that already enable individualizing the care of PBC patients are reviewed—and how emerging biomedical technologies might improve the ability to individualize management of PBC patients in the future is speculated on. The premise throughout is that individualized care for PBC, current or future, should achieve the following major objectives:

- Identification of disease variants that may require different management, such as PBC with autoimmune features or the premature ductopenic variant

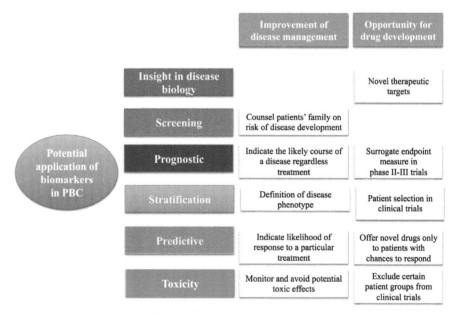

Fig. 1. Potential application of biomarkers in PBC.

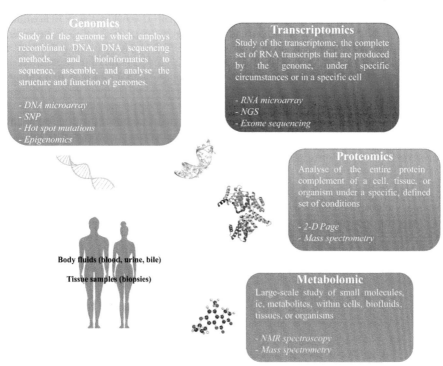

Fig. 2. Example of omics platforms available to study PBC. DNA, deoxyribonucleic acid; NGS, next-generation sequencing; NMR, nuclear magnetic resonance; RNA, ribonucleic acid.

- Stratification of patients according to different disease trajectories that might require different forms of surveillance, such as portal hypertensive progression; hepatocellular failure-type progression, or progression to HCC
- Stratification based on the risk of disease progression
- Stratification based on the likelihood of response to, and side-effects from, different therapeutic options.

In each case, stratification should ideally reflect the underlying mechanism because this informs ongoing development or repurposing of pharmacotherapies. Beyond these major objectives, the authors anticipate that PM initiatives will identify hitherto unknown disease subphenotypes.

STRATIFICATION OF DISEASE VARIANTS

Clinical variants with different disease course have been described. It remains unclear whether these clinical entities are distinct conditions (resulting from unique pathologic processes) or extremes of phenotype (resulting from shared pathologic processes). Either way, it is important to identify patients with variant syndromes because they have different disease trajectories and benefit from different management. PM initiatives should provide insight, if carefully designed.

Primary Biliary Cholangitis with Features of Autoimmune Hepatitis

Also known as PBC/autoimmune hepatitis (AIH) overlap syndrome, primary biliary cholangitis with features of autoimmune hepatitis is a variant of PBC in which there are characteristics of both PBC and AIH. Features of AIH coexist in 8% to 10% of patients with PBC.[2] There is ongoing debate about the nature of PBC with AIH features, whether it is simply the presence of 2 disorders (ie, PBC and AIH) in one individual, a distinct condition with characteristics of PBC and AIH, or one end of the spectrum of hepatic activity in PBC. One reason for ongoing debate is that interface hepatitis, a hallmark of AIH, is also common in PBC, albeit less florid and without other, characteristic histologic features of AIH, such as rosetting and emperipolesis.

It is important to recognize PBC with AIH features because patients with this variant are likely to benefit from combined treatment with ursodeoxycholic acid (UDCA) and classic immunosuppression. Without immunosuppression, it is associated with earlier development of liver fibrosis and cirrhosis.[3] A diagnosis of PBC with AIH features should be considered in any PBC patient with moderately to highly elevated transaminases, with or without raised IgG. The diagnosis should also be considered in PBC patients with inadequate response to treatment with UDCA treatment after 6 months to 12 months showing elevated transaminases[2] (other than elevated alkaline phosphatase [ALP]). The diagnosis is currently made according to Paris criteria[4] endorsed by the European Association for the Study of the Liver (EASL)[2] (**Box 1**). It follows that a liver biopsy is mandatory to make a diagnosis. For those who satisfy the Paris criteria, international guidelines on PBC[2] recommend treatment with immunosuppression (combined or sequential treatment with corticosteroids and azathioprine) in the short term and medium term. A potential problem with the Paris criteria, however, is that they were developed without tests of specificity or sensitivity. This is not a criticism: there is no gold standard against which the Paris criteria may be tested. They might, however, be specific at the cost of sensitivity, meaning they may fail to identify all patients who could benefit from immunosuppression in addition to UDCA. The most recent EASL guidelines on AIH[5] recommend immunosuppressive treatment of AIH patients at lower cutoffs for transaminase or IgG levels and a modified histologic activity index as low as 4 of 18 points. A trial of glucocorticosteroids may, therefore, be

---

Box 1
Diagnostic criteria of primary biliary cholangitis–autoimmune hepatitis overlap syndrome

PBC criteria

ALP >2 × ULN or GGT >5 × ULN

AMA >1:40

Liver biopsy specimen showing florid bile duct lesions

AIH criteria

ALT >5 × ULN or a positive test for anti–smooth muscle antibodies

IgG >2 × ULN

Liver biopsy showing moderate or severe periportal or periseptal lymphocytic piecemeal necrosis

Diagnostic criteria of PBC-AIH overlap syndrome of which at least 2 of 3 accepted criteria for PBC and AIH, respectively, should be present. Histologic evidence of moderate to severe lymphocytic piecemeal necrosis (interface hepatitis) is mandatory for the diagnosis.

Data from Chazouillères O, Wendum D, Serfaty L, et al. Primary biliary cirrhosis-autoimmune hepatitis overlap syndrome: clinical features and response to therapy. Hepatology 1998;28(2):296–301.

warranted in PBC patients with prominent interface hepatitis demonstrated on liver biopsy, even if they do not fulfill the Paris criteria for diagnosis of overlap.

The authors' practical approach is to focus the treatment on the disease that seems to be the predominant entity. The authors suggest treating with immunosuppression if histology shows moderate to severe interface hepatitis, regardless of biochemical (transaminases) activity. Also, the authors suggest not overdiagnosing overlap presentations, given the common presence of mildly to moderately raised transaminases associated with cholestasis (likely a surrogate marker of the interface hepatitis that the authors observe associated with the florid duct lesions of PBC) and that generally responds well to choleretic agents.

Better characterization of PBC with features of AIH is a priority for PM initiatives. The aim is to identify PBC patients who would benefit from immunosuppression, ideally at diagnosis and ideally without recourse to a liver biopsy. Transcriptomic analysis of liver tissue might identify transcriptional biomarkers that can then be sought in circulation. RNA sequencing is not well suited for diagnostic use due to its complexity, computational intensity, limited throughput, and need for expert technicians. In addition, it is challenging to perform RNA sequencing analyses with small amounts of tissue, especially formalin-fixed paraffin-embedded (FFPE) biopsies, which is a limiting factor in large-scale studies. Transcriptomic analysis can be performed on FFPE biopsies using the NanoString (South Lake Union, Seattle, WA, USA) nCounter platform analyzing total mRNA level of hundreds of genes. This might highlight the expression of regulatory genes encoding essential inflammatory chemokines, interleukin, complement that might offer a signature of treatment response to immunosuppressive therapy.[6] Tissue markers should then be correlated with circulating markers. An approach that might yield suitably accurate circulating biomarkers includes immunoassays based on Luminex (Austin, Texas) xMAP (multianalyte profiling) technology that enable simultaneous detection and quantitation of multiple secreted proteins (cytokines, chemokines, growth factors, and so forth).[7] This high-throughput technology produces results comparable to ELISA but with greater efficiency, speed, and dynamic range, allowing a correlation of the composition of the portal tract infiltrate and transcriptomics readout with peripheral immune-phenotype before and after immunosuppression therapy.

The relevant studies will not, however, be easy. PBC with AIH features is a rare variant of a rare disease; therefore, recruiting an adequately powered sample will be difficult. Potential biomarkers must be tested against the current standard, which, as discussed previously, might be flawed. The study would require liver biopsy of PBC patients without AIH features; this is unlikely to be popular among support groups. Potential biomarkers must be tested against biochemical and histologic response to immunosuppression.

Premature Ductopenic Variant

The premature ductopenic variant is a poorly described variant of PBC, with only 4 cases reported in the literature.[8] It is defined histologically by extreme ductopenia disproportionate to the extent of liver fibrosis. Although the extent of fibrosis may be limited initially, progression to cirrhosis might be inevitable in the long term. Laboratory tests show a marked elevation of cholestatic markers (ALP and gamma glutamyl transferase [GGT]). The bilirubin may be elevated without features cirrhosis or portal hypertension. Owing to markedly decreased quality of life, LT is generally required within a few years of presentation.

Whether this is a disease variant or an extreme form of PBC is unknown. When this variant is suspected, a liver biopsy is required to confirm the diagnosis. This may be useful to inform prognosis and guide management. Patients with this variant typically develop jaundice early in the disease course. As a result, they may satisfy listing criteria for LT before they have cirrhosis and liver failure. Provided the symptoms of cholestasis are adequately controlled, however, LT may be safely deferred. Conversely, pruritus is severe and notoriously difficult to control in this variant. For PBC patients known to have premature ductopenia, it may be appropriate to progress rapidly through the stepwise treatment of cholestatic pruritus and consider LT for quality of life sooner rather than later.

There is no specific therapy for the premature ductopenic variant. Anecdotally, response to UDCA is often poor. The efficacy of obeticholic acid and off-label medications, such as fibrates and budesonide, is untested. Clinicians may be hesitant to offer obeticholic acid, which may exacerbate pruritus, to a patient with severe itch. This has to be weighed, however, against the potential benefit of bile duct regeneration and future symptoms improvement. However this approach has not been proved yet.

PM might have a major role to define this severe variant and highlight pathways of treatment.

In the hypothesis that these patients have different bile acid (BA) pools that are increased in their hydrophobicity beyond the capacity of UDCA to moderate or atypical patterns of handling of UDCA itself, a first approach might be to study the phenotype and quantity of circulating BA and liver tissue BA using mass spectrometry–based targeted metabolomics approach. A major challenge, however, is to select patients with this rare condition for study; this implies a major collaborative national or international effort to identify patients with severe itch and jaundice who should then undergo liver biopsy for confirmation diagnosis.

STRATIFICATION OF PATIENTS BY DIFFERENT DISEASE TRAJECTORIES

Preliminary data suggest there may be different patterns of disease progression in PBC. The Japanese Society of Hepatology describes 3 clinical types (**Fig. 3**). A majority of patients progress gradually and remain in the asymptomatic stage for longer than a decade (gradual progressive type). Some patients who progress to portal hypertension presenting without jaundice (portal hypertension type) and others progress rapidly to jaundice and ultimately hepatic failure (jaundice/hepatic failure type). The jaundice/hepatic failure type tends to affect relatively younger patients compared with the other 2 types. Patients with the jaundice/hepatic failure–type PBC are often positive for anti-gp210 antibody, whereas those with the portal hypertension–type PBC have anticentromere antibodies. The latter antibodies are characteristic of systemic sclerosis (SSc) but are also found in PBC patients without coexistent SSc.[9–11] The only two, old, studies describing this clinical entity looking at the underlying pathologic damage suggest that portal hypertension is initially of presinusoidal type and then as the disease progresses is joined by a sinusoidal component.[12,13] Alternatively, given the strong association with anticentromere antibodies, the mechanism might be that of noncirrhotic portal hypertension occurring in SSc and other connective tissue diseases. As a form of noncirrhotic portal hypertension, this type of progression of PBC is generally recognized by (1) the presence of unequivocal signs of portal hypertension; (2) the absence of cirrhosis, advanced fibrosis, or other causes of chronic liver diseases; and (3) the absence of thrombosis of the hepatic veins or of the portal vein at imaging. In these patients, the liver function is usually preserved; the treatment is based on the monitoring and prevention of complications of portal hypertension, with only few patients requiring LT for unmanageable portal hypertension or liver

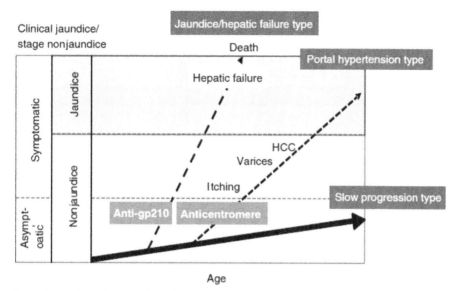

Fig. 3. Potential trajectories based on the autoantibody profile in PBC. (*From* Working Sub-group (English version) for Clinical Practice Guidelines for Primary Biliary Cirrhosis. Guidelines for the management of primary biliary cirrhosis: the Intractable Hepatobiliary Disease Study Group supported by the Ministry of Health, Labour and Welfare of Japan. Hepatol Res 2014;44 Suppl S1:71–90; with permission.)

failure. A target proteomic approach looking at markers on inflammation and/or fibrosis and their dynamic over time might be appropriate to better define different disease trajectories.

STRATIFICATION OF PATIENTS BY RISK OF DISEASE PROGRESSION
Stage of Disease

Measures of liver fibrosis, that is, the stage of disease, are relevant in prognostication because in PBC; as in other liver diseases, they predict treatment response and liver failure.[14,15] Liver biopsy is the gold standard to assess liver fibrosis. Its invasiveness with significant potential complications and the poor patient acceptance, however, coupled with its inherent shortcomings related to sampling error have led to an exponential interest in the identification and use of noninvasive markers of liver fibrosis. To be included in clinical practice, noninvasive markers should predict treatment response, survival, and the risk of cancer and portal hypertension.

Pathologic features

Liver biopsy for staging of PBC lost favor after the publication of a study by Garrido and Hubscher[16]: in this study, the investigators evaluated fibrosis using Menghini needle from simulated needle biopsy in fields approximately the size of conventional needle biopsy and from whole-section scanning in areas with little and extensive fibrosis. They showed considerable variation in the stage of fibrosis across each of 50 explanted PBC livers, evaluated using the staging system of Ludwig and colleagues.[17] There have been no subsequent studies to verify or challenge this observation. There is less variability in staging using the new system of Nakanuma.[18] In this system, the stage of disease is based on the degree of fibrosis, bile duct loss, and cholestasis assessed by deposition of orcein-positive granules, whereas the grade of necroinflammatory activity is based on cholangitis, interface hepatitis, and lobular hepatitis. The accumulation of orcein-positive granules occurs evenly across the PBC liver, which means that staging using the Nakanuma system is more reliable.[19,20] Even so, the widespread availability of noninvasive measures of fibrosis means that liver biopsy for staging of PBC is somewhat obsolete. Liver biopsy does, however, remain useful in certain settings. Nowadays, the main indications are to confirm the diagnosis of PBC when PBC-specific antibodies are absent and confirm a diagnosis of PBC with AIH features. Liver biopsy is also useful to confirm ductopenia and assess the relative contribution of each liver injury when a comorbid liver disease is present, such as nonalcoholic steatohepatitis. In patients with inadequate response to UDCA, liver biopsy may provide the explanation. For example, it may identify a previously unsuspected variant syndrome, steatohepatitis, or interface hepatitis of moderate or greater severity.

Liver biopsy could undoubtedly inform risk stratification in PBC. For example, the Nakanuma[18] stage and grade have been shown to correlate with clinicolaboratory features. Recent data have shown an association between interface hepatitis, bridging fibrosis, and cirrhosis and long-term outcomes in PBC independently from UDCA treatment, confirming historical data.[14,15] Furthermore, the presence of ductopenia/bile duct loss has been reported to be a predictor of PBC progression.[21] These data suggest that liver biopsy could be as important for treatment stratification in PBC as it is in AIH and other liver conditions—but the balance of risk versus benefit and patient acceptability need to be considered. This is exactly the area of unmet need that PM should address.

Ideally, analysis of circulating byproducts (eg, epigenetic factors, such as microRNAs, cell-free DNA, glucose, and fatty acid and amino acid metabolites from high-throughput omics profiling, among others), namely liquid biopsy, could provide access to molecular information related to the severity of portal inflammation, biliary damage, cholestasis, and fibrosis and thus improve patients' stratification and allow evaluation of disease biology dynamically over time. To develop such noninvasive surrogate test of liver pathology, a major effort would be required to select a cohort of PBC patients who undergo deep phenotyping of liver tissue samples and biofluids (such as serum, plasma, peripheral blood mononuclear cells, and urine) at different time points. Building up a well-sized cohort in such a rare condition and performing follow-up liver biopsies are challenging. Nonetheless, this is a promising horizon toward which further research efforts should be directed.

Non-invasive markers of fibrosis

Liver stiffness measure (LSM) by transient elastography, aspartate aminotransferase (AST)-to-platelet ratio index (APRI), and enhanced liver fibrosis (ELF) represent alternative and potentially complementary approaches to assessing liver fibrosis and are associated with minimal discomfort and hazard to the patient when compared with biopsy.

LSM has been regarded as a good marker to exclude or confirm severe fibrosis or cirrhosis in PBC. The largest study (N = 103) demonstrated high specificity and sensitivity (>90%) of transient elastography in distinguishing severe fibrosis from cirrhosis in PBC patients.[22] A threshold of LSM greater than 9.6 kPa (F4) at diagnosis was associated with a 5-fold increase in the risk of future liver decompensation or LT. The results were not as strong when it came to intermediate fibrosis (F2: sensitivity 0.67, specificity 1.0). This may be due to the presence of inflammation and cholestasis that could overestimate the measurement.[22]

Investigators also show a predictive role of longitudinal assessment of LSM: a progression of greater than or equal to 2.1 kPa/y in the overall cohort was associated with 8-fold increased risk of liver decompensation, LT, or death.[22] Before proposing regular assessments of LSM as standard practice, however, for example, on an annual basis, these data would require external validation in a large cohort, in longitudinal fashion. Also, whether the risk estimate is independent of the achievement of treatment response has to be clarified.

There is convincing evidence for the use of APRI in prognostication of PBC. In a recent study of 386 PBC patients, the APRI measured at baseline or after 1 year of therapy with UDCA independently predicted LT-free survival. Measured at baseline, APRI greater than 0.54 best discriminated good versus poor prognosis. Measured after 1 year of treatment, APRI greater than 0.54 identified a subgroup of patients at risk of disease progression despite meeting the Paris I, Paris II, Barcelona, and Toronto definitions of UDCA response.[23]

The ELF score, calculated from serum measurements of hyaluronic acid, tissue inhibitor of metalloproteinase 1, and procollagen type III N-terminal propeptide, is another noninvasive marker proposed in PBC. There is only 1 multicenter study (N = 161) looking at the ELF score in PBC. ELF showed a good ability to stratify patients into groups of differing prognoses. Prediction of decompensations was good, with an area under a receiver operating characteristic curve (AUC) ranging between 0.68 and 0.78 based on how many years before the first event the serum was collected; however, no calibration, that is, agreement between predicted versus observed events, was provided.[24]

The development of the ELF score is paradigmatic of the potentiality to transfer biomarkers (proteomic markers, in this case) from discovery to clinical practice; it also highlights the pitfalls and limitations of this. Despite encouraging results, ELF score has not been adopted with enthusiasm in clinical practice in PBC, and overall in hepatology, and its use is currently limited to clinical trials where fibrosis is an endpoint (eg, https://clinicaltrials.gov/ct2/show/NCT01672853). The main limitation for its use include the high cost of the equipment and the need for regular recalibration and trained operators to ensure accuracy and reproducibility of the results. There are also concerns regarding its biological meaning and interpretation: for instance, it is unclear whether ELF is a marker of disease severity or disease stage; fluctuations over time have not been studied and this prevents its application as dynamic biomarker; also, stratified analysis for influence factors, such as gender, age and ethnicity, are lacking.[25] More data on ELF score application in patients with PBC are needed to make firm recommendations on its use in this condition A head-to-head comparison with the most robust, currently available prognostic tests, such as the continuous scoring systems (UK-PBC and GLOBE scores) and the transient elastography, would be of interest.

Treatment Response Profile

First-line treatment of PBC is UDCA.[26] Although a majority of patients have an improvement of the liver biochemistry after this therapy, 20% to 40% of patients have insufficient or no response to UDCA. Since 2016, obeticholic acid has been approved by the Food and Drug Administration and European Medicines Agency as a second-line treatment in association with UDCA in nonresponders to first-line therapy or in those intolerant to UDCA monotherapy. Moreover, several molecules targeting pathways involved in cholestasis or immune-related mechanisms might soon be available. It follows the importance of risk-stratification of patients' management based on the treatment response profile to allocate the best treatment to the right patient and improve the overall management.

Age and gender

Age and gender were shown to influence response to treatment with UDCA in PBC in the UK-PBC national cohort.[27] Gender was not confirmed, however, to be a predictor of treatment response in the international cohort of the Global PBC Study Group.[28]

Younger age at diagnosis was strongly and independently associated with response to UDCA, with an approximately linear relationship between age and the probability of response; rates ranged from 90% for patients greater than 70 years to 50% for those younger than age 30. The authors suggest that the relationship between age at diagnosis and likelihood of UDCA response was explicable by the effect of hormones, such that high estrogen levels increase resistance to effective treatment.[27] Furthermore, age and gender seemed to correlate with symptoms. Young girls were more likely to have fatigue and pruritus than older and male patients. The Newcastle group showed that fatigue is associated with a reduced survival.[29] Whether this translates in a worse outcome for young women is not clear.

Liver biochemistry

It is well established that the liver function tests (LFTs) on treatment with UDCA strongly predict LT-free survival in PBC.[30] This observation has prompted the development of several prognostic models based on the UDCA response that may be used to stratify patients according to their risk of developing chronic liver failure.

UDCA biochemical response can be assessed using either a qualitative definition based on binary variables or quantitative scoring systems computed from continuous parameters.[2] All these definitions and scores have been developed to be used only after 1 year of UDCA therapy to stratify according to treatment response.

Qualitative definitions Qualitative definitions use thresholds of the LFTs, such as bilirubin, transaminases, and ALP, after 6 months to 24 months of treatment with UDCA on a stable, optimized dose (13–15 mg/kg/d) to dichotomize patients into responders or nonresponders. The best-known of these binary definitions are reported in **Box 2**. Their accuracy in predicting death or LT has been validated externally[27] and they have all been proposed in the recent Clinical Practice Guidelines of EASL 2017.[2] Where binary definitions are used for risk stratification, it is advised to use a definition with higher sensitivity but lower specificity. Possibly for this reason, the POISE trial definition of UDCA nonresponse (total bilirubin >1 × upper limit of normal [ULN] or ALP $\geq$1.67 × ULN) seems to have become the commercial standard, included in the eligibility criteria or endpoints of the phase I/II study of FFP104 by Fast Forward Pharmaceuticals (Utrecht, Netherlands); phase II study of LJN452 by Novartis (Basel, Switzerland), and phase II study of MBX-8025 by CymaBay (Newark, California, USA) Therapeutics (for details, see https://clinicaltrials.gov/). EASL advocates ALP less than 1.5 × ULN as the threshold at which long-term risk becomes clinically meaningful compared with a control healthy population.[2]

The main advantage of dichotomous definition is that they are easy to use. Such definitons do, however, have limitations because they could potentially lead to loss of important predictive information. Most importantly, they imply there are only 2 levels of risk, which is inaccurate. There is a continuous relationship between the individual LFT and the risk of liver death or LT.[31] Thus, dichotomous definitions fail to quantify intermediate levels of risk. Furthermore, they ignore the relationship between risk and time. They do not indicate whether the high-risk patient will need an LT tomorrow or 15 years in the future.

Box 2
Biochemical response criteria for risk stratification in ursodeoxycholic acid–treated primary
biliary cholangitis patients and characteristics of the cohorts where they were developed

Response Definitions and Prognostic Models	Definition and Parameters Evaluated	Type of Prediction	Number of Patients	Centers
Paris I, 2008	ALP <3 × ULN, AST <2 × ULN and bilirubin ≤1 mg/dL after 1 y	Dichotomous	292	Single center
Barcelona, 2006	>40% decrease of ALP or normalization after 1 y	Dichotomous	192	Single center
Toronto, 2010	ALP ≤1.67 × ULN after 2 y	Dichotomous	69	Single center
Paris II, 2011	ALP ≤1.5 × ULN, AST ≤1.5 × ULN and bilirubin ≤l mg/dL after 1 y	Dichotomous	165	Single center
Rotterdam, 2009	Normalization of abnormal bilirubin and/or albumin after 1 y	Dichotomous	375	Single center
GLOBE score, 2015	Age, bilirubin, albumin, ALP, platelets	Continuous	2488	15 tertiary centers
UK-PBC score, 2016	Bilirubin, alanine aminotransferase (ALT)/AST ALP, platelets, albumin	Continuous	1916	155 secondary and tertiary centers

Quantitative scoring systems Proposed by the UK-PBC Research Group and the Global PBC Study Group,[28,31] quantitative scoring systems enable hepatologists to overcome the limitations of the binary risk stratification. In particular, these models quantify an individual's risk in relation to time. In comparison with the binary definition of response that only evaluate parameters of disease activity, they include surrogate markers of disease stage. Both UK-PBC and GLOBE outperform the Paris I definition.[32]

Each risk score includes the LFTs after treatment with UDCA as well as surrogate measurements of disease stage (see **Box 2**). In addition, the GLOBE score includes the age at diagnosis. In both risk scores, all the predictive variables are continuous—and treated as such. The UK-PBC risk score estimates the risk of LT or liver-related death occurring within 5 years, 10 years, or 15 years. The GLOBE score predicts LT-free survival at 3 years, 5 years, 10 years, and 15 years. Both risk scores were shown to outperform previous models, with C statistics at 15 years in the validation cohorts of 0.90 and 0.82, respectively.

In clinical practice, the UK-PBC and GLOBE scores should be most useful to identify patients who would obtain greatest benefit from further risk-reduction using second-line therapy. This is timely with several potential disease-modifying agents for PBC in phase II or III clinical trials. The UK-PBC and GLOBE scores may also be used to identify low-risk patients, for whom follow-up in primary care may be appropriate. There are no clear-cut thresholds that should prompt addition of second-line therapies or de-escalation of follow-up back to primary care. These thresholds vary from one patient to the next, influenced by the patient profile (age, fibrosis stage, and severity of itch, among others), side effects, and cost-effectiveness of a specific agent.

To date, metabolomics analysis of various classes of blood metabolites has been proposed only to define distinct profiles in patients with PBC. It would also allow, however, classifying patient responsiveness to therapies. The circulating metabolome capturing different metabolites classes (eg, BAs, aminoacids, acylcarnitines, Krebs cycle intermediates, lipids species, among the others), some of which in key biochemical pathways are known to be involved in PBC responsiveness, might be able to be defined by open (untargeted) and close (targeted) approaches. These might be integrated in the predicting model of treatment response to UDCA the authors recently proposed to develop enhanced predictive approaches for identification of high-risk patients earlier in the disease and facilitating application of enhanced therapy in a more timely fashion.[33]

Primary Biliary Cholangitis–Specific Autoantibody Profile

The anti-gp210 targets glycoprotein 210 of the nuclear pore complex. It is reportedly associated with more aggressive disease. In 3 studies from Italy and Japan, the presence of anti-gp210 antibodies was associated with more advanced disease, suggesting that anti-gp210 antibodies might be related to hepatocellular failure-type progression.[32] More recently, antibodies against hexokinase (HK1) and a nuclear protein involved in the metabolism of collagen (KL-p) have been shown sensitive and specific for detection of PBC and could be useful in diagnosis in Anti-mitochondrial M2 antibody (AMA-M2) negative, gp210 antibody negative, and sp100 antibody-negative patients. Furthermore, investigators found a correlation between the presence of antibodies anti-HK1 and disease progression, with lower transplant-free survival.[34] The PBC-specific antinuclear antibodies (ANAs) are still of limited validity in clinical practice because studies showing their prognostic role are limited and only retrospective. Longitudinal, large-scale studies using time-to-event data are needed to confirm their role as reliable markers of prognosis.

PERSPECTIVES OF PRECISION MEDICINE IN PRIMARY BILIARY CHOLANGITIS

To facilitate the identification of high-risk individuals for cost-effective disease monitoring and second-line therapies, mounting efforts have been put forth to develop risk prediction models, including biochemical variables with good accuracy and calibration regarding survival. The next step is the identification and incorporation of novel biomarkers, including genetic and molecular biomarkers, to allow identification of disease variants and trajectory, and to estimate the risk of disease progression and the likelihood of treatment response, paving the way for PM in PBC.

The PM initiative ongoing in PBC, as in many other fields of medicine, promises a new era of health care with targeted disease treatment and management. This features a longitudinal study of national and international cohorts of 1000 or more people with large quantity of data and biospecimens necessary to conduct a wide range of studies, with the aim of customizing interventions based on a person's profile.

Conducting a large study cohort study is challenging from several aspects: identification of financial resources needed for implementing such a large-scale project; time required to obtain meaningful results — this is a major problem in PBC due to its indolent nature, where prospective studies of outcomes would span decades to allow for a robust number of endpoints to occur; obtaining permission for data sharing and the need for researchers to recontact/consent participants; concerns about privacy, security, and access to individual data and health records; and coordination, transparency, and governance.

PM is expected to benefit from combining genetic and molecular studies with high-throughput methods, that is, genomics, transcriptomics, proteomics, and metabolomics, among others. These methods permit the determination of thousands of molecules within a tissue or biological fluid that can configure the signature of a disease. The use of these methods is demanding in terms of the design of the study, acquisition, storage, analysis, and interpretation of the data.

When carried out within the adequate medical context, genetic screens are powerful tools for identifying new genes and variations within genes that are involved in specific physiopathologic processes. An example in hepatology is the variant of patatin-like phospholipase domain-containing protein 3 gene (PNPLA3) that has been associated with the susceptibility and histologic severity of nonalcoholic fatty liver disease (NALFD).[35] PNPLA3 has been proposed as a novel biomarker for (gene-based) classification of NALFD and should be considered in the diagnostic work-up of this disease.

Genetic information will likely help advance the field of pharmacogenomics. Many single-nucleotide polymorphisms (SNPs) have been used to predict outcomes of specific pharmacologic agents. Some SNPs are used to predict whether an individual is susceptible to side effects from a certain class of drugs. Several groups, including the authors', are trying to create simpler tools that combine genetic and molecular data along with clinical and demographic parameters to predict treatment response to UDCA. In theory, this could be used at the outset to decide whether to escalate treatment of high-risk patients, offering second-line treatment at the outset.

An example of how genomics can be brought to real practice is the 100,000 Genomes Project, which was launched in 2012 in the United Kingdom. This project is performing whole-genome sequencing of 100,000 genomes from 70,000 individuals with rare diseases, their families, and patients with cancer. The main aim of this program is to set up a genomic medicine service for National Health Service patients with potential benefits in disease prevention, management, and treatment. It will also stimulate the development of diagnostics, devices, medicines, and treatments based on a new understanding of the genetic and molecular basis of disease. Finally, it will build partnerships between National Health Service, academia, and industry.

Genomic technologies have made feasible investigating the expression of thousands of genes, that is, transcriptomics, at a time using large sets of samples. The clinical application of transcriptomics profiling to reveal novel gene expression signatures is challenging in a complex disease like PBC for the following reasons. PBC might result from a large number of different genes and biological pathways and several phenotypes; therefore, large cohorts of well-characterized patients are necessary to obtain genomic signatures of clinical relevance. Also, pathogenic (that may be immune-related) and prognostic genes signatures (that may be related to fibrosis progression rather than severity of biliary inflammation) might contain a large number of genes and the prediction algorithms may be complex and not easy to transfer to routine clinical practice. Finally, there is the problem of false-positive tests inherent to all high-throughput techniques where large data sets are analyzed. That said, when used correctly, transcriptomics technologies may be translated into scoring systems that can reproducibly predict clinical outcomes. An example in hepatology is the development of a simple risk score classifier based on the expression of a small number of genes that can predict in a reproducible manner overall survival of patients after surgical resection for HCC.[36]

Another branch of omics-based technology is the high-throughput identification and quantification of small-sized molecules, that is, metabolomics. There is increased interest in understanding which metabolic differences between normal and diseased tissues can lead to the development of more selective and effective treatments. The main aim of metabolomics research is the discovery of specific metabolic profiles in serum, urine, feces, tissues, and other biological materials that are associated with disease features, response to specific treatments, or survival. Blood is the most commonly collected (as serum or plasma) and stored biological fluid in epidemiologic studies and has been the most often used sample in metabolomics analyses to date. Because blood components are under tight homeostatic regulation, the extent of variation in blood metabolite concentration is limited. Urine samples represent a good alternative to blood and have greater capture of exogenous compounds, such as microbiota, drugs, and diet, and urine composition can vary a lot, especially in disease states. A 24-hour collection is preferred over spot urine collection because it provides a complete picture of cumulative metabolite excretion over a 24-hour period. However, 24-hour samples are difficult to collect for epidemiologic studies.

The development of metabolomics-based diagnostic and prognostic tests has the same problems inherent to all high-throughput techniques, that is, the detection of true relationships between a group of metabolites and disease, minimizing the risk of false-positive associations. An additional complication in metabolomics, compared with other omics-based methods, is the preparation and storage of the samples, due to large differences in solubility and stability among metabolites. This is particularly important in relation to epidemiologic studies because samples regularly undergo freeze-thaw cycles that may unpredictably affect the analytical results. Metabolic profiling can run in either targeted or untargeted mode. Targeted profiling separates a limited number of specific metabolites of known identity and is a more hypothesis-driven approach. In PBC, such an approach might be focused on markers of BA physiology, inflammation, and fibrosis. Untargeted approaches are applied to capture metabolic classes that escape target analysis (eg, Krebs cycle intermediates, short-chain fatty acids, nucleotides). Untargeted analysis does not require an a priori hypothesis and can be used to discover novel metabolic associations and disease pathways. Data density is high, however, and because analysis is not optimized for specific metabolites, metabolite identification and quantification may be difficult. Several targeted attempts to identify a metabolomics signature are ongoing in PBC; these highlighted altered metabolic pathways associated with glucose, fatty acid, and amino acid metabolites.[37,38] Effort is required to associate the metabolomics profile with clinical features, such as disease subphenotypes, symptoms, disease course, treatment response, and survival.

Before initiating such studies, it is of primary importance to have a robust hypothesis, which dictates the entire omics workflow and greatly influences the study outcomes. The hypothesis dictates which technologies to choose from (eg, genomic and transcriptomic approaches to study the immunologic signature of the disease; metabolomics approaches on plasma and urine to study the cholestatic component; and proteomic approach to identify markers of the different patterns of fibrosis progression in PBC), the sample to study (eg, circulating cells vs infiltrating cells and whole blood cells vs peripheral blood mononuclear cells), and which approaches to use (eg, targeted vs untargeted metabolomics study) to carry on the study. As a next step, integration of omics data (transomics) is useful, complementary, and more informative than if single omics stood alone, despite being challenging.

Omics-based research to develop PM, however, requires more than just accumulating data. First of all, it is necessary to develop standard protocols that yield consistent results in different laboratories so that data can be built into a single repository. Another problem is the integration of all the data generated by omics-based screens (such as RNAs, proteins, metabolites, protein-protein interactions, protein-lipid interactions, protein-nucleic acid interactions, and so on). Finally, practical application will necessitate the creation of tools by which omics information can be filtered and made readily accessible to clinicians who will incorporate it into medical decision making at the point of care. A key component to advance PM from the academic setting to the point of care in the community is the incorporation of genetic and molecular databases directly into a universal electronic medical record (EMR) system. An effective EMR system prompts practitioners to follow certain diagnostic or treatment algorithms based on an individual's information and reference genomic/molecular datasets stored in the EMR.

PM, when fully realized, has great potential to change the way patients are managed with PBC today. Knowing the genetic and/or molecular variations linked to specific disease phenotype might influence the way disease is screened for drugs are selected and disease progression is surveyed. Ideally, all patients who enter a health care system in the future will have their DNA/molecular profile routinely sequenced and analyzed at admission and entered into a database to enhance patient care. The cost of obtaining, analyzing, storing, and integrating this information will have to be balanced with the potential overall savings to the health care system.

SUMMARY

In view of forthcoming availability of novel drugs that might have a positive impact on morbidity and mortality of patients with PBC and thanks to the rise of high-throughput omics technologies, the PBC field is now moving more quickly toward clinical translation to support PM. PM development has a great potential to change the standard of care in diagnostics, therapeutics, and clinical trials in this disease. In the future, a diagnostic work-up of PBC patients may include information on genetic variants and molecular signature that may define a particular subtype of disease and provide an estimate of treatment response and survival. To reach this point, specific interventions are needed, such as sequencing more genomes, creating bigger biobanks, and linking biological information to health data in EMR. This hopefully will help to shed light on the pathogenic mechanisms of this condition and translate knowledge into new therapies and care pathways.

REFERENCES

1. Collins FS, Varmus H. A new initiative on precision medicine. N Engl J Med 2015; 372(9):793–5.
2. Hirschfield GM, Beuers U, Corpechot C, et al. EASL clinical practice guidelines: the diagnosis and management of patients with primary biliary cholangitis. J Hepatol 2017;67(1):145–72.
3. Poupon R, Chazouilleres O, Corpechot C, et al. Development of autoimmune hepatitis in patients with typical primary biliary cirrhosis. Hepatology 2006; 44(1):85–90.
4. Chazouillères O, Wendum D, Serfaty L, et al. Primary biliary cirrhosis-autoimmune hepatitis overlap syndrome: clinical features and response to therapy. Hepatology 1998;28(2):296–301.
5. European Association for the Study of the Liver. EASL clinical practice guidelines: autoimmune hepatitis. J Hepatol 2015;63(4):971–1004.

6. Millar B, Wong LL, Green K, et al. Autoimmune hepatitis patients with poor treatment response have a distinct liver transcriptome: implications for personalised therapy. J Hepatol 2017;66(1):S364.

7. Ercole A, Magnoni S, Vegliante G, et al. Current and emerging technologies for probing molecular signatures of traumatic brain injury. Front Neurol 2017;8:450.

8. Vleggaar FP, van Buuren HR, Zondervan PE, et al, Dutch Multicentre PBC Study Group the DMP Study. Jaundice in non-cirrhotic primary biliary cirrhosis: the premature ductopenic variant. Gut 2001;49(2):276–81.

9. Liberal R, Grant CR, Sakkas L, et al. Diagnostic and clinical significance of anti-centromere antibodies in primary biliary cirrhosis. Clin Res Hepatol Gastroenterol 2013;37(6):572–85.

10. Nakamura M, Kondo H, Tanaka A, et al. Autoantibody status and histological variables influence biochemical response to treatment and long-term outcomes in Japanese patients with primary biliary cirrhosis. Hepatol Res 2015;45(8):846–55.

11. Nakamura M, Kondo H, Mori T, et al. Anti-gp210 and anti-centromere antibodies are different risk factors for the progression of primary biliary cirrhosis. Hepatology 2007;45(1):118–27.

12. Navasa M, Parés A, Bruguera M, et al. Portal hypertension in primary biliary cirrhosis. J Hepatol 1987;5(3):292–8.

13. Kew MC, Varma RR, Dos Santos HA, et al. Portal hypertension in primary biliary cirrhosis. Gut 1971;12(10):830–4.

14. Corpechot C, Abenavoli L, Rabahi N, et al. Biochemical response to ursodeoxycholic acid and long-term prognosis in primary biliary cirrhosis. Hepatology 2008; 48(3):871–7.

15. Carbone M, Sharp SJ, Heneghan MA, et al. P1198: histological stage is relevant for risk-stratification in primary biliary cirrhosis. J Hepatol 2015;62:S805.

16. Garrido MC, Hubscher SG. Accuracy of staging in primary biliary cirrhosis. J Clin Pathol 1996;49(7):556–9. Available at: http://www.ncbi.nlm.nih.gov/pubmed/8813953. Accessed January 15, 2018.

17. Ludwig J, Dickson ER, McDonald GS. Staging of chronic nonsuppurative destructive cholangitis (syndrome of primary biliary cirrhosis). Virchows Arch A Pathol Anat Histol 1978;379(2):103–12. Available at: http://www.ncbi.nlm.nih.gov/pubmed/150690. Accessed January 15, 2018.

18. Nakanuma Y, Zen Y, Harada K, et al. Application of a new histological staging and grading system for primary biliary cirrhosis to liver biopsy specimens: interobserver agreement. Pathol Int 2010;60(3):167–74.

19. Desmet VJ. Histopathology of cholestasis. Verh Dtsch Ges Pathol 1995;79: 233–40. Available at: http://www.ncbi.nlm.nih.gov/pubmed/8600686. Accessed January 15, 2018.

20. Goldfischer S, Popper H, Sternlieb I. The significance of variations in the distribution of copper in liver disease. Am J Pathol 1980;99(3):715–30. Available at: http://www.ncbi.nlm.nih.gov/pubmed/7386600. Accessed January 15, 2018.

21. Kumagi T, Guindi M, Fischer SE, et al. Baseline ductopenia and treatment response predict long-term histological progression in primary biliary cirrhosis. Am J Gastroenterol 2010;105(10):2186–94.

22. Corpechot C, Carrat F, Poujol-Robert A, et al. Noninvasive elastography-based assessment of liver fibrosis progression and prognosis in primary biliary cirrhosis. Hepatology 2012;56(1):198–208.

23. Trivedi PJ, Bruns T, Cheung A, et al. Optimising risk stratification in primary biliary cirrhosis: AST/platelet ratio index predicts outcome independent of ursodeoxycholic acid response. J Hepatol 2014;60(6):1249–58.

24. Mayo MJ, Parkes J, Adams-Huet B, et al. Prediction of clinical outcomes in primary biliary cirrhosis by serum enhanced liver fibrosis assay. Hepatology 2008; 48(5):1549–57.

25. Lichtinghagen R, Pietsch D, Bantel H, et al. The Enhanced Liver Fibrosis (ELF) score: normal values, influence factors and proposed cut-off values. J Hepatol 2013;59(2):236–42.

26. Poupon R, Poupon R, Calmus Y, et al. Is ursodeoxycholic acid an effective treatment for primary biliary cirrhosis? Lancet 1987;329(8537):834–6.

27. Carbone M, Mells GF, Pells G, et al. Sex and age are determinants of the clinical phenotype of primary biliary cirrhosis and response to ursodeoxycholic acid. Gastroenterology 2013;144(3):560–9.e7.

28. Lammers WJ, Hirschfield GM, Corpechot C, et al. Development and validation of a scoring system to predict outcomes of patients with primary biliary cirrhosis receiving ursodeoxycholic acid therapy. Gastroenterology 2015;149(7): 1804–12.e4.

29. Jones DE, Al-Rifai A, Frith J, et al. The independent effects of fatigue and UDCA therapy on mortality in primary biliary cirrhosis: results of a 9year follow-up. J Hepatol 2010;53(5):911–7.

30. Leuschner U, Fischer H, Kurtz W, et al. Ursodeoxycholic acid in primary biliary cirrhosis: results of a controlled double-blind trial. Gastroenterology 1989;97(5): 1268–74. Available at: http://www.ncbi.nlm.nih.gov/pubmed/2551765. Accessed January 16, 2018.

31. Carbone M, Sharp SJ, Flack S, et al. The UK-PBC risk scores: derivation and validation of a scoring system for long-term prediction of end-stage liver disease in primary biliary cholangitis. Hepatology 2016;63(3):930–50.

32. Yang F, Yang Y, Wang Q, et al. The risk predictive values of UK-PBC and GLOBE scoring system in Chinese patients with primary biliary cholangitis: the additional effect of anti-gp210. Aliment Pharmacol Ther 2017;45(5):733–43.

33. Carbone M, Nardi A, Carpino G, et al. Pre-treatment risk stratification in primary biliary cholangitis: A predictive model to guide first-line combination therapy. 50(1):21–2.

34. Reig A, Garcia M, Shums Z, et al. The novel hexokinase 1 antibodies are useful for the diagnosis and associated with bad prognosis in primary biliary cholangitis. J Hepatol 2017;66(1):S355–6.

35. Sookoian S, Pirola CJ. Meta-analysis of the influence of I148M variant of patatin-like phospholipase domain containing 3 gene (PNPLA3) on the susceptibility and histological severity of nonalcoholic fatty liver disease. Hepatology 2011;53(6): 1883–94.

36. Nault J-C, De Reyniès A, Villanueva A, et al. A hepatocellular carcinoma 5-gene score associated with survival of patients after liver resection. Gastroenterology 2013;145(1):176–87.

37. Hao J, Yang T, Zhou Y, et al. Serum metabolomics analysis reveals a distinct metabolic profile of patients with primary biliary cholangitis. Sci Rep 2017; 7(1):784.

38. Bell LN, Wulff J, Comerford M, et al. Serum metabolic signatures of primary biliary cirrhosis and primary sclerosing cholangitis. Liver Int 2015;35(1):263–74.

Family Health History
The First Genetic Test in Precision Medicine

Robin L. Bennett, MS, CGC

KEYWORDS

- Family history • Medical family history • Pedigree • Pedigree nomenclature
- Donor gametes • Transgender

KEY POINTS

- Genetic and genomic testing should always be interpreted in the context of the patient's medical and family history.
- There are many methods of recording family history and there are a growing number of programs compatible with the electronic medical record.
- All health practitioners should know how to record a medical family history in the form of a pedigree, using standard pedigree nomenclature, and to provide a basic interpretation of this information.
- There are recommendations for pedigree symbols for complex personal and family relationships (eg, same-sex couples, pregnancies conceived with donor gametes, adoption, transgender, consanguinity).
- Simple red-flags of family history include a diagnosis at an earlier age than typical (50 years is a good age to remember for common adult-onset disorders), bilateral disease in paired organs, multifocal disease (eg, 2 primary cancers), and 2 or more closely related relatives on the same side of the family with the condition (especially if diagnosed at a young age).

INTRODUCTION

There are a plethora of genetic tests to consider in the evaluation and management of patients. A genetic test may be diagnostic, presymptomatic, or a screening test for healthy persons. Genetic tests are done on different tissues, such as blood or saliva (germline) or other tissues (somatic). These tests may be offered throughout the life-cycle: for pregnancy planning (preconception), prenatal (during a pregnancy), newborn screening, in childhood, and throughout adulthood. An underlying theme of all of these genetic tests and approaches is that genetic testing should always be

This article originally appeared in *Medical Clinics*, Volume 103, Issue 6, November 2019.
Disclosure: The author has nothing to disclose.
Division of Medical Genetics, Department of Medicine, University of Washington, University of Washington Medical Center, Box 357720, 1959 Northeast Pacific Street, Seattle, WA 98195-7720, USA
E-mail address: robinb@uw.edu

interpreted in the context of the patient's medical and family history. A patient's medical family history is the first genetic test; it is a gateway for determining the approach to considering the need for genetic testing and the interpretation of the test results.[1–3] Family history can be provided by the patient in advance of the visit and confirmed by the practitioner or gathered at the clinic visit.

CORE INFORMATION TO INCLUDE IN MEDICAL FAMILY HISTORY

A medical family history is the compiling of key medical and demographic information about the patient and closely related biological relatives. Information is included about at least the first-degree relatives (children, full siblings, parents) and second-degree relatives (half-siblings, both sets of grandparents, and aunts and uncles). Third-degree relatives may also be included (first cousins, half-aunts and uncles). A 3-generation family history is considered minimum, but a more extensive family history may be required depending on the age of the person. For example, if a 40-year-old man is concerned about a family history of colon cancer in his sister and his paternal uncle, the history would likely include information about his children, siblings and their children (his nieces and nephews), his parents and their siblings (his aunts and uncles on both sides of the family), and his grandparents (at least on his father's side of the family). This approach compares with family history for an adolescent, which would likely be limited to health information about siblings, parents, aunts and uncles and their children, and grandparents (3 generations). Core health and demographic information to document for patients and their close relatives is noted in **Box 1**.

RED FLAGS OF MEDICAL FAMILY HISTORY

A major outcome from recording a patient's medical family history is to determine whether the clinician should be doing anything differently for this patient than usual

---

Box 1
Key health and demographic information to document in a family health history for the patient and closely related relatives

- Age (or year of birth)
- Age at death and cause of death (year if known)
- Siblings (distinguish whether half or full siblings)
- Children (note whether with separate partners)
- Miscarriages (particularly for a preconception or pregnancy consultation)
- Parents and grandparents
- Major health conditions, and the age at diagnosis (eg, cancer, aneurysm)
- Major surgeries (eg, cardiac, hysterectomy, oophorectomy, mastectomy, prostatectomy)
- Environmental exposures (eg, tobacco, alcohol, drugs)
- Occupational exposures (eg, asbestos exposure, mining)
- Country of ancestral origin for both sets of grandparents (if known)
- Whether a person's parents are closely related (first cousins or more closely related)

The date the information was collected, who provided the information, and who recorded the information should be noted.

and whether there are red flags in this family history that suggest the patient is at higher-than-average risk for a disease/disorder. Gathering this type of information does not need to be complicated. Early age of disease onset is one of the easiest alerts to remember to consider a hereditary condition; 50 years of age is a conservative cutoff for many common diseases (eg, cancer and heart disease). Another simple clue to think genetic is when 2 or more closely related relatives have the same condition on the same side of the family. A person who has more than 1 major health condition (eg, 2 primary cancers, hearing loss and retinal disease, 2 major vascular events, a seizure disorder and intellectual disability) may have a hereditary condition. A summary of the "signposts" in family history to think genetic are reviewed in **Box 2**.

ANCESTRY AND FAMILY HISTORY

Recording countries of origin for patients is important in genetic diagnosis and interpretation of genetic and genomic testing and should always be noted on a family history. Certain genetic disorders are more common in some populations because of founder mutations from a small pool of common ancestors. For example, there are 2 common pathogenic mutations in *BRCA1* (c.5266dupC and c.68_69delAG) and 1 in *BRCA2* (c. 5946delT) in the Ashkenazi population (Jews with ancestors from eastern Europe); thus 1 in 40 men and women of this ancestry is at risk to carry one of these pathogenic mutations. In Iceland there is a common pathogenic mutation in *BRCA2* (999del5) that is found in 0.6% of the population and is observed in 10.4% of women with breast cancer and 38% of men with breast cancers.[4] In Finland there is a spectrum of more than 30 mostly autosomal recessive disorders that occur more often in this population because of founder pathogenic mutations (http://findis.org/heritage. html, accessed March 13, 2019). Knowing the person's ancestry can help guide the approach to genetic testing. For example, a person who has a family history of breast or ovarian cancer might first be tested for the 3 common founder mutations seen in the Ashkenazi population before proceeding to full gene sequencing (which saves costs).

Knowing ancestry can also guide informed consent for genetic testing. However, most of the genetic population studies on normal and pathogenic variants for inherited disorders have been based on individuals of European ancestry. Therefore, individuals who are from underrepresented populations (eg, African, Asian, Latino, Native American, First Nation) have a higher likelihood of the identification of a genetic variant of

---

Box 2
Signposts of medical and family history that suggest an inherited disorder

- Common disorders that occur at younger ages than typical
- A person with more than 1 major health condition or medical event
- Two or more relatives on the same side of the family with a health condition (particularly if earlier than typical age of onset)
- Bilateral disease in paired organs
- Two primary cancers (eg, breast and ovarian cancer, 2 primary colon cancers, prostate and colon cancer)
- Unusual presentation of the condition (eg, male breast cancer, lung cancer in a nonsmoker)
- Sudden death in a person who seemed healthy
- Medical problems in the offspring of parents who are consanguineous (first cousins or closer)

uncertain significance than a person of European ancestry.[5] Although variants of uncertain significance (VUS) may be found in any person, patients from these populations should be forewarned of the higher likelihood of identification of a VUS in advance of any genetic testing. Likewise, the identification of carrier status for autosomal recessive disorders varies by ancestry (eg, the likelihood of identifying a common mutation in the cystic fibrosis gene, *CFTR*, is higher in persons of European ancestry than in persons of African ancestry).

OTHER IMPORTANT ELEMENTS

Individuals who are closely related (eg, first cousins) are at slightly increased risk to have children with a recessive disorder (because of inheriting a pathogenic mutation from a common ancestor).[6,7] Although the risk to develop a significant medical problem in the first years of life is low for the offspring of first cousins (a few percent higher than for nonconsanguineous couples), this information is important to note for genetic risk assessment, and a referral to genetic counseling may be important (particularly for couples who are pregnant or considering a pregnancy).

Age at time of diagnosis is also an important piece of information. For example, if a person has a first-degree relative with colon cancer at age 40 years, screening for colon cancer would be offered to the patient 10 years younger (age 30 years) even in light of that patient having a negative genetic test.

RECORDING A FAMILY HISTORY: A PEDIGREE IS A USEFUL TOOL

Any new patient to primary or specialty care should have key family history documented. Whether the collection method is through a standard paper table or checkbox that is scanned into the medical record, or through a graphical pedigree that is hand drawn or generated by a software program, the most important focus is to gather this information in the first place. There is a growing movement with the electronic medical record (EMR) and patient health portals to have patients generate the family history for the medical record and perhaps even to share this information electronically with their relatives. Welch and colleagues[8] summarize and review many of the electronic patient-facing family health history tools.

Recording a graphical family history in the form of a pedigree is a skill that all practitioners should be familiar with. The health information collected can be targeted by specialty (eg, cardiology, neurology, ophthalmology, oncology) or broader (eg, a first prenatal, pediatric, or primary care visit). With a pedigree, pages of health information can be compressed to 1 visual document through the association of simple symbols: squares, circles, diamonds, triangles, and lines. The square (male) or circle (female) can be shaded to track a condition (eg, aneurysm, cancer, seizures).

A pedigree has many advantages compared with a table format: the key health information can be tracked by the shading of the pedigree symbols so that patterns of inheritance can be more easily recognized. Autosomal dominant patterns showing transmission of disease from one generation to the next with both men and women affected are clearly visible. A preponderance of men affected in a pedigree might suggest an X-linked pattern of inheritance. If only 1 generation is affected, this may disclose autosomal recessive inheritance. If a person has family health information that does not identify conditions that run in the family, standard preventive health screening is likely the appropriate strategy.

Often the approach to genetic and genomic testing is to test the person who is most likely to have a positive test and then to provide cascade testing to other relatives, starting with first-degree relatives of the one who had a positive test. A pedigree is a visual tool to help determine who is the best person to test in the family and which other relatives should be tested.

All health professionals should be able to interpret the major symbols that are used to form a pedigree. Standard symbols for pedigree nomenclature, developed through a peer review process, are now considered the international standard, are included in major software pedigree drawing programs, and are being incorporated into the main EMR programs[9,10]; they are included in the American Medical Association Manual of Style, 10th Edition (http://www.amamanualofsyle.com/view/10.1093/jama/9780195176339.0, accessed March 13, 2019). Commonly used pedigree symbols are shown in **Figs. 1–3**.

When family history is recorded from a scanned health form or in simple text, often only positive health information is recorded. For example, the medical record may state "positive for grandmother and aunt with colon cancer." This information lacks important details, such as the age the relatives were diagnosed with cancer, whether they are living, or even whether they are on the same side of the family. In contrast, the clinician may report family history is negative or unremarkable. This information gives no clue as to the breadth of health information collected or the framework of the family structure. Is this information collected on a 50-year-old person and the person's 4 siblings, parents who are living in their 70s, and grandparents who died in their 90s, or is it on a 50-year-old person who is estranged from 1 or more parent and knows nothing about the extended family health history? A pedigree would provide the clinician with this information at a glance.

INCLUSIVE FAMILY HISTORY

Collecting family history is rarely straightforward. Blended families are common. It is important for genetic risk assessment to distinguish biological from nonbiological relatives (eg, step-siblings or a person who has been adopted). There may be misattributed paternity in a family that may not have been disclosed. A person may know little about a relative because of estrangement. A person may have been conceived by a donor gamete, or a surrogate may be involved with carrying a pregnancy. Gender identity may be nonconforming or a person may be transitioning gender. Many of these ways of representing relationships and identify are addressed in the National Society of Genetic Counselors 2008 recommendations.[1,10]

For individuals who are transgender, the gender identity can be used with the transition noted below the symbol (eg, male-transition-female would be a circle with MTF noted). A diamond can also be used for a person who is gender nonconforming or for a person who is transgender (and the transition noted as female to male, or male to female).

In all cases, it is important to be respectful of the person's identity and the family relationships.

THE FAMILY HISTORY INTERVIEW

When gathering information about a person's family history, whether in an electronic format or by a hand-drawn pedigree, it is useful to begin with the consultand (the person seeking medical attention), or the proband (the affected individual who brings the family to medical attention). An arrow is used to point out this person as a point of reference because the family history radiates out from this point to relatives by ascent (the parents, siblings, grandparents, and prior generations) and descent (the children and grandchildren). Adding names or initials can be helpful to keep track of who is who in the family. For healthy relatives who are related distantly, it is acceptable to record

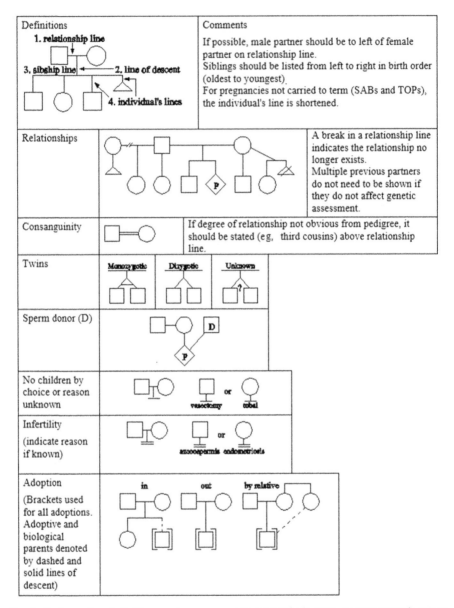

Fig. 1. Pedigree line definitions and common pedigree symbols. SAB, spontaneous abortion; TOP, termination of pregnancy. (*Adapted from* Bennett RL, French KS, Resta RG, et al. Standardized human pedigree nomenclature: update and assessment of the recommendations of the National Society of Genetic Counselors. J Genet Couns 2008;17(5):428; with permission.)

the number of relatives within a symbol (eg, a square labeled with a 3 would be 3 men, or a circle labeled with a 4 would represent 4 women).[10]

Asking open-ended questions is the best way to obtain a range of health information. A query of, "Describe the major medical problems that affect your parents" is

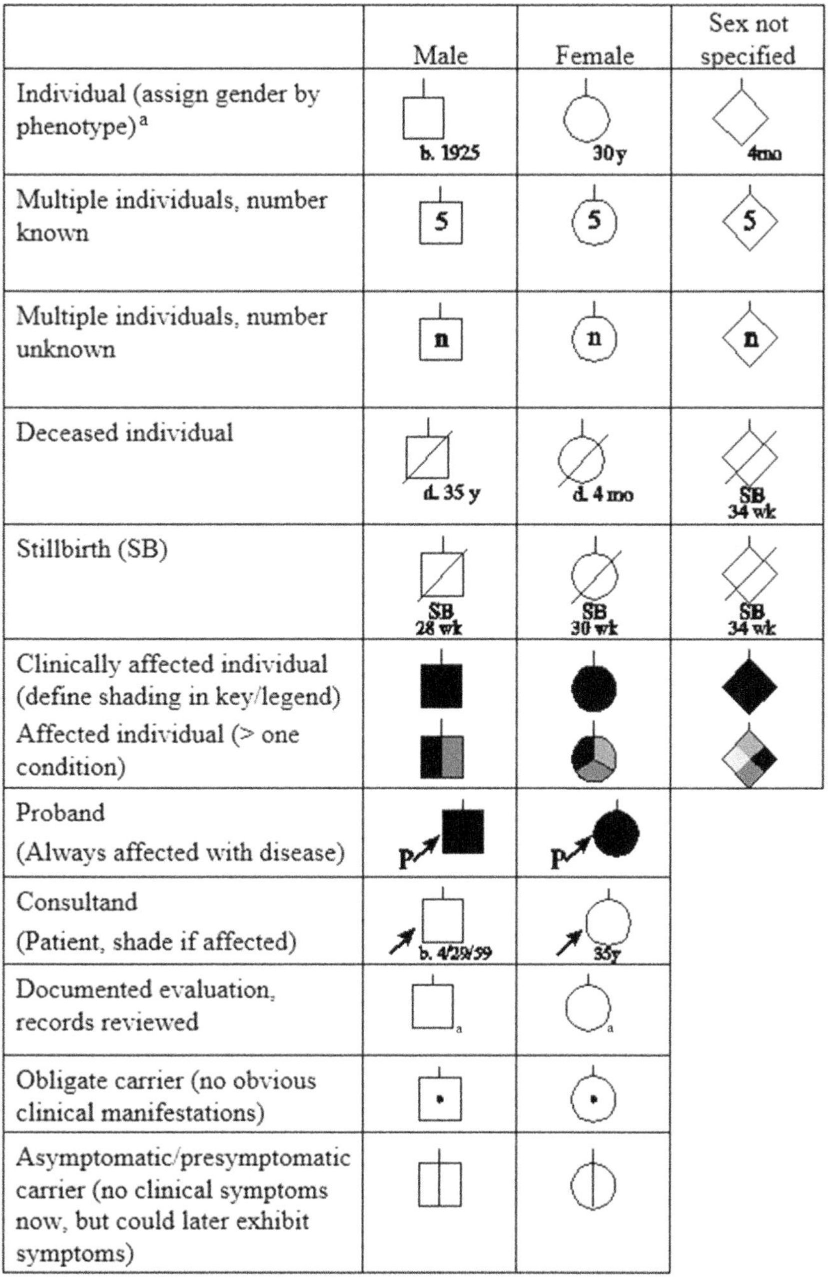

	Male	Female	Sex not specified
Individual (assign gender by phenotype)[a]	☐ b. 1925	◯ 30y	◇ 4mo
Multiple individuals, number known	☐ 5	◯ 5	◇ 5
Multiple individuals, number unknown	☐ n	◯ n	◇ n
Deceased individual	☒ d. 35 y	⊘ d. 4 mo	◇ SB 34 wk
Stillbirth (SB)	☐ SB 28 wk	⊘ SB 30 wk	◇ SB 34 wk
Clinically affected individual (define shading in key/legend) Affected individual (> one condition)	■ ■	● ●	◆ ◆
Proband (Always affected with disease)	P ⬈ ■	P ⬈ ●	
Consultand (Patient, shade if affected)	⬈ ☐ b. 4/28/59	⬈ ◯ 35y	
Documented evaluation, records reviewed	☐a	◯a	
Obligate carrier (no obvious clinical manifestations)	☐ •	◯ •	
Asymptomatic/presymptomatic carrier (no clinical symptoms now, but could later exhibit symptoms)	⊟	⊖	

Fig. 2. Additional pedigree symbols. [a] A diamond can be used for a person who is gender nonconforming and the sex at birth noted in text below the symbol. A diamond can also be used for a person who is transgender and the sex at birth noted or male-transition-female (MTF) or female-transition-male (FTM), as appropriate. The identifying gender symbol can also be used (eg, a square and FTM, or a circle and MTF). (*Adapted from* Bennett RL, French KS, Resta RG, et al. Standardized human pedigree nomenclature: update and assessment of the recommendations of the National Society of Genetic Counselors. J Genet Couns 2008;17(5):427; with permission.)

more likely to provide relevant information than "So, your parents are healthy?" It is helpful to have a systematic approach of asking questions starting with the patient, then extending to children (and grandchildren if appropriate), siblings, and then each parent and their siblings and parents. Specialty physicians ask questions in the targeted areas such as history of cancer or heart disease. For more general family health history, a "head-to-toe" review-of-systems approach targeting the whole family helps with organization (eg, problems with hearing, vision, heart, skeletal). At the end of the interview, it can be helpful to wrap up with, "Are there any conditions that you think run in your family? Is there anything else that I have not asked about your family's health that you think it is important for me to know?"[1]

FAMILY HISTORY IS A SNAPSHOT OF A FAMILY'S EXPERIENCE OF HEALTH AND DISEASE AND PROVIDES AN OPPORTUNITY TO ESTABLISH RAPPORT

Family history often contains emotionally charged information. Some diseases are not discussed openly in families. A person may be bereaved by the recent death of a relative. Feelings of chronic grief may be experienced if multiple relatives have died of a condition. The patient's family history can help the practitioner anticipate a patient's concerns. For example, if the patient is approaching the age that other relatives have been diagnosed or died of a condition, the patient may be anxious. As with any sensitive information, empathic interviewing skills are required and important life events should be acknowledged (eg, "That must have been difficult for you.").

Patients are more likely to comply with recommendations if they have a relationship with the clinician. Obtaining family health information is an excellent way to establish rapport with a patient. Patients are the experts on their family information, and this can

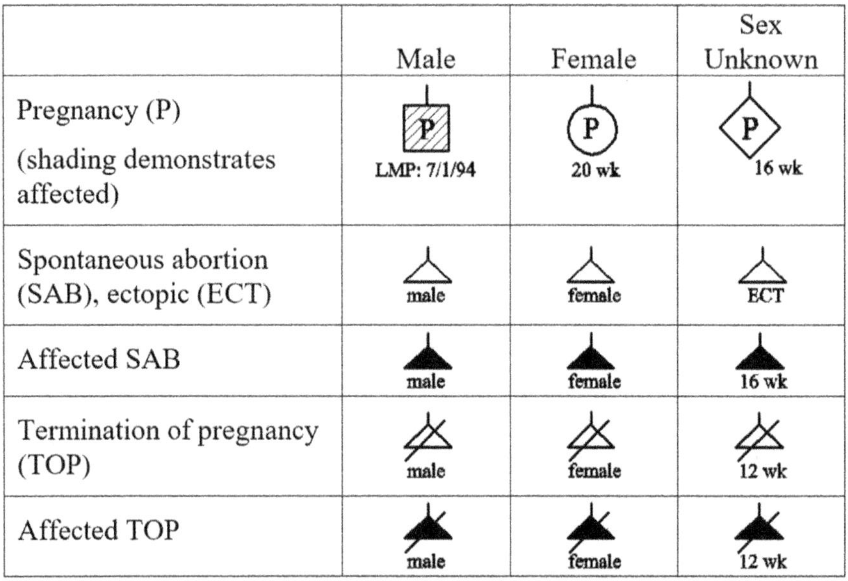

	Male	Female	Sex Unknown
Pregnancy (P) (shading demonstrates affected)	P LMP: 7/1/94	P 20 wk	P 16 wk
Spontaneous abortion (SAB), ectopic (ECT)	male	female	ECT
Affected SAB	male	female	16 wk
Termination of pregnancy (TOP)	male	female	12 wk
Affected TOP	male	female	12 wk

Fig. 3. Pedigree symbols related to pregnancy, miscarriage, and termination of pregnancy. (*Adapted from* Bennett RL, French KS, Resta RG, et al. Standardized human pedigree nomenclature: update and assessment of the recommendations of the National Society of Genetic Counselors. J Genet Couns 2008;17(5):427; with permission.)

be empowering for the patients. In this role as expert, the patients are more likely to be active participants in decisions about their health care. Patients are likely to feel listened to in the process of taking a family history, and this may even decrease patient anxiety.[1]

FAMILY HISTORY EVOLVES OVER TIME

When a medical family history is recorded, it is important to note the date the information was recorded and by whom; was this information recorded by the patient and reviewed by the practitioner or used from another clinic visit? Medical decision making is based on the information provided at that time; different decisions may be made with new information. Families change: relatives are born, die, and are diagnosed with diseases. Updates to family history (as new information is provided or at periodic visits) are important.

FAMILY HISTORY, GENETICS, GENOMICS, AND THE ELECTRONIC MEDICAL RECORD

The integration of family history information in the context of a patient's medical conditions and incorporation of genetic and genomic results is complex. An ideal state might seem to connect all relatives with a universal health record that would update as new information is known. For example, if someone's sister has a new diagnosis of breast cancer and has a pathogenic mutation in the BRCA1 gene, this information could be automatically uploaded into the person's file so that health providers would know what testing was needed. The practitioner may even receive an alert with clinical decision support, such as referral to a genetic counselor and/or for a genetic test.

Complications surrounding what may seem simple on the surface arise quickly. What about automatic disclosure of information that might be stigmatizing[11] (eg, mental illness, termination of pregnancy for a genetic indication, even a diagnosis of cancer that has not been shared with other relatives)? Can a person consent to sharing information with some relatives and not others? What about a child conceived by a donor sperm or donor egg; should the information about the health of the gamete donor be linked to that child's EMR and updated as health changes (for either the child or the gamete donor)? Should certain genetic information be specially protected (eg, presymptomatic test results for Huntington disease)? How is discrepant information dealt with in the EMR (eg, a man's pedigree says his father died at 50 years of age but his sister's pedigree notes he died at age 45 years; that age at diagnosis may denote different eligibility for genetic testing or recommendations for health screening).

SUMMARY

Family health history remains an essential tool in the application of genetic medicine. Even as genetic and genomic tools increase in availability, accuracy, and utility, the personal medical and family history continues to be the fulcrum on which interpretation of precision genomic medicine turns. The opportunities for family history in the electronic health history are vast, but the nuances of family structures and privacy must be seriously considered and respected. Medical and family history information can now potentially be collected and sorted from birth (or even prenatally) to grave. As more data accumulate on patients, their family histories, and concomitant genetic information, it is important that the critically important information for patient care be available in contrast with information overload. Dialogue between practitioners, specialists, genetics providers, software developers, laboratories, researchers, public health specialists, and patient advocacy organizations is necessary to continue to bring the power of medical family history and genomic health to fruition.

REFERENCES

1. Bennett RL. The practical guide to the genetic family history. 2nd edition. New York: Wiley Liss; 2010.
2. Pyeritz RE. The family history: the first genetic test, and still useful after all those years? Genet Med 2012;14:3–9.
3. Guttmacher AE, Collins FS, Carmona RH. The family history-more important than ever. N Engl J Med 2004;351:2333–6.
4. Tulinius H, Olafsdottir GH, Sigvaldason H, et al. The effect of a single BRCA2 mutation on cancer in Iceland. J Med Genet 2002;39:457–62.
5. Popely A, Fullerton SM. Genomics is failing on diversity. Nature 2016;538:161–4.
6. Bennett RL, Motulsky AG, Bittles AH, et al. Genetic counseling and screening of consanguineous couples and their offspring: recommendations of the National Society of Genetic Counselors. J Genet Couns 2002;11:97–119.
7. Hamamy HA, Antonarakis SE, Cavalli0Sforza LL, et al. Consanguineous marriages, pearls and perils: Geneva International Consanguinity Workshop Report. Genet Med 2011;13:998–1005.
8. Welch BM, Wiley K, Pflieger L, et al. Review and comparison of electronic patient-facing family health history tools. J Genet Couns 2018;27:381–91.
9. Bennett RL, Steinhaus KA, Uhrich SB, et al. Recommendations for standardized pedigree nomenclature. Am J Hum Genet 1995;56:745–52.
10. Bennett RL, French KS, Resta RG, et al. Standardized human pedigree nomenclature: update and assessment of the recommendations of the National Society of Genetic Counselors. J Genet Couns 2008;17:424–33.
11. Bennett RL. Pedigree parables. Clin Genet 2000;58:241–9.

Precision Medicine
Genomic Profiles to Individualize Therapy

Oscar E. Streeter Jr, MD[a],*, Phillip J. Beron, MD[b],
Prashant Natarajan Iyer, BE (Chem), MTPC, SCPM[c]

KEYWORDS

- Precision medicine • Big data • Genomic profiling • Immunotherapy
- Checkpoint inhibitors • Hyperthermia • Radiogenomics • Machine learning

KEY POINTS

- Precision medicine is generally understood to be the application of genotypic and Omics biomarkers to determine the most appropriate, outcome-driven treatment or therapy for individual patients.
- Information technology (IT)-enabled big data management and health care are becoming and will be required tools in the clinical kit to properly manage and leverage the complex data that result from genomic, clinic, financial, and behavioral data to benefit individualize patient care and outcomes by predicting for multiple stratified populations.
- Immunotherapy in 2017 has been most effective in checkpoint inhibitor medications.
- One of the novel immunomodulators is hyperthermia (HT) that is most effective in combination with radiation therapy (RT) or chemotherapy.

Precision medicine is an evolving term whose definition is changing as the influence of genomic and population big data biomarkers are becoming well understood.

WHAT IS PRECISION MEDICINE?

Precision medicine is generally understood as the application of genotypic and Omics biomarkers to determine the most appropriate, outcome-driven treatment of or therapy for individual patients. The authors agree with this definition but would like to extend it — in line with a more comprehensive and clinically relevant view, that is, precision medicine is the determination and delivery of the "right therapy to the right

This article originally appeared in *Otolaryngologic Clinics*, Volume 50, Issue 4, August 2017.
Disclosure Statement: O.E. Streeter and P.J. Beron have no disclosures. P.N. Iyer: Oracle Corporation, employer.
[a] The Center for Thermal Oncology, 2001 Santa Monica Boulevard, Suite 1190, Santa Monica, CA 90404, USA; [b] Department of Radiation Oncology, UCLA Health System, 200 UCLA Medical Plaza, Suite B265, Los Angeles, CA 90095, USA; [c] Healthcare Solutions, Oracle Corporation, 5805 Owens Drive, Pleasanton, CA 94588, USA
* Corresponding author.
E-mail address: ostreeter@thermaloncology.com

Clinics Collections 8 (2020) 29–37
https://doi.org/10.1016/j.ccol.2020.07.003
2352-7986/20/

patient at the right time."[1] The authors' view of precision medicine acknowledges a few realities that must be addressed via any multidisciplinary approach that combines people, behaviors, social determinants of health (a patients zip code has as much influence on their health as their genetic code), and their phenotypic data (**Fig. 1**). An integrated definition, such as the one used in this article, also addresses prevailing concerns about cost, access, and outcomes for individual patients and multidimensional stratified populations.

The authors posit that the definition of precision medicine that will enable oncology, chronic/acute care, and prevention/wellness must not only address the availability of genomics sequencing data and biomarkers but also do more on health variables that are constantly being defined. Although genomics at the point of care is fundamental to precision medicine, care at the bedside (in the facility or at home) also requires the acquisition, management, integration, clinician validation, and use of data from disparate sources, such as

1. Clinical care (imaging, electronic medical records [EMRs], computerised physician order entry [CPOE], clinical narratives, and sensor/device data)
2. Research (clinical research, trials, publications, results of data discovery, and secondary use)
3. Financial (cost, charges, affordability, income disparities, and credit scores)
4. External and patient-reported data that encompasses patient self-reported data on the Web and via smartphones; family and disease histories/lore that are not in the history and physical examination; environmental variables; behavior/sentiment data; and, increasingly, income/educational/cognitive disparities.

These data sources are varied, voluminous, and processed at high velocities (**Fig. 2**). There also is a corresponding need in the context of therapy and procedures to examine the veracity and value of data and information in enabling and supporting precision medicine. Supporting the natural evolution of precision medicine requires an understanding of the new world of big data technologies, analytics, and machine learning. It also needs recognition that a patient's data will no longer be created

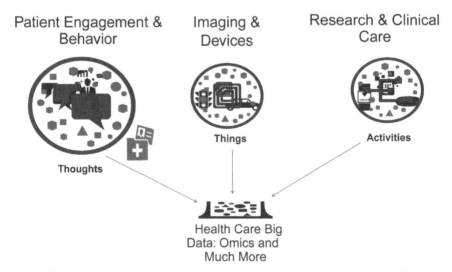

Fig. 1. Big data collection requires a central repository; processes need to be developed across institutions.

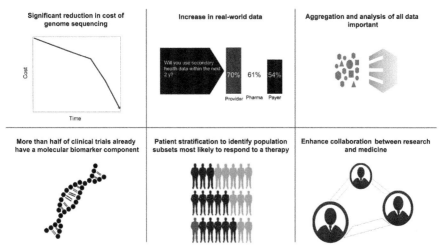

Fig. 2. The growth of big data.

and used inside a facility's 4 walls or in its EMRs. In this new world of health care datafication, important patient (and other) information will be sourced from secondary use that involves integrated order-results workflows that are driven by

1. Incorporating molecular and clinical annotation by additional collaborators—molecular pathologists, consulting physicians, primary care providers, and other specialists
2. Machine learning–based, large-scale, affordable, and automated analysis of images, speech, video, and large text (clinical narratives, discharge summaries, and progress notes)
3. New data from smart devices, home monitors, telemedicine, medical images, and social networks (life and viral networks)
4. Separation of signal from noise—and incorporating actionable analytics, clinician feedback loops and approval, and annotation into clinical system workflows

IT-enabled big data management and health care should be a required tool in the clinical kit to properly manage and leverage the complex data that result from genomic, clinical, financial, and behavioral data that brings the biggest benefit to individual patients, their outcomes, and applying the new clinical guidelines and newly created knowledge by extrapolating or predicting for multiple stratified populations that can be expanded to cover new analytics dimensions beyond the diagnosis or disease, including

1. Demographics—gender, race, ethnicity, zip code, and so forth
2. Real-time, location-specific influences—suspended particulate (smog, forest fires, and disasters) or other carcinogens (eg, asbestos, human activities such as fracking)
3. Social determinants of health—examples are activities of daily living (ADL), physical activity, diet, education, and income
4. Patient outcomes, including the effect of a procedure or therapy on survival, recovery, and health management

Addressing key health determinants simultaneously at the population and individual levels and the integration of clinical/Omics/other relevant data are critical in delivering precision medicine. Relating individuals to both research cohorts and stratified populations by taking advantage of the latest software technologies—prescriptive analytics, big data integration, and machine learning—provide opportunities to create or use knowledge that has not existed before or is undiscovered.

Applying precision medicine into the clinical workflow generates preventative and diagnostic solutions to advance human care—bringing new targeted therapies, improved patient outcomes, and cost savings.[1]

GENOMIC PROFILING

To understand this evolving technology of genomic profiling,[2] a few terms need to be defined. Base pairs are 2 nucleotides on opposite complementary DNA or RNA strands that are connected by hydrogen bonds. Sequencing is a method of detecting single bases as they are incorporated into DNA template strands. Whole-exome sequencing is a technique for sequencing all the expressed genes in a genome.

Next-generation sequencing is the application of genome sequencers that with a single run of material can analyze more than 1.8 terabases (the amount of genetic sequence data equivalent to 10^{12} base pairs). The cost of sequencing has fallen approximately 10-fold over the last few years, with improved accuracy and speed, bringing the cost to less than $2000 with targeted, although limited at this point, improvement in care at the bedside. It is now available to most patients covered by insurance. Genomic data analysis is where newly identified sequences are aligned to a reference genome.

The first and best example of the success of precision medicine in oncology is imatinib mesylate (Gleevec, Novartis Pharma Services AG, Basel, Switzerland) used to treat chronic myeloid leukemia (CML) with the *BCR-ABL* translocation. CML is due to a clonal evolution, starting with the acquisition of the 9(9;22) (q34;q11) translocation (Philadelphia chromosome), which creates a fusion between the *BCR* and *ABL1* genes. Imatinib mesylate controls CML because it is an inhibitor of *ABL* family kinases, including the *BCR-ABL* fusion gene.[3]

Most squamous cell carcinomas of the head and neck respond to standard drug therapy. When the clonal composition of the pretreatment biopsy is compared over time, however, after drug treatment, there may be changes in clonal-mutation prevalence.[4] Sequencing reveals large changes in the abundance of specific clones that may give clues as to which genotypes may confer resistance and may be sensitive to intervention. Therefore, local recurrence or new metastatic sites should be biopsied and sequenced to determine which drug or other intervention may improve response. Therefore, surgeons play a key role in requesting the pathologist send both the primary tumor and recurrent/metastatic tumor for sequencing. An example of this process used in a multidisciplinary clinic is the Weill Cornell Medical College Institute for Precision Medicine. The process starts with clinical examination and consent, followed by metastatic tumor biopsy and whole-exome sequencing/biobanking of tissue for future reference. Results are discussed in a tumor board, with communication to the patient and referring physicians to guide treatment, and used to fuel translational research and development of new diagnostics and therapeutics.[5] A trial currently accruing patients that best demonstrates the application of precision medicine in oncology is the recently opened National Cancer Institute Molecular Analysis for Therapy Choice (NCI-MATCH) clinical trial. This precision medicine trial explores treating patients based on the molecular profile of tumors with the inclusion criteria of adult patients, solid tumors (including rare tumors and lymphomas), and tumors that no longer respond to standard treatment, with an accrual goal of approximately 3000 cancer patients screened with a tumor biopsy. Biopsied tumor tissue is submitted for gene sequencing to identify initially 143 gene mutations that may respond to a specific therapy (the list of gene mutations is expanding with new discoveries). If a patient's tumor has a genetic abnormality that matches one targeted by a drug used in the trial, the patient becomes eligible to join the treatment portion of NCI-MATCH. This is an important trial found at the Web site, clinicaltrials.gov, and includes a listing of the mutations examined and drugs useful for each mutation. It is an excellent resource for physicians in the clinics helping to individualize therapy and is constantly updated. As of the fall of 2016, more than 1000 clinical sites, across America, are participating in this trial. It is a federally sponsored trial and free to eligible patients with an estimated primary completion date of June 2022.[6]

Head and neck squamous cell carcinoma (HNSCC) is an immunosuppressive disease that when recurrent or metastatic responds to immunotherapy, such as checkpoint inhibitors that are available currently.[7] Ongoing trials are considering combining current immunotherapies with cancer vaccines. An open-access article by Robert Ferris provides a review of immunologic principles related to head and neck cancer, including the concept of cancer immunosurveillance and immune escape.[8] The authors recommend this article because it has figures describing immune escape and antigen presentation allowing recognition of tumor cells by immune system. Most importantly are tables listing the mechanisms of immune escape in HNSCC, monoclonal antibodies under investigation in HNSCC, and a detailed table of immunotherapy trials in HNSCC. Most clinicians will be working with checkpoint inhibitors and a brief discussion of this immunotherapy is warranted and illustrated in a free-access *JAMA Oncology* patient page.[9] Immune checkpoint inhibitor drugs can target either tumor cells or T cells. They block normal proteins on cancer cells or the proteins on T cells that respond to those "normal proteins."

The checkpoint inhibitors prevent tumor cells from attaching to T cells, allowing the T cells to stay activated. A response to immune checkpoint inhibitor treatment results in a brief increase in tumor size (pseudoprogression) due to the increase in the number of activated T cells that enter the tumor.

To evaluate genetic mutation changes in tumors when there may not be enough tissue for mutation analysis in a primary or metastatic biopsy or to monitor tumor response, there is an increasing use of analyzing cell-free DNA mutations (cfDNAs) in the plasma and circulating tumor cells (CTCs) in the buffy coat of a centrifuged peripheral blood draw (**Figs. 3** and **4**).[10,11] Every month there are more Clinical Laboratory Improvement (CLIA) certified tests for tumors in specific organs. Commercial companies have developed blood sampling techniques to profile and monitor for programmed death ligand-1 (PD-L1) expression, an important biomarker in immune-oncology treatment decision making and will play an increasing role in the treatment of head and neck cancers.

HYPERTHERMIA AS A NOVEL IMMUNE MODULATOR

HT is also a form of precision medicine. Because HT over the past 2 decades has been limited in the United States due to a lack of available equipment and trained practitioners who can deliver this modality between the temperature range of 41°C and 43°C, there is limited understanding of its role in stimulating a nontoxic immune response in practically all tumors. An important phase III trial reported long-term results comparing RT alone with RT plus HT to metastatic lymph nodes in stage IV head and neck patients.[12] This study was conducted in 1985 to 1986 to improve

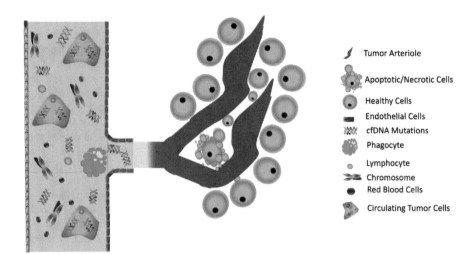

Fig. 3. Illustration of the origin of cfDNAs and CTCs from a milieu of apoptotic and necrotic fragments from tumors and other cellular fragments. (*Courtsey of* Oscar Streeter, MD, The Center for Thermal Oncology, Santa Monica, California.)

the outcome of fixed and inoperable (N3) metastatic lymph nodes in HNSCC in 41 patients with 46 metastatic lymph nodes. Because of the striking results of the combined modality arm, the study was prematurely closed because of ethical reasons with a 5-year actuarial probability of nodal control of 24.2% for the radiation-only arm versus 68.6% in the RT plus HT arm. The actuarial survival of the 2 groups at 5 year favors the RT plus HT arm of 53.3% versus 0% (*P* = .02). Although metastatic disease

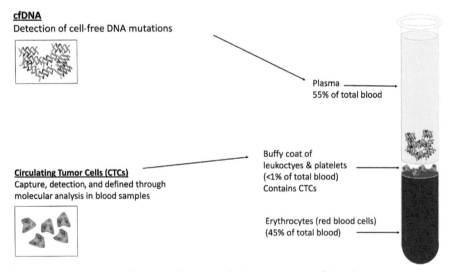

Fig. 4. Liquid biopsies. After centrifugation of a blood sample, cfDNA from shed tumors is detected from the plasma component of the supernatant, whereas CTCs are captured from the buffy coat component.

developed in 19% of the patients, it was reduced in the RT plus HT arm to 12.5% vs 24% in the RT-alone arm. It is now known that HT not only has a direct cytotoxic effect but stimulates a natural immune response in the fever range of 39°C to 41°C by activation of heat shock proteins, generating important immune actions and increasing blood flow, effective in primary and metastatic disease.[13] The mechanisms of how HT can be used in metastatic disease as immunotherapy is because of the following effect on heated tumor cells: (1) an increase in the surface expression of MICA, a NKG2D ligand, and major histocompatibility class 1 (MHC 1), making the tumor cells more sensitive to lysis by natural killer (NK) cells and CD8+ T cells, respectively, and (2) the release of heat shock proteins (HSPs), which activate NK cells and antigen-presenting cells (APCs). HSPs contain potential tumor antigens, and APCs take up the HSP-antigen complex and cross-present the antigen to CD8+ T cells; (3) release of exosomes, which contain potential tumor antigens, and APCs take up the antigen and cross present the antigen to CD8+ T cells; (4) immune cells, such as NK cells, CD8+ T cells and dendritic cells, in the tumor also get heated and become activated; and (5) tumor vasculature becomes more permeable and may increase expression of the intercellular cell adhesion molecule (ICAM)-1, a protein expressed by the cancer cell with one function to facilitate signal transduction immune response. ICAM-1 also facilitates better immune trafficking between tumor cells and draining lymph nodes.

RADIOGENOMICS

Although the use of big data in health care research is still in its infancy, the potential of combining big data with information from comparative effectiveness research and EMR data with machine learning in the future will help with decision making on what type of therapy is best for individual patients, including informing individual patients of potential complications and risk of secondary cancers based on their genomic

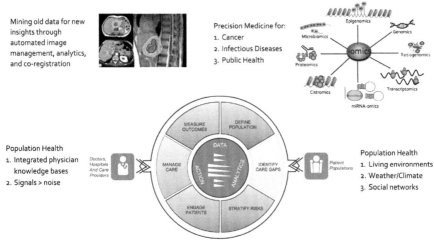

Key takeaways:
1. Precision medicine and population health are two sides of the same coin.
2. In healthcare, it is not always about searching for the needle in the haystack.
3. Big data analytics in precision medicine allows us to burn the hay to find the needle.

Fig. 5. Precision medicine applications.

profile.[14] The challenges associated with implementing big data analytics in radiation oncology or in medical oncology are (1) validity of the training data set, (2) availability of public health and computer science experts, (3) silo ownership of the data, and (4) and the critical need to shift from deductive to inductive reasoning using new statistical and probabilistic tools from the field of machine learning (**Fig. 5**).

WHAT IS MACHINE LEARNING?

Machine learning approaches problems as a doctor progressing through a residency would, starting with patient observation, using algorithms that sift through variables, and looking for combinations that reliably predict outcome. Ongoing research at Harvard Medical School and at the Perelman School of Medicine and Wharton School, University of Pennsylvania, have demonstrated that machine learning algorithms can predict death in metastatic cancer patients. This is accomplished by not only looking at known outcomes for a specific stage of cancer, but other variables such as infections during treatment, use of a wheelchair as well as other variables that are not ordinarily considered in determining prognosis. Obermeyer and Emanuel[15] predict prognostic algorithms will come into use in the next 5 years with several more years of prospective validation.

SUMMARY

Although there has been significant progress in the ability to sequence a person's genome in 1 sequencing process, the ability to aggregate all these data into a useful instrument to treat a single patient with cancer is a big data problem that will not be solved by any single institution. That type of computing power and transmitting that information across different platforms require a new type of thinking in medicine, the idea that the institution does not own the data, patients do, and must be part of a larger database tool that currently is in its infancy. For head and neck cancer patients, what can be used today is looking for a mutation that has a therapeutic target and understanding that the tumor will undergo clonal evolution and eventually become resistant. Also, a counterintuitive benefit for patients that is just as important is the ability to identify therapies of low value and avoiding adverse reactions.

REFERENCES

1. Oracle Health Sciences. Precision medicine: providing the right therapy to the right patient at the right time. 2016. Available at: http://www.oracle.com/us/industries/health-sciences/precision-medicine-info-2692756.pdf. Accessed October 1, 2016.
2. Green ED, Guyeer MS, National Human Genome Research Institute. Charting a course for genomic medicine from base pairs to bedside. Nature 2011; 470(7333):204–13.
3. Mohamed AN, Pemberton P, Zonder J, et al. The effect of imatinib mesylate on patients with Philadelphia chromosome-positive chronic myeloid leukemia with secondary chromosomal aberrations. Clin Cancer Res 2003;9(4):1333–7.
4. Aparicio S, Caldas C. The implications of clonal genome evolution for cancer medicine. N Engl J Med 2013;368(9):842–51.
5. Beltran H, Eng K, Mosquera JM, et al. Whole-exome sequencing of metastatic cancer and biomarkers of treatment response. JAMA Oncol 2015;1(4):466–74.
6. National Cancer Institute. NCI-MATCH: targeted therapy directed by genetic testing in treating patients with advanced refractory solid tumors or lymphomas

(ClinicalTrials.gov Identifier: NCT02465060). 2015. Available at: https://clinicaltrials.gov/ct2/results?term=nct02465060. Accessed September 28, 2016.

7. Lalami Y, Awada A. Innovative perspectives of immunotherapy in head and neck cancer. From relevant scientific rationale to effective clinical practice. Cancer Treat Rev 2016;43:113–23.

8. Ferris RL. Immunology and immunotherapy of head and neck cancer. J Clin Oncol 2015;33(29):3293–304.

9. West H. Immune checkpoint inhibitors. JAMA Oncol 2015;1(1):115.

10. Diaz LA Jr, Bardelli A. Liquid biopsies: genotyping circulating tumor DNA. J Clin Oncol 2014;32(6):579–86.

11. Economopoulo P, Agelaki S, Perisanidis C, et al. The promise of immunotherapy in head and neck squamous cell carcinoma. Ann Oncol 2016;27(9):1675–85.

12. Valdagni R, Amichetti M. Report of long-term follow-up in a randomized trial comparing radiation therapy and radiation therapy plus hyperthermia to metastatic lymph nodes in Stage IV head and neck patients. Int J Radiat Oncol Biol Phys 1994;28(1):163–9.

13. Toraya-Brown S, Fiering S. Local tumor hyperthermia as immunotherapy for metastatic cancer. Int J Hyperthermia 2014;30(8):531–9.

14. Trifiletti DM, Showaalter TN. Big data and comparative effectiveness research in radiation oncology: synergy and accelerated discovery. Front Oncol 2015;5(274):1–5.

15. Obermeyer Z, Emanuel EJ. Predicting the future - big data, machine learning, and clinical medicine. N Engl J Med 2016;375(13):1216–9.

The Future of Biomarkers

Jean-Louis Vincent, MD, PhD*, Elisa Bogossian, MD,
Marco Menozzi, MD

KEYWORDS

- Precision medicine • Phenotypes • Biomarker panels • Sensitivity • Specificity

KEY POINTS

- New biomarkers are being developed that will facilitate the move toward personalized medicine.
- Combinations of biomarkers are more likely to be of use than single biomarkers.
- Developments in omics will add new biomarkers to the traditional protein and cytokine markers.

CASE PRESENTATION IN THE INTENSIVE CARE UNIT IN 2040

Mr X, a postoperative patient on the general surgical floor, develops a temperature of more than 38°C. In just 2 minutes, his bedside sepsis panel alerts that he has an infection. In just 7 minutes, the presence of *Klebsiella* is identified from a blood sample and its antibiotic sensitivities provided. Appropriate antibiotics are started according to a computerized algorithm. The antibiotic doses given are higher than usual because tests suggest he has increased renal clearance of drugs. Nevertheless, his bedside renal panel indicates he is at high risk of developing renal failure likely to require renal replacement therapy (RRT) in the next few days, so immediate transfer to the intensive care unit (ICU) is organized. His urine output then starts to fall, and his blood volume biomarker level indicates a risk of fluid overload showing that he needs close monitoring, especially because his acute respiratory destress syndrome (ARDS) risk panel is also in the red zone. These results suggest RRT should be started, even before his creatinine levels increase significantly (in any case, creatinine levels are no longer trusted very much; there are better markers now). The new lung protective agent will also be prescribed, even though this drug is costly.

This article originally appeared in *Critical Care Clinics*, Volume 36, Issue 1, January 2020.
Disclosure Statement: The authors have no conflicts of interest to declare.
Department of Intensive Care, Erasme Hospital, Université libre de Bruxelles, Route de Lennik 808, Brussels 1070, Belgium
* Corresponding author.
E-mail address: jlvincent@intensive.org

INTRODUCTION

Markers of disease have been used for centuries, but it was only really in the 1980s that the term, *biomarker*, came into widespread use. Biomarkers can range from simple physiologic measurements of, for example, pulse and blood pressure, to highly complex and expensive molecular or imaging variables. Since the early 1980s, biomarker research across all fields of medicine has increased dramatically and this expansion shows no sign of slowing down as new technology assists in facilitating the development of new biomarkers and assessing their place in modern medicine. In some fields, for example, oncology, biomarkers have played a key role in defining distinct disease entities that respond to specific treatments, enabling precision medicine to be applied to individual patients. In the critical care arena, progress has been much slower, partly because much critical illness, for example, ARDS and sepsis, is syndromic and heterogeneous rather than consisting of clearly defined, homogeneous disease states.[1,2] With increasing availability of data from large patient databases and improved technology to analyze and identify potential biomarkers, huge advances will be seen in this field in the future.

GENERAL BIOMARKER APPLICATIONS

Importantly, biomarkers can have multiple applications. The US Food and Drug Administration (FDA) and the National Institutes of Health have recently listed 7 categories of biomarker: susceptibility/risk, diagnostic, monitoring, prognostic, predictive, pharmacodynamic/response, and safety[3] (**Table 1**). There may be some overlap between categories and any 1 biomarker may meet the criteria for several different categories. The fictional case history at the beginning of this article demonstrates some of these uses, with biomarkers for diagnosis, prediction, therapeutic response, and prognosis. This article explores 2 of the key applications for biomarkers in the ICU, focusing on how each will likely evolve in the future.

Table 1
Categories of biomarker with some possible examples from critical care medicine

Category[a]	Example of Use…	…To Guide/Assess in This Context
Susceptibility/risk	ARDS, risk of respiratory arrest	Early endotracheal intubation
Diagnostic	Infection	Early and adequate antibiotic therapy
Monitoring	Fluid status	Fluid management
Prognostic	Risk of multiple organ failure /death	ICU admission
Predictive	Good outcome	ICU discharge
Pharmacodynamic/response	Serial sepsis biomarkers	Duration of antibiotic therapy
Safety	Chloride levels	Stop saline infusions

[a] Categories as proposed by the US Food and Drug Administration and the National Institutes of Health Biomarker Working Group.

Data from FDA-NIH Biomarker Working Group. BEST (Biomarkers, EndpointS, and other Tools) Resource: Glossary. Available at: https://www.ncbi.nlm.nih.gov/books/NBK338448/pdf/Bookshelf_NBK338448.pdf. Accessed 9/7/19.

Diagnostic Biomarkers

A diagnostic biomarker is used to identify or confirm the presence of a disease or condition.[4] The number of available diagnostic markers is vast, enabling identification of diseases ranging from myocardial infarction to prostate cancer to lactose intolerance. Some of these tests are highly sensitive for the condition in question, others much less so. The same applies to specificity. New diagnostic biomarkers are being developed on a daily basis as understanding of disease pathogenesis improves and ability to reliably detect and measure even very low concentrations of substances increases. The challenge is to ensure that such biomarkers are correctly validated and relevant. Moreover, diagnostic biomarkers are of limited interest if the information they provide is not associated with the ability to offer appropriate treatment of the condition in question or to influence clinical decision making so that patient outcomes can be improved. This is particularly true in critical care medicine.

Diagnostic markers also can be used to assess disease severity, which can be helpful when evaluating the need for aggressive therapies, such as a surgical intervention or a costly medication. Assessing severity also can help in deciding whether a patient in an emergency department should be oriented toward the ICU or the general floor. This type of biomarker use may be especially important in the middle of the night, when doctors are often less experienced or may not be fully awake. Increasingly, artificial intelligence and machine-learning systems will combine biomarker information with other elements, for example, patient age and medical history, to provide accurate patient triage based on known outcomes.[5]

Given the high morbidity and mortality associated with sepsis and the recognized importance of early appropriate management, availability of a biomarker able to accurately diagnose sepsis would be a major breakthrough. Over the years, many candidate markers of sepsis have been identified, proposed, and studied[6]; however, none is perfect and can unequivocally and reliably differentiate all patients with sepsis from those without. Even procalcitonin (PCT) and C-reactive protein, the 2 most widely studied sepsis biomarkers, have many limitations.[7] A major problem is the lack of a gold standard against which biomarkers can be tested: there is and will always be a gray zone between demonstrated, suspected, possible, and unlikely infections.[8]

Will there be better sepsis markers in the future? Unfortunately, given the highly complex nature of the sepsis response and the heterogeneity of the patients sepsis can affect, it is unlikely that 1 biomarker will be found that can definitively separate septic from nonseptic patients. Rather than relying on single biomarkers, combinations or panels of biomarkers probably will be used in the future. As an example, SeptiCyte (Immunexpress, Seattle, WA) is a test based on the expression of 4 key genes involved in the host response to infection: *CEACAM4*, *LAMP1*, *PLAC8*, and *PLA2G7*. Septicyte is the first host response gene expression assay authorized by the FDA for the diagnosis of sepsis in ICU patients. In a clinical trial,[9] the assay was able to differentiate sepsis from sepsis-like states on the first day of ICU admission with good sensitivity and specificity, combined in an area under the receiver operating characteristic curve of approximately 0.85. It performed better than other markers of sepsis, including PCT.[9] Nevertheless, the test results currently take an average of 6 hours to become available, limiting its usefulness to guide initiation of treatment. Clearly these time delays will be much shorter in the future.

In another approach, Langelier and colleagues[10] used metagenomics next-generation sequencing to develop pathogen, microbiome diversity, and host gene expression metrics to differentiate critically ill patients with lower tract respiratory infections from those without. Combining the 3 metrics together resulted in a negative predictive value of 100%. Combining bacterial and host characteristics will be a key feature of future biomarkers.

Importantly, markers of sepsis should be distinguished from tests to identify the presence of microorganisms. There is no doubt that rapidly identifying the presence of microorganisms will be possible in the near future,[11–13] without having to rely on time-consuming microbiological cultures. As these tests are refined and they are more widely used, the time needed to obtain a result will decrease from several hours to minutes, and the price, which remains a strong limitation to their use today, will go down. Nevertheless, the distinction between colonization and infection may never be entirely clear. Hence, it is likely that combinations of sepsis markers, to assess the presence of sepsis and its severity, with microbiological tests, to choose the correct antibiotic, will always be needed.

Response Biomarkers

Therapeutic response biomarkers are vitally important because they can help guide treatment decisions to optimize patient outcomes. Monitoring of biomarker levels over time after treatment start can help determine whether the treatment is effective or needs to be reviewed and altered. This approach is widely used in many medical conditions, including chronic hypertension and diabetes. In critical illness, response biomarkers will be increasingly used to guide antibiotic duration in sepsis, to decide when to start and stop RRT or to determine ongoing fluid needs.

Antibiotic doses and durations in patients with sepsis are largely determined from data in noncritically ill populations. Yet critically ill patients frequently have acute hepatic and renal dysfunction, which can influence drug metabolism and clearance; capillary leak and fluid resuscitation, which can alter volumes of distribution; and comorbid conditions that can also alter antibiotic response. Moreover, the rapid and multiple changes in physiologic alterations during critical illness make it difficult to predict how a patient will respond to a particular dose. Antibiotic doses, therefore, need to be individualized much more than is currently the case. This will be facilitated in the future by more rapid and widely available drug-level monitoring.

The duration of therapy is also important. Giving antibiotics for an arbitrary planned duration of 4 days, 7 days, or 10 days exposes patients to risk of inadequate or excessive treatment as well as increased risks of adverse events when treatment is prolonged and promotion of the development of resistance. Again, durations should be personalized based on identified pathogens and individual clinical response. Some patients will recover quickly even from bad infections, whereas others remain febrile and acutely ill for longer periods of time. Changes in levels of biomarkers over time may help adjust the duration of antibiotic therapy in individual patients. This approach has already been studied with several biomarkers, notably PCT and C-reactive protein. In a multicenter randomized controlled trial in the Netherlands, patients who received antibiotics for presumed infection were randomized to PCT-guided (advice to discontinue antibiotics if PCT decreased by 80% or more of its peak value or to less than or equal to 0.5 μg/L) or standard-of-care antibiotic discontinuation.[14] Antibiotic duration was lower in the PCT-guided group (absolute difference 1.22; 95% CI, 0.65–1.78; $P<.0001$) and mortality rates also were lower in this group. Importantly, however, although use of PCT to guide initiation of antibiotics in stable patients with respiratory tract infections was associated with reduced antibiotic durations with no increase in mortality,[15,16] in critically ill patients, use of PCT for initiation or escalation of antibiotics had no impact on antibiotic durations and was associated with worse outcomes.[17] In a meta-analysis of 15 studies in critically ill patients, Lam and colleagues[18] reported no difference in short-term mortality for studies using PCT to guide antibiotic initiation but lower mortality in studies using PCT to guide antibiotic discontinuation. Current recommendations for patients with sepsis suggest use of PCT only to guide antibiotic discontinuation.[19] PCT has now been approved by the FDA for use by clinicians to help guide antibiotic management decisions in patients with sepsis or lower respiratory tract infections. This strategy will be increasingly used in the future and should help decrease the emergence of multidrug resistant organisms, a major concern worldwide.

The use of biomarkers can also help identify the need to re-explore a source of sepsis. Hence, the evaluation of the time course of a biomarker will help assess patient course. Persistence of high levels of sepsis markers suggests that treatment is not effective and should trigger further reevaluation of the patient and repeated exploration for a possible source.[20]

THE FUTURE OF ORGAN-SPECIFIC BIOMARKERS

Biomarkers can provide important information related to organ function in critically ill patients in terms of diagnosis, prediction, prognosis, and treatment guidance and response (**Table 2**). As for sepsis, when considering organ function, the ability to diagnose organ dysfunction early is paramount so that treatments, if available, can be started promptly. Current markers are often limited by delay in appearance as well as problems with sensitivity and specificity. Combinations of multiple markers in the future are likely to be more accurate than single markers.

Cerebral Function

Brain injury can be the result of direct and indirect brain injury, but, whatever the cause, cerebral biomarkers will increasingly be used to predict which patients will survive with a good as opposed to a bad neurologic outcome.[21,22] Accurate prediction of prognosis will help provide appropriate treatment, limit premature withdrawal of life-sustaining therapy in patients who may go on to survive with good outcomes, help inform discussions with relatives, and potentially reduce the economic burden on society.[23]

Several biomarkers have already been studied for this purpose, including neuron-specific enolase and S-100B protein, but many can be produced by extracerebral sources so are not specific to cerebral injury or can be influenced by other factors. MicroRNAs are so-called functional biomarkers that play an important role in the pathophysiology of organ dysfunction. Importantly, some microRNAs are tissue-specific, potentially making them valuable biomarkers of injury to the tissue in question.[23,24] Recently, Tissier and colleagues[25] analyzed gene expression profiles in comatose survivors of out-of-hospital cardiac arrest and, using functional enrichment analysis, identified differential expression of more than 300 genes, involved in innate and adaptative immunity, in patients with unfavorable compared with those with favorable outcomes. The transcriptomic signature was able to predict outcome already at hospital admission. Although single tests will never alone be sufficient to lead to a decision to withhold/withdraw life-sustaining therapy in these patients, as part of the total information available, they can help inform these difficult decisions.

Respiratory Function

Important future roles for biomarkers in patients with acute respiratory failure will be to accurately determine whether or when to start mechanical ventilation or extracorporeal membrane oxygenation (ECMO), how to adjust ventilatory conditions for an individual patient, and when and how to wean the patient from mechanical ventilation.

Table 2
Examples of future applications of biomarkers per organ system

Organ System	Signal	Potential Therapeutic Implications
Cerebral	Encephalopathy Cell alterations	Cerebral/metabolic support Adapted monitoring Therapeutic limitation

Pulmonary	Overdistension/parenchymal
	  alterations
	Respiratory muscle and
	  diaphragmatic dysfunction
		Decrease tidal volume
		Adjust PEEP level
		Start ECMO/ECCO2R
		Start corticosteroids
		Need for lung transplantation

Cardiovascular	Risk of myocardial ischemia Altered cell oxygen supply	Need for PTCA Antiplatelet agent Myocardial protective substance Need for LVAD/transplant
Renal	Altered perfusion Impending injury	Fluids (albumin?) Renal protective agents Specific vasoactive agent Start RRT Expect long-term failure

Coagulation	Subtle coagulopathy
	Endothelial activation
		Adjust (anti)hemostatic agents
		Give an anticoagulant/endothelial
		  protective agent
		  (thrombomodulin?)

Gastrointestinal	Dysfunction	Withhold enteral nutrition Give a specific nutrient
Hepatic	Dysfunction	Liver protective agent Need for liver transplantation
Metabolic, cellular	Deficiencies	Add proteins, amino acids Add vitamins and other trace elements

Abbreviations: ECCO2R, extracorporeal CO_2 removal; LVAD, left ventricular assist device; PTCA, percutaneous transluminal coronary angioplasty.

Recently, latent class analysis has identified patients with ARDS who have different subphenotypes, based in part on differences in concentrations of the inflammatory biomarkers interleukin (IL)-6, IL-8, soluble tumor necrosis factor receptor 1 and plasminogen activator inhibitor 1. The 2 groups were found to respond differently to different fluid management strategies[26] and to different positive end-expiratory pressure (PEEP) settings[27] and had different responses to simvastatin treatment.[28]

Cardiovascular Function

Biomarkers will help evaluate more rapidly the presence myocardial function and the need for intervention, including some myocardial protection. Acute aortic syndromes, which are particularly challenging to diagnose, also will be more easily recognized, probably by combinations of several biomarkers.[29]

In circulatory shock, biomarkers will increasingly be used to evaluate the need for fluid therapy. For example, natriuretic peptides can reflect the degree of myocardial fiber distension and, therefore, potentially indicate adequate fluid status or fluid overload. Use of natriuretic peptides is already widespread in the diagnosis of heart failure,[30] but their usefulness in critically ill patients is unclear.[31] The combination of biomarkers with the colloid osmotic pressure and bioimpedance techniques could help identify and quantitate fluid overload.[32]

In addition to what some people call macrohemodynamic alterations, the role of the microcirculation in critical illness has gained interest in recent years as techniques have been developed that enable its assessment. Importantly, in patients with shock, microcirculatory changes persist even when global hemodynamic parameters seem to have normalized, making normalization of the microcirculation a potentially important resuscitation target. Markers of endothelial damage, such as endothelial progenitor cells and endothelial microparticles, have been associated with outcomes[33,34] and may help determine the best therapeutic support for the microcirculation and to monitor treatment success in the future.[33]

Renal Function

Evaluation of renal hemodynamics will help select the right drug, for example, angiotensin II in certain patients to increase postglomerular perfusion. Although not yet possible with sufficient accuracy,[35] renal biomarkers will be developed to decide when to start and when to stop RRT, thus avoiding unnecessary treatments in some and providing maximum benefit in others. They also can help predict long-term renal outcomes, which is important for organizational and sometimes ethical decisions. Several new biomarkers, urinary-based or blood-based, of renal dysfunction have been proposed in recent years and been shown to have various degrees of accuracy in prediction and prognosis, including insulin-like growth factor binding protein 7 and tissue inhibitor of metalloproteinase 2, neutrophil gelatinase–associated lipocalin, and kidney injury molecule-1. Combinations of these biomarkers are likely to be most useful[36] but some work remains to determine which panels are most effective for each purpose and to develop rapid point-of-care assays that can be used at the bedside.

Hemostatic Function

Biomarkers of coagulopathy can include markers of platelet activation and function, for example, platelet-derived microparticles.[37] Markers of endothelial cell dysfunction can also indicate development and prognosis of coagulopathy. Panels of different biomarkers will enable the underlying cause of the coagulopathy to be identified enabling appropriate treatment.

Gastrointestinal Function

The importance of adequate nutrition in ICU patients is well recognized but the ability to provide correct nutrition to individual patients is currently limited. Biomarkers of gastrointestinal function will enable in evaluating the potential benefits but also the likely risks of enteral feeding more accurately. Instead of the vague current recommendation that enteral nutrition should be withheld in the presence of profound shock,[38] quantifying the precise degree of gut impairment and its evolution over time will be possible, enabling feeding to be started in a timely manner.

Biomarkers will also enable the diagnosis of certain conditions, for example, acute mesenteric ischemia, to be made noninvasively instead of surgically,[39] thus reducing risks associated with surgery and anesthesia and making diagnosis, and therefore treatment initiation, more rapid.

Hepatic Support

Few interventions are currently available that can improve liver function, but new liver support systems and drugs for hepatic protection are being developed. Current markers of liver dysfunction or injury, including bilirubin and liver enzymes, are elevated late in the disease course, and biomarkers that can identify liver dysfunction early are needed.

THERANOSTICS

The term, *theranostics*, refers to the use of techniques, including biomarkers and phenotypes, to guide therapeutic interventions. This approach is widely used in cancer therapy and in rheumatoid arthritis.[40] In the field of sepsis, it is highly unlikely that sepsis drugs that are effective in all patients will be developed, because of the complexity of the condition, with an immune response that changes over time and varies among individuals. Rather, a theranostic approach will increasingly be used. For example, corticosteroids in septic shock will be guided by genetic expression signatures or metabolic response.[41,42] Corticosteroids in patients with ARDS may be guided by a mediator in the bronchoalveolar fluid. In a multicenter study by Steinberg and colleagues,[43] mortality rates were lower in patients with ARDS treated with methylprednisolone who had high bronchoalveolar procollagen type III levels compared with those who had lower levels. A randomized controlled trial is currently ongoing to assess whether procollagen II can indeed be used to guide corticosteroid use in persistent ARDS (Procollagen-3 Driven Corticosteroids for Persistent Acute Respiratory Distress Syndrome; ClinicalTrials.gov Identifier: NCT03371498).

In a retrospective analysis, Seymour and colleagues[44] identified 4 clinical phenotypes of sepsis based on clinical characteristics and organ dysfunction patterns. The different phenotypes were associated with different outcomes and different measures of host-response measured using biomarkers of coagulation, inflammation, and endothelial and renal injury. Importantly, in simulation models, estimated treatment effects of early goal-directed therapy, activated protein C, and eritoran varied according to the relative frequencies of the 4 phenotypes, suggesting these phenotypes could potentially identify groups of patients more likely to respond to these interventions. As discussed previously, latent class analysis has identified subphenotypes of ARDS that respond differently to different management strategies.[26–28]

SUMMARY

The numbers of biomarkers in critical care medicine is increasing rapidly, but there is a real need to improve analysis and validation. Groups, such as the Operation Brain Trauma Therapy,[45] a multicenter preclinical therapy and biomarker screening consortium, will help speed progress in this field, and big data analytics and machine learning will facilitate translation of research to clinical application.[46]

Although it is not impossible that a biomarker will be 100% sensitive and 100% specific for a certain condition or application, it is clear that the vast majority of biomarkers will not attain this ideal. Combined panels of biomarkers, therefore, will increasingly be used[9,36] rather than focusing on single compounds, especially as technology enables multiple markers to be assessed simultaneously from 1 blood sample or sensor at point of care and costs begin to decrease (**Table 3**). Importantly, biomarkers should not be used alone to make diagnostic, prognostic, or treatment decisions but rather to guide them, combined with physician expertise and clinical judgment.[47] The focus on traditional markers, for example, proteins and cytokines, has begun to move toward newer omics markers,[48] using transcriptomics, metabolomics, and genomics. The potential for use of biomarkers to advance the move toward personalized medicine is exciting. As new biomarkers appear and are validated, panels with have to be altered accordingly and increasingly it will be possible to accurately predict and diagnose conditions and complications, target treatments for individual patients and

Table 3
General evolution of biomarker characteristics over time

Characteristic	Present	Future
Sensitivity	Very good	Very good (even better)
Specificity	Very good	Very good (even better)
Reproducibility	Very good	Very good (even better)
Cost	High	Low
Practicality	Complex methods	Simplified test
Delay in obtaining the results	Long	Short

monitor doses and treatment durations, and prognosticate short-term and long-term outcomes. The future of biomarkers will be one of constant evolution.

REFERENCES

1. Ware LB. Biomarkers in critical illness: new insights and challenges for the future. Am J Respir Crit Care Med 2017;196:944–5.
2. Sweeney TE, Khatri P. Generalizable biomarkers in critical care: toward precision medicine. Crit Care Med 2017;45:934–9.
3. FDA-NIH Biomarker Working Group. BEST (biomarkers, EndpointS, and other tools) resource: glossary. Available at: https://www.ncbi.nlm.nih.gov/books/NBK338448/pdf/Bookshelf_NBK338448.pdf. Accessed July 7, 2019.
4. Califf RM. Biomarker definitions and their applications. Exp Biol Med (Maywood) 2018;243:213–21.
5. Raita Y, Goto T, Faridi MK, et al. Emergency department triage prediction of clinical outcomes using machine learning models. Crit Care 2019;23:64.
6. Pierrakos C, Vincent JL. Sepsis biomarkers: a review. Crit Care 2010;14:R15.
7. Vincent JL, Van NM, Lelubre C. Host response biomarkers in sepsis: the role of procalcitonin. Methods Mol Biol 2015;1237:213–24.
8. European Society of Intensive Care Medicine. The problem of sepsis. An expert report of the European Society of Intensive Care Medicine. Intensive Care Med 1994;20:300–4.
9. Miller RR III, Lopansri BK, Burke JP, et al. Validation of a host response assay, SeptiCyte LAB, for discriminating sepsis from systemic inflammatory response syndrome in the ICU. Am J Respir Crit Care Med 2018;198:903–13.
10. Langelier C, Kalantar KL, Moazed F, et al. Integrating host response and unbiased microbe detection for lower respiratory tract infection diagnosis in critically ill adults. Proc Natl Acad Sci U S A 2018;115:E12353–62.
11. Vincent JL, Brealey D, Libert N, et al. Rapid Diagnosis of Infection in the Critically Ill (RADICAL), a multicenter study of molecular detection in bloodstream infections, pneumonia and sterile site infections. Crit Care Med 2015;43:2283–91.
12. Jagtap P, Singh R, Deepika K, et al. A flowthrough assay for rapid bedside stratification of bloodstream bacterial infection in critically ill patients: a pilot study. J Clin Microbiol 2018;56 [pii:e00408-18].
13. Zhang C, Zheng X, Zhao C, et al. Detection of pathogenic microorganisms from bloodstream infection specimens using TaqMan array card technology. Sci Rep 2018;8:12828.

14. de Jong E, van Oers JA, Beishuizen A, et al. Efficacy and safety of procalcitonin guidance in reducing the duration of antibiotic treatment in critically ill patients: a randomised, controlled, open-label trial. Lancet Infect Dis 2016;16:819–27.

15. Christ-Crain M, Stolz D, Bingisser R, et al. Procalcitonin guidance of antibiotic therapy in community-acquired pneumonia: a randomized trial. Am J Respir Crit Care Med 2006;174:84–93.

16. Schuetz P, Christ-Crain M, Thomann R, et al. Effect of procalcitonin-based guidelines vs standard guidelines on antibiotic use in lower respiratory tract infections: the ProHOSP randomized controlled trial. JAMA 2009;302:1059–66.

17. Jensen JU, Hein L, Lundgren B, et al. Procalcitonin-guided interventions against infections to increase early appropriate antibiotics and improve survival in the intensive care unit: a randomized trial. Crit Care Med 2011;39:2048–58.

18. Lam SW, Bauer SR, Fowler R, et al. Systematic review and meta-analysis of procalcitonin-guidance versus usual care for antimicrobial management in critically ill patients: focus on subgroups based on antibiotic initiation, cessation, or mixed strategies. Crit Care Med 2018;46:684–90.

19. Rhodes A, Evans LE, Alhazzani W, et al. Surviving sepsis campaign: international guidelines for management of sepsis and septic shock: 2016. Crit Care Med 2017;45:486–552.

20. Schmit X, Vincent JL. The time course of blood C-reactive protein concentrations in relation to the response to initial antimicrobial therapy in patients with sepsis. Infection 2008;36:213–9.

21. Annborn M, Nilsson F, Dankiewicz J, et al. The combination of biomarkers for prognostication of long-term outcome in patients treated with mild hypothermia after out-of-hospital cardiac arrest-A pilot study. Ther Hypothermia Temp Manag 2016;6:85–90.

22. Isenschmid C, Kalt J, Gamp M, et al. Routine blood markers from different biological pathways improve early risk stratification in cardiac arrest patients: results from the prospective, observational COMMUNICATE study. Resuscitation 2018; 130:138–45.

23. Devaux Y, Stammet P. What's new in prognostication after cardiac arrest: micro-RNAs? Intensive Care Med 2018;44:897–9.

24. Devaux Y, Dankiewicz J, Salgado-Somoza A, et al. Association of circulating microRNA-124-3p levels with outcomes after out-of-hospital cardiac arrest: a substudy of a randomized clinical trial. JAMA Cardiol 2016;1:305–13.

25. Tissier R, Hocini H, Tchitchek N, et al. Early blood transcriptomic signature predicts patients' outcome after out-of-hospital cardiac arrest. Resuscitation 2019; 138:222–32.

26. Famous KR, Delucchi K, Ware LB, et al. Acute respiratory distress syndrome subphenotypes respond differently to randomized fluid management strategy. Am J Respir Crit Care Med 2017;195:331–8.

27. Calfee CS, Delucchi K, Parsons PE, et al. Subphenotypes in acute respiratory distress syndrome: latent class analysis of data from two randomised controlled trials. Lancet Respir Med 2014;2:611–20.

28. Calfee CS, Delucchi KL, Sinha P, et al. Acute respiratory distress syndrome subphenotypes and differential response to simvastatin: secondary analysis of a randomised controlled trial. Lancet Respir Med 2018;6:691–8.

29. Yildiz M, Oksen D, Behnes M, et al. Contribution and value of biomarkers in acute aortic syndromes. Curr Pharm Biotechnol 2017;18:495–8.

30. Chow SL, Maisel AS, Anand I, et al. Role of biomarkers for the prevention, assessment, and management of heart failure: a Scientific Statement from the American Heart Association. Circulation 2017;135:e1054–91.
31. Matsuo A, Nagai-Okatani C, Nishigori M, et al. Natriuretic peptides in human heart: novel insight into their molecular forms, functions, and diagnostic use. Peptides 2019;111:3–17.
32. Massari F, Scicchitano P, Iacoviello M, et al. Serum biochemical determinants of peripheral congestion assessed by bioimpedance vector analysis in acute heart failure. Heart Lung 2019;48(5):395–9.
33. Tapia P, Gatica S, Cortes-Rivera C, et al. Circulating endothelial cells from septic shock patients convert to fibroblasts are associated with the resuscitation fluid dose and are biomarkers for survival prediction. Crit Care Med 2019;47:942–50.
34. van Ierssel SH, Jorens PG, Van Craenenbroeck EM, et al. The endothelium, a protagonist in the pathophysiology of critical illness: focus on cellular markers. Biomed Res Int 2014;2014:985813.
35. Klein SJ, Brandtner AK, Lehner GF, et al. Biomarkers for prediction of renal replacement therapy in acute kidney injury: a systematic review and meta-analysis. Intensive Care Med 2018;44:323–36.
36. Kashani K, Al-Khafaji A, Ardiles T, et al. Discovery and validation of cell cycle arrest biomarkers in human acute kidney injury. Crit Care 2013;17:R25.
37. Melki I, Tessandier N, Zufferey A, et al. Platelet microvesicles in health and disease. Platelets 2017;28:214–21.
38. Singer P, Blaser AR, Berger MM, et al. ESPEN guideline on clinical nutrition in the intensive care unit. Clin Nutr 2019;38:48–79.
39. Treskes N, Persoon AM, van Zanten ARH. Diagnostic accuracy of novel serological biomarkers to detect acute mesenteric ischemia: a systematic review and meta-analysis. Intern Emerg Med 2017;12:821–36.
40. Kaneko Y, Takeuchi T. Targeted antibody therapy and relevant novel biomarkers for precision medicine for rheumatoid arthritis. Int Immunol 2017;29:511–7.
41. Wong HR, Atkinson SJ, Cvijanovich NZ, et al. Combining prognostic and predictive enrichment strategies to identify children with septic shock responsive to corticosteroids. Crit Care Med 2016;44:e1000–3.
42. Antcliffe DB, Burnham KL, Al-Beidh F, et al. Transcriptomic signatures in sepsis and a differential response to steroids. From the VANISH randomized trial. Am J Respir Crit Care Med 2019;199:980–6.
43. Steinberg KP, Hudson LD, Goodman RB, et al. Efficacy and safety of corticosteroids for persistent acute respiratory distress syndrome. N Engl J Med 2006;354:1671–84.
44. Seymour CW, Kennedy JN, Wang S, et al. Derivation, validation, and potential treatment implications of novel clinical phenotypes for sepsis. JAMA 2019;321:2003–17.
45. Kochanek PM, Dixon CE, Mondello S, et al. Multi-center pre-clinical consortia to enhance translation of therapies and biomarkers for traumatic brain injury: Operation Brain Trauma Therapy and beyond. Front Neurol 2018;9:640.
46. Vincent JL, Creteur J. Big data are here to stay. Anaesth Crit Care Pain Med 2019;38:339–40.
47. Vincent JL, Teixeira L. Sepsis biomarkers. Value and limitations. Am J Respir Crit Care Med 2014;190:1081–2.
48. Rello J, van Engelen TSR, Alp E, et al. Towards precision medicine in sepsis: a position paper from the European Society of Clinical Microbiology and Infectious Diseases. Clin Microbiol Infect 2018;24:1264–72.

Pharmacogenomics
Prescribing Precisely

Dyson T. Wake, PharmD[a], Nadim Ilbawi, MD[b],
Henry Mark Dunnenberger, PharmD[a], Peter J. Hulick, MD, MMSc[c],*

KEYWORDS

- Pharmacogenomic • Pharmacogenetic • Medication optimization
- Precision medicine • Adverse effects • Personalized medicine • Patient safety

KEY POINTS

- Pharmacogenomics (PGx) is the use of patient-specific genetic variations to guide medication selection.
- Genetic variations can cause changes in number or function of metabolic enzymes, drug receptors and transporters leading to increased risks of adverse effects or decreased therapeutic efficacy.
- With notable exceptions, PGx testing is best used to assess the risk of general suboptimal response rather than the potential for specific side effects or allergies.
- Guidelines exist to help clinicians understand how to use PGx results when they are available.
- PGx testing is a powerful tool but does not override the need for clinical assessment and judgment.

INTRODUCTION

The use of pharmacogenomics (PGx) and other genetic tools to guide medication selection and improve patient care is on the rise. The US Food and Drug Administration (FDA) currently provides information for 284 biomarkers in 214 medications, including multiple boxed warnings that recommend PGx testing before initiating therapy. Several companies are now marketing genetic testing directly to consumers.[1,2]

This article originally appeared in *Medical Clinics*, Volume 103, Issue 6, November 2019.
Disclosure Statement: P.J. Hulick, D.T. Wake and N. Ilbawi: None. H.M. Dunnenberger: Consultant for Admera Health and Veritas Genetics.
[a] Pharmacogenomics, Mark R. Neaman Center for Personalized Medicine, NorthShore University HealthSystem, 2650 Ridge Avenue, Evanston, IL 60201, USA; [b] Department of Family Medicine, NorthShore University HealthSystem, 6810 North McCormick Boulevard, Lincolnwood, IL 60712, USA; [c] Center for Medical Genetics, Mark R. Neaman Center for Personalized Medicine, NorthShore University HealthSystem, University of Chicago, Pritzker School of Medicine, 1000 Central Street Suite 610, Evanston, IL 60201, USA
* Corresponding author.
E-mail address: phulick@northshore.org

Clinics Collections 8 (2020) 51–64
https://doi.org/10.1016/j.ccol.2020.07.005
2352-7986/20/© 2020 Elsevier Inc. All rights reserved.

However, education to providers on how best to incorporate these results, or whether a test is appropriate for their patient, has not kept pace with these new developments.[3,4]

Clinicians have noted interest in several potential benefits of PGx testing, including guidance on initiating new medications, mutually informed decision making, and a reduction of the "medication odyssey" to find a suitable regimen.[5] However, several studies have found that providers may have concerns about their ability to accurately interpret PGx results and optimally incorporate them into therapeutic decisions.[6] An important factor to consider is the time necessary to incorporate PGx counseling into the patient visit. Recent reviews of primary care providers' responsibilities have found difficulty with meeting the current preventative medicine recommendations alone in standard visit windows; let alone additional PGx concerns and questions.[7] However; it is also possible that through avoidance of adverse effects and optimization of patients' medication regimens, PGx guidance could *increase* the time available to providers and improve engagement with patients.

The goal of this article was to answer the most important questions a provider may have while first investigating PGx testing:

- Which patients are likely to receive benefits from PGx testing?
- How does one choose between PGx tests?
- How does a provider translate PGx results into meaningful clinical recommendations?
- Finally, what changes are anticipated in the PGx landscape in the coming years and how can providers stay abreast of this progress?

BACKGROUND

PGx is the understanding and extrapolation of variations in the patient's underlying DNA into therapeutic recommendations or more simply use of a patient's specific DNA variations to guide medication selection. Definitions for genetic terms can be found in **Table 1**. A variation occurs when one or more of the nucleotides are altered: switched, inserted, or deleted. The focus is on how such variation can cause alteration in metabolism or sensitivity to certain medications.

PGx variation is most typically captured by the "star" (*) system. A *1 is most often assigned to the default reference allele (haplotype) or wild-type/fully functional allele. When other haplotypes are present, other designations are assigned (eg, *2, *3). It is important to note that the *1 allele designation is often based on the subpopulation originally studied and may not represent the most common allele in every population. A laboratory will assign a *1 designation if no other variants are detected on their assay, thus a *1 designation does *not* preclude the possibility that other alleles affecting function are present. This is an important factor in deciding on a testing laboratory.

Somatic versus germline variation is an important distinction. Germline variations are found in DNA throughout the patient's body, including gamete cells, and can be inherited. Somatic variations occur in a specific body area and may spread further throughout the body through cell division, but are not present in gamete cells and cannot be inherited. PGx testing focuses on germline variations that exist within the patient since birth. One exception is the application of genomics-guided cancer treatment, which can be based on somatic changes in the tumor.

Another important dichotomy is reactive versus preemptive testing. Reactive testing is testing done in response to a clinical need. In contrast, preemptive PGx testing is completed before a specific need for the information.[8] The benefit of a preemptive test is the avoidance of delay in utilizing the PGx test to guide therapy. With a shift

Table 1
Definitions of common terms

Term	Definition
Allele	One of 2 or more versions of a gene or single nucleotide polymorphism (SNP) at a given position on a chromosome.
Chromosome	A DNA structure composed of several genes.
Deoxyribonucleic acid (DNA)	A double helix structure created by patterns of 4 nucleotides: adenine (A), thymine (T), guanine (G), and cytosine (C).
Diplotype	Specific combination of 2 haplotypes. Each haplotype is of either maternal or paternal inheritance.
Gene	The DNA instructions for the formation of a protein.
Genome	An organism's entire genetic code.
Genotype	The patient's genetic code at the specific sites being assayed.
Haplotype	A specific combination of SNPs or variations in the DNA sequence occurring on the same chromosome
Phenotype	The expression of the patient's genetic code for a given gene. This can be defined at many levels, including enzymatic activity of the protein produced by a gene to a broader clinical implication, which might be a phenotype explained by the influence of multiple genes, as in warfarin metabolism.
Prodrug	A medication that is metabolized into a more active form after administration.
Single nucleotide polymorphism (SNP)	A variation or mutation in DNA that results in the change of one nucleotide for another or the addition or removal of a nucleotide

toward preemptive testing, the focus for most providers will move to what should be done with genetic information rather than when it should be collected.

IN WHICH PATIENTS SHOULD A PROVIDER CONSIDER PGx TESTING?

PGx guidance is available in many areas of medicine, including psychiatry, cardiology, and pain management (**Table 2**).[9–13] Antidepressant medications represent a prime opportunity for the use of PGx as there are multiple equivalent therapeutic options. The American Psychiatric Association guideline for treatment of major depressive disorder (MDD) recommends that any of a dozen alternatives are all equally "correct" medications and it is left to patient and provider to eventually find the best option.[14] Many patients have inadequate response to their initial therapy and subsequent recommendations largely consist of choosing another "first-line" option. PGx clinical guidelines are available to inform the use of tricyclic antidepressants (TCAs) and selective serotonin reuptake inhibitors (SSRIs) based on CYP2D6 and CYP2C19 activity.[11,12] Recent studies have shown decreases in adverse effects and improvement in depression scores in patients who have PGx-guided antidepressant therapy.[15,16] Therefore, patients considering initiating a new antidepressant medication may benefit from the use of PGx testing.

Table 2
Commonly prescribed medications with pharmacogenomic guidance

Depression/Anxiety	Pain	Cardiovascular	Miscellaneous
• Selective serotonin reuptake inhibitors (SSRIs) • Tricyclic antidepressants (TCA) • Venlafaxine • Aripiprazole	• Codeine • Hydrocodone • Oxycodone • Tramadol	• Warfarin • Clopidogrel • Metoprolol • Carvedilol	• Proton pump inhibitors (PPIs) • Simvastatin • Phenytoin • Tacrolimus • Abacavir

These medications are described in pharmacogenomics (PGx) guidelines or have Food and Drug Administration labeling regarding a PGx interaction.

PGx is especially enticing when considering the time span involved. SSRIs can take 4 to 6 weeks to demonstrate full therapeutic response.[17] The patient and provider could spend several months managing dose adjustments, appointments, and new prescriptions before determining that a single medication is ineffective. PGx testing could allow the provider to more rapidly determine if a lack of response represents an insufficient trial or belies an inherent issue with the medication.

The applicability of PGx testing depends in part on the potential severity of the reaction. Abacavir is used in the treatment of human immunodeficiency virus and has the potential to cause severe cutaneous adverse reactions (SCAR).[18] Although this risk is generally low, the HLA-B*57:01 variant is associated with a significantly increased risk of SCAR with abacavir. As a result, abacavir is not only contraindicated in those known to be positive for HLA-B*57:01, but FDA labeling recommends "All patients should be screened for the HLA-B*5701 allele prior to initiating therapy."[18]

Another area of extensive research is the use of PGx to guide the appropriate dosing of the anticoagulant warfarin. Beyond factors such as concomitant medications, other health conditions, and dietary vitamin K intake, genetic variations have been found to alter warfarin therapy.[19] Alterations in CYP2C9 can impair the metabolism of warfarin and changes in VKORC1 may increase a patient's sensitivity to warfarin therapy.[10,20]

PGx guidance based on these initial gene links led to interesting variability in the results of 2 major studies. The European Pharmacogenetics of Anticoagulant Therapy (EU-PACT) trial found PGx guidance was associated with greater time in therapeutic international normalized ratio range than standard dosing.[21] Concurrently the Clarification of Optimal Anticoagulation through Genetics (COAG) trial found PGx guidance did not improve warfarin control and in fact was associated with less effective management for black patients.[22] The juxtaposition of these results highlights the need to match PGx tests to the patient. Tests in these studies primarily interrogated for CYP2C9*2 and *3. Although these represent the most prominent loss of function alleles in White patients this is not the case for all populations. In Black patients, the most common loss of function allele is CYP2C9*8.[10] The EU-PACT trial was composed of more than 98% white patients, whereas more than 25% of those in the COAG study were black. Using a panel based on White genetic proportions to guide dosages of black patients led to more harm than benefit. Current guidelines recommend against the use of PGx guidance in patients of African ancestry if the assay covers only CYP2C9*2 and *3. The most recent guidelines incorporate CYP4F2 (which metabolizes vitamin K) and other variations relevant in specific patient populations.[10]

The use of codeine has recently been restricted to adult patients following new evidence for increased risks of adverse effects in the pediatric patient population. Case reports have demonstrated the potential for serious adverse reactions in infants of breastfeeding mothers who have consumed codeine.[23] A major component of these restrictions is that codeine is a prodrug and is activated into morphine largely by CYP2D6.[24] Genetic variations can significantly increase a patient's CYP2D6 enzymatic activity and cause a corresponding increase in the proportion of morphine leading to elevated risks for adverse effects. Similar reactions may be seen in other CYP2D6-mediated pain medications, such as tramadol, oxycodone, and hydrocodone.[13] PGx guidance has also demonstrated improvements in reduction of pain intensity for patients with reduced CYP2D6 enzyme activity.[25]

Several studies have demonstrated that a vast majority of patients have at least 1 clinically actionable variant that could affect prescribing. A 2014 study of more than 10,000 patients by Vanderbilt University found that 91% of patients had at least 1 clinically significant variation in the 5 genes tested.[26] Another group using a wider PGx panel found that more than 97% of patients had a least 1 variation linked to drug response and a median of 3 such variations.[27] Without a precise delineation of which patients should or should not receive testing, it is best to understand factors that may increase or decrease the potential value of PGx testing.

Studies have found patients are highly interested in PGx testing.[5,28] In particular, patients are interested in the opportunity to use PGx guidance in reducing side effects and guiding therapeutic selections.[29] Barriers to wider use also have been reported, such as concerns for cost or insurance reimbursement.[30] In addition, some surveys have indicated that patients are concerned with who may have access to the results.[31]

For all its benefits, PGx testing may not be right for every patient. Some questions or concerns cannot be answered by current PGx testing, and patients should be counseled to ensure that they are properly informed of what the tests can and cannot provide (**Table 3**).[27]

When evaluating whether PGx results should be used in a patient's care, there are 3 tenets that must be investigated:

1. The strength of literature supporting the interaction
2. The likelihood and severity of the clinical impact of the interaction
3. The risks associated with alternative therapies

PGx testing does not apply to every medication. Hundreds of medications have been investigated for links to genetic variants, but newer medications and those used by smaller patient populations may not have been examined yet. For other medications, there may exist only a small set of cases and studies focusing on narrow populations or with inconclusive results. Because of this lack of clarity, several organizations give a rating for the strength of evidence supporting a given PGx interaction.[32,33] The severity of the potential interaction may also sway the provider or patient's desire to incorporate PGx guidance.

In addition, providers must consider that any change in therapy is also associated with its own risks. If PGx guidance leads to the use of a second-line agent, providers should be cognizant that this could entail risk of therapeutic failure if the new agent is generally less effective or tolerated. Providers may also find themselves prescribing medications with which they have less familiarity or agents not covered by the patient's insurance.

Another important consideration is that PGx testing is not able to determine the "perfect" medication for the patient. A "clean" PGx result does not indicate that the medication will not cause side effects or that it will be therapeutically effective; it only means that no adverse PGx interaction was discovered. Such patients would still be expected to have the normal risk of side effects with treatment and the normal risk of

Table 3
What pharmacogenomics (PGx) can and cannot do

PGx Can...	PGx Cannot...
• Identify medications with increased risk of adverse effects	• Predict all adverse reactions to medication
• Identify medications with increased risk of therapeutic failure	• Predict the risk of a *specific* side effect for all medication
• Help narrow therapeutic selection	• Determine the risk of future diagnosis with a disease or of sequalae
• Assist in predicting dosage for some medications	• Serve as a "magic bullet" that delivers a perfect regimen with no risks

therapeutic failure. Thus, PGx testing should be thought of more as a tool to reveal potential complications of therapy rather than to reveal the one best option for treatment.

HOW ARE PGx TESTS ORDERED?

PGx testing can be performed as either a single-gene assay or as a panel of dozens or more genes.[34] Early testing was primarily composed of assays of a handful of variants in a single gene, targeted at the most common and most impactful variants. Economies of scale and new technologies have allowed large increases in the number of genes and variations covered with nominal increases in cost. PGx testing via panels is becoming more common with companies now offering substantial panels at similar costs of a single gene test. Most PGx tests analyze a subset of variants (also called single nucleotide variants, or SNPs) known to be relevant for determining PGx haplotypes of clinical significance. This is in contrast to sequencing the entire gene to look for variations across the entire gene.

When determining which test or panel will best serve the patient or population, it is important to consider indications with therapeutic overlap. For instance, if testing is desired for *CYP2D6* and *CYP2C19* due to the possibility of initiating therapy with antidepressants, then it also may be prudent to consider whether PGx guidance for medications to treat cardiovascular and pain conditions will be of value to the patient.[10–12,35] A panel test may represent a nominal cost increase over the single-gene assay but deliver dividends by ensuring that commonly coprescribed medications are also reviewed.

PGx panels themselves are not homogeneous and can vary significantly in breadth and scope.[34,36] Most panels will cover several of the most well-studied and impactful genes. Panels can have different combinations of SNPs even for the well-studied, impactful genes, and this can contribute to why one laboratory may report a *1 designation versus a different laboratory that reports a more refined haplotype. Other genes may be included based on the creator's review of literature or expectation for future research. A panel purporting to have a large number of genes may not necessarily provide additional value to the patient, as not all variants provide equal clinical utility.

In fact, some variants can be incredibly rare outside of certain populations but may be fairly common within that group. For instance, the variant of HLA-B*15:02 that is associated with increased risk of SCAR in patients prescribed carbamazepine has an allele frequency of 0.04% in patients of European ancestry but a frequency of 6.88% in those of east Asian ancestry.[37] One panel may provide more value to a patient if it interrogates variations that are more closely in line with his or her ancestry.

It is also important to investigate what other alternative or special assays are provided by the panel. Multiple copies of the *CYP2D6* gene (such as duplications) occur in in approximately 1 in 8 patients and this number may be even larger in Black and Asian patients.[38] Duplication of the gene can cause increased enzymatic activity and may be clinically significant. However, not all panels can test for the presence or extent of gene duplications.

Beyond the contents of the panel are factors related to the ordering and use of the panel. Does it require a cheek-swab, saliva sample, or blood draw, and are any of these a potential issue for the patient? Will the results be available in a therapeutically necessary window? The manner in which the results are returned can differ drastically between laboratories. Some panels provide little beyond raw genetic data, some provide hard copies of interpreted PGx results and recommendations, and others are fully integrated into the electronic health record and allow for the use of sophisticated clinical decision support (CDS) tools.

Finally, it is also important to consider the potential cost of PGx testing. Patients have greatly varied means and desires to pay for PGx testing. Some are cost-insensitive and willing to pay substantial amounts upfront. For others, providers may need to be cognizant of which testing companies offer sliding scale pricing or other assistance.

HOW TO USE/INTERPRET PGx TESTING?

The goal of PGx testing is incorporation into your routine therapeutic decision process. One important aspect to remember about PGx testing, and indeed about any particular tool or test, is that it is only one piece of the larger patient picture. PGx testing should be used in conjunction with all other relevant factors, such as renal function, concomitant medications, and interacting disease states to determine the final risk-benefit analysis of treatment. A "normal" PGx result should not generally be used as justification to initiate a medication to which the patient previously experienced a severe adverse reaction just as a result indicating a patient may be at increased risk of therapeutic failure should not necessarily lead to cessation of currently effective therapy.

Depending on the gene and protein in question, different result structures and terminology may be used.[39] Some genes may be described in terms of the metabolic activity, some by their general function, and others as simply present or absent. Understanding why these descriptions are used is important in comprehending the underlying effect that the results represent.

The gene variants, called alleles, may be denoted using star allele nomenclature. Each star allele is denoted by an asterisk and then a number (eg, *1, *2, *17) and represents 1 or more SNPs that are inherited together. Star alleles are assigned activity levels, with *1 typically used to denote "wild-type" or the absence of any discovered variations. As this is a diagnosis of exclusion, the breadth of the panel may alter which patients are reported as *1.

Pairs of these star alleles, called diplotypes, are categorized into phenotypes describing their enzymatic activity; from poor to ultrarapid metabolism, as shown in **Table 4**. A normal metabolizer (NM), historically called an extensive metabolizer, typically has the expected or "average" amount of enzymatic activity and would be expected to have the normal chance of therapeutic failure and adverse events.[9,39] Intermediate (IM) and poor metabolizers (PM) have less enzymatic activity than the "average" patient; leading to increased exposure to the medication (or slower conversion of a prodrug to its active form). Conversely, rapid metabolizers (RMs) and ultrarapid metabolizers (UMs) have increased activity.

Some gene results describe the general function of genes such as with SLCO1B1 (related to simvastatin), VKORC1 (related to warfarin), and OPRM1 (related to opioids).[39] Results for these genes may be reported as normal, intermediate, or poor function. Similar to the results of the metabolic enzymes, a normal function result indicates that the patient has the expected amount of function and typically does not require dose adjustment. Those described as intermediate or poor function have reduced functional activity, with poor representing the more profound loss of activity.

Results for genes such as human leukocyte antigens (HLA) may be described as "positive" or "negative."[39] HLAs are important pieces of immune function and patients with an actionable variant for one of these genes are at increased risk for severe adverse reactions with specific medications. Patients who are positive for HLA-B*58:01 are at an increased risk of hypersensitivity to allopurinol and those positive for HLA-B*15:02 are at increased risk for SCARs if treated with carbamazepine or oxcarbazepine.[40,41] For these genes, the proportional amount of activity provided by the gene is less important than the presence of the variant itself.

Beyond the terminology, the manner in which the results are presented or formatted can vary significantly between reports. Some are presented as raw genetic information and others as the final therapeutic recommendation. Reports may use proprietary iconography to describe the results with certain symbols indicating patients with expected increased risk of either side effects or therapeutic failure. Other reports may use a "traffic light" style representation with 3 main categories indicating medications expected to have normal risk (green), to be used with caution (yellow) or avoided (red). Results displayed in either format may cause a provider to oversimplify PGx results and ignore additional clinical considerations. A report may have any or all of these methods of conveying information and as each such system is different, care should be taken to fully understand the implications of each categorization.

PHARMACOGENOMIC RESOURCES

Because of the constantly shifting nature of genetic medicine, it is important to know how to stay apprised of further developments in the recommendations for testing or interpretation of results. Online resources have been created to ease this burden. The Clinical Pharmacogenetics Implementation Consortium (CPIC) and Dutch Pharmacogenomics Working Group provide guidelines with background evidence in support of their therapeutic recommendations.[9,33] The Genetic Testing Registry provides overviews regarding available genetic testing companies.[42] The Pharmacogenetic Knowledgebase (PharmGKB) provides a curated database of gene variations and their links to medications.[43] This may represent a good source for delving into upcoming or less known PGx interactions.

Primary literature may represent a great tool for specialists to stay abreast of relevant changes but may be too time-consuming for more general practitioners. There are several organizations (**Table 5**) that provide contact with programs using PGx and updates on the current state of evidence.[33,44] Collaboration or discussion with these groups can ensure that everyone is providing care at the highest level possible.

However, these resources may still require significant time to use and do not represent a sustainable solution for most providers. CDS systems are paramount for systemic adoption of PGx.[6,45] These tools can provide flags or alerts when a medication with potentially actionable PGx associations is ordered and direct the provider to either incorporate existing results into their decision process or facilitate the ordering of a PGx test.

CASE EXAMPLE

A 25-year-old woman who is in your clinic has a recent diagnosis of MDD and no other health concerns. She is currently taking no prescription medications and reports

Table 4
Definition of phenotypes

Phenotype	Description	Effect on Medication Response
Ultrarapid Metabolizer (UM)	Significantly increased enzymatic activity	Medications metabolized by these enzymes would be expected to be eliminated at an increased rate. Affected medications would have reduced half-lives and have less time for the medication to fulfillits therapeutic objective. Patients would be at an increased risk of therapeutic failure due to the lower effective dose they would experience.
Rapid Metabolizer (RM)	Elevated enzyme activity but less than ultrarapid	Medications that are prodrugs activated by this enzyme would be expected to have a greater proportion of the active moiety. In this case, patients would be at increased risk of adverse effects due to the higher effective dose they would experience
Normal Metabolizer (NM)	The normal or expected amount of enzymatic activity	These patients are expected to have the normal or average amount expected risk of side effects and therapeutic response. In general, these patients do not require dose adjustment.
Intermediate Metabolizer (IM)	Decreased enzymatic activity	Medications metabolized by these enzymes would be expected to be eliminated at a decreased rate. Affected medications would have increased half-lives and remain active in the body longer, patients would be at increased risk of adverse effects due to the higher effective dose they would experience.
Poor Metabolizer (PM)	Minimal or absent enzymatic activity	Medications that are prodrugs activated by this enzyme would be expected to have a diminished proportion of

(continued on next page)

Table 4 (continued)		
Phenotype	Description	Effect on Medication Response
		the active moiety. In this case, patients would be at an increased risk of therapeutic failure due to the lower effective dose they would experience.

having "bad experiences with meds" in the past. She is hesitant to initiate an antidepressant medication but also reports that she has heard of genetic testing that can determine which medication she should use if she must begin one. She wishes to know more about this "DNA test."

PGx testing may decrease the trial and error necessary to find the correct medication and may alleviate some hesitancy from the patient to attempt pharmacotherapy. However, it is also important to counsel the patient on the current limitations of testing. Although the test may provide some delineation between suboptimal choices and those with the most promise, it is unlikely that the test will be able to highlight a single, best medication regimen. After counseling, she decides to proceed with PGx testing.

Several months later, the patient is ready to try pharmacotherapy. The results of the PGx test show that she is a CYP2D6 UM and a CYP2C19 IM. She wants to know what this means for her and which medications would be best. Her insurance will cover paroxetine, sertraline, or bupropion. After reviewing the CPIC and PharmGKB resources (see **Table 5**) you note paroxetine is metabolized by CYP2D6 and would be expected to have reduced efficacy in this patient, as it is eliminated more rapidly. Sertraline is metabolized by CYP2C19 and in patients with greatly reduced activity this can lead to increased rates of adverse effects. In general, CYP2C19 IMs retain sufficient enzymatic activity to process sertraline and current CPIC guidelines recommend initiating the normal starting dose of medication. Bupropion has no current PGx guideline recommendations.

You discuss these aspects with her and the general pros and cons of sertraline and bupropion. She indicates that her aunt takes sertraline and has not had any issues, Her aunt may have a different pharmacogenomic profile, so family history must be used cautiously. You decide to proceed with a trial of sertraline therapy at the normal starting dose.

The same patient, now 47, remains a loyal patient at your clinic. She has MDD for which she continues to take sertraline, as well as hypertension, hyperlipidemia, and atherosclerosis. She is scheduled to undergo percutaneous coronary intervention (PCI) in the next month and will be started on antiplatelet therapy. She calls and says that "The surgery doc says I have the wrong genes for the medication they were going to put me on" and wishes to understand more about the reaction. You discover that the team planned to initiate clopidogrel post PCI but received an alert based on her PGx test results.

Clopidogrel is a prodrug that is activated in the body primarily through CYP2C19. Patients with reduced CYP2C19 activity are at risk for reduced activation and thus reduced antiplatelet effect. CPIC guidelines recommend against the use of clopidogrel in CYP2C19 IM and PM. Prasugrel or ticagrelor are alternatives that do not

Table 5
Brief descriptions of pharmacogenomics organizations

Organization	Abbreviation	Brief Description
Clinical Pharmacogenetics Implementation Consortium	CPIC	Creates clinical guidelines for the incorporation of PGx results into clinical decisions
Implementing GeNomics In pracTicE	IGNITE	Investigates and provides resources for the implementation of PGx into clinical practice
Electronic Medical Records and Genomics Network	eMERGE	Funded by the National Institutes of Health (NIH) to create and disperse information on the utilization of electronic health records to facilitate genetic medicine
Pharmacogenomics Knowledgebase	PharmGKB	NIH-funded repository of genetic variations and links to medications

demonstrate this reduced therapeutic efficacy. You discuss these elements with your patient and suggest that the surgery team consider the use of either antiplatelet alternative.

This is an example of the inherent benefits of preemptive testing. Although *CYP2C19* and clopidogrel have a demonstrated link, this PGx information may not be immediately available for many patients at the time of need and it may be detrimental to delay the procedure until PGx testing is performed. This patient was initially tested because of a concern regarding antidepressants. However, cardiovascular concerns are common in patients with MDD and those same genes also both provide guidance for cardiovascular medications, such as clopidogrel, metoprolol, and flecainide.[46] Other genes covered by her panel may assist with cholesterol medication selection, initiation of warfarin, or with selection of antipsychotic therapies if such comorbidities arise. PGx testing truly delivers life-long results that continue to benefit the patient's medication selection.

HOW MIGHT PGx TESTING CHANGE IN THE NEAR FUTURE?

One possible paradigm shift in the near future may be a greater use of next generation sequencing (NGS). Although current tests look for the presence of a few specific variants within a gene, NGS may return the patient's entire DNA sequence for the gene. This may allow for the detection of rare variations and better understanding of genetic function. But this deluge of new data also will create issues for researchers and clinicians, as there will be large quantities of "variants of unknown significance" without clear guidance. CDS also may need to be redesigned to allow the storage and use of the new structure of data.

The maintenance of existing CDS architectures and the formation of new programs for delivering data will represent a significant opportunity in the coming years. Several health systems have begun using CDS tools to integrate PGx data into the clinical decision process and provide information to providers at the time when it is most valuable. Such CDS tools will be paramount as PGx tests become more common and new formats for results and testing arise. Focus may also be applied to the development of patient-facing apps and portals through which the patient may interface with his or her providers and receive counseling on the results.

SUMMARY

As powerful as PGx may be, it is important to remember that it is just another tool that providers may use to improve their patients' care. It will not always be the best tool for the job and results should not override a provider's expertise. PGx itself is only one part of the larger paradigm shift that is personalized medicine.

In that same vein, providers should have a plan in place for what to do with results before the test is ordered. This is both to ensure that the clinical question being asked is one that PGx testing can answer and that the patient is able to receive the benefits of testing. It is not uncommon for the rationale for testing to be patient curiosity or general information gathering and such cases are reasonable as long as both the patient and provider properly understand the results returned.

The techniques of PGx testing and the manner in which results are dispersed will continue to evolve. CDS resources to store and interpret genetic medicine will become more prevalent and more powerful but the changes should focus on improving the integration of PGx testing into clinical workflows rather than just more sophisticated analysis for the sake of data.

Regardless of which laboratory results or data analysis tool is used, the end result always should be what is most beneficial to the patient. And as each patient is an individual with his or her own perspectives just as varied as the genetics described here, it is important to match the treatment to the patient's goals just as much as to the test results.

REFERENCES

1. Bloss CS, Schork NJ, Topol EJ. Direct-to-consumer pharmacogenomic testing is associated with increased physician utilisation. J Med Genet 2014;51(2):83–9.
2. FDA. FDA authorizes first direct-to-consumer test for detecting genetic variants that may be associated with medication metabolism. 2018. Available at: https://www.fda.gov/NewsEvents/Newsroom/PressAnnouncements/ucm624753.htm. Accessed February 1, 2019.
3. Rohrer Vitek CR, Abul-Husn NS, Connolly JJ, et al. Healthcare provider education to support integration of pharmacogenomics in practice: the eMERGE Network experience. Pharmacogenomics 2017;18(10):1013–25.
4. Lemke AA, Hutten Selkirk CG, Glaser NS, et al. Primary care physician experiences with integrated pharmacogenomic testing in a community health system. Per Med 2017;14(5):389–400.
5. Lemke AA, Hulick PJ, Wake DT, et al. Patient perspectives following pharmacogenomics results disclosure in an integrated health system. Pharmacogenomics 2018;19(4):321–31.
6. Unertl KM, Field JR, Price L, et al. Clinician perspectives on using pharmacogenomics in clinical practice. Per Med 2015;12(4):339–47.
7. Yarnall KS, Pollak KI, Ostbye T, et al. Primary care: is there enough time for prevention? Am J Public Health 2003;93(4):635–41.
8. Weitzel KW, Cavallari LH, Lesko LJ. Preemptive panel-based pharmacogenetic testing: the time is now. Pharm Res 2017;34(8):1551–5.
9. Swen JJ, Nijenhuis M, de Boer A, et al. Pharmacogenetics: from bench to byte–an update of guidelines. Clin Pharmacol Ther 2011;89(5):662–73.

10. Johnson JA, Caudle KE, Gong L, et al. Clinical pharmacogenetics implementation consortium (cpic) guideline for pharmacogenetics-guided warfarin dosing: 2017 update. Clin Pharmacol Ther 2017;102(3):397–404.
11. Hicks JK, Bishop JR, Sangkuhl K, et al, Clinical Pharmacogenetics Implementation Consortium. Clinical Pharmacogenetics Implementation Consortium (CPIC) guideline for CYP2D6 and CYP2C19 genotypes and dosing of selective serotonin reuptake inhibitors. Clin Pharmacol Ther 2015;98(2):127–34.
12. Hicks JK, Sangkuhl K, Swen JJ, et al. Clinical pharmacogenetics implementation consortium guideline (CPIC) for CYP2D6 and CYP2C19 genotypes and dosing of tricyclic antidepressants: 2016 update. Clin Pharmacol Ther 2017;102(1):37–44.
13. Crews KR, Gaedigk A, Dunnenberger HM, et al. Clinical Pharmacogenetics Implementation Consortium guidelines for cytochrome P450 2D6 genotype and codeine therapy: 2014 update. Clin Pharmacol Ther 2014;95(4):376–82.
14. Practice guideline for the treatment of patients with major depressive disorder (revision). American Psychiatric Association. Am J Psychiatry 2000;157(4 Suppl):1–45.
15. Hall-Flavin DK, Winner JG, Allen JD, et al. Utility of integrated pharmacogenomic testing to support the treatment of major depressive disorder in a psychiatric outpatient setting. Pharmacogenet Genomics 2013;23(10):535–48.
16. Olson MC, Maciel A, Gariepy JF, et al. Clinical impact of pharmacogenetic-guided treatment for patients exhibiting neuropsychiatric disorders: a randomized controlled trial. Prim Care Companion CNS Disord 2017;19(2).
17. Frazer A, Benmansour S. Delayed pharmacological effects of antidepressants. Mol Psychiatry 2002;7(Suppl 1):S23–8.
18. ZIAGEN [Package Insert]. Research Triangle Park, NC: GlaxoSmithKline; 2015.
19. Cho SM, Lee KY, Choi JR, et al. Development and comparison of warfarin dosing algorithms in stroke patients. Yonsei Med J 2016;57(3):635–40.
20. Johnson JA, Gong L, Whirl-Carrillo M, et al. Clinical pharmacogenetics implementation consortium guidelines for CYP2C9 and VKORC1 genotypes and warfarin dosing. Clin Pharmacol Ther 2011;90(4):625–9.
21. Pirmohamed M, Burnside G, Eriksson N, et al. A randomized trial of genotype-guided dosing of warfarin. N Engl J Med 2013;369(24):2294–303.
22. Kimmel SE, French B, Kasner SE, et al. A pharmacogenetic versus a clinical algorithm for warfarin dosing. N Engl J Med 2013;369(24):2283–93.
23. Kelly LE, Rieder M, van den Anker J, et al. More codeine fatalities after tonsillectomy in North American children. Pediatrics 2012;129(5):e1343–7.
24. Thorn CF, Klein TE, Altman RB. Codeine and morphine pathway. Pharmacogenet Genomics 2009;19(7):556–8.
25. Smith DM, Weitzel KW, Elsey AR, et al. CYP2D6-guided opioid therapy improves pain control in CYP2D6 intermediate and poor metabolizers: a pragmatic clinical trial. Genet Med 2019. [Epub ahead of print].
26. Van Driest SL, Shi Y, Bowton EA, et al. Clinically actionable genotypes among 10,000 patients with preemptive pharmacogenomic testing. Clin Pharmacol Ther 2014;95(4):423–31.
27. Dunnenberger HM, Biszewski M, Bell GC, et al. Implementation of a multidisciplinary pharmacogenomics clinic in a community health system. Am J Health Syst Pharm 2016;73(23):1956–66.
28. Patel HN, Ursan ID, Zueger PM, et al. Stakeholder views on pharmacogenomic testing. Pharmacotherapy 2014;34(2):151–65.
29. Haga SB, Mills R, Moaddeb J, et al. Patient experiences with pharmacogenetic testing in a primary care setting. Pharmacogenomics 2016;17(15):1629–36.

30. Bielinski SJ, St Sauver JL, Olson JE, et al. Are patients willing to incur out-of-pocket costs for pharmacogenomic testing? Pharmacogenomics J 2016; 17(1):1–3.
31. Haga SB, O'Daniel JM, Tindall GM, et al. Survey of US public attitudes toward pharmacogenetic testing. Pharmacogenomics J 2012;12(3):197–204.
32. Whirl-Carrillo M, McDonagh EM, Hebert JM, et al. Pharmacogenomics knowledge for personalized medicine. Clin Pharmacol Ther 2012;92(4):414–7.
33. Caudle KE, Klein TE, Hoffman JM, et al. Incorporation of pharmacogenomics into routine clinical practice: the Clinical Pharmacogenetics Implementation Consortium (CPIC) guideline development process. Curr Drug Metab 2014;15(2): 209–17.
34. Vo TT, Bell GC, Owusu Obeng A, et al. Pharmacogenomics implementation: considerations for selecting a reference laboratory. Pharmacotherapy 2017;37(9): 1014–22.
35. Scott SA, Sangkuhl K, Stein CM, et al. Clinical Pharmacogenetics Implementation Consortium guidelines for CYP2C19 genotype and clopidogrel therapy: 2013 update. Clin Pharmacol Ther 2013;94(3):317–23.
36. Bousman C, Maruf AA, Muller DJ. Towards the integration of pharmacogenetics in psychiatry: a minimum, evidence-based genetic testing panel. Curr Opin Psychiatry 2019;32(1):7–15.
37. Phillips EJ, Sukasem C, Whirl-Carrillo M, et al. Clinical Pharmacogenetics Implementation Consortium Guideline for HLA genotype and use of carbamazepine and oxcarbazepine: 2017 update. Clin Pharmacol Ther 2018;103(4): 574–81.
38. Hosono N, Kato M, Kiyotani K, et al. CYP2D6 genotyping for functional-gene dosage analysis by allele copy number detection. Clin Chem 2009;55(8): 1546–54.
39. Caudle KE, Dunnenberger HM, Freimuth RR, et al. Standardizing terms for clinical pharmacogenetic test results: consensus terms from the Clinical Pharmacogenetics Implementation Consortium (CPIC). Genet Med 2017;19(2):215–23.
40. Hershfield MS, Callaghan JT, Tassaneeyakul W, et al. Clinical Pharmacogenetics Implementation Consortium guidelines for human leukocyte antigen-B genotype and allopurinol dosing. Clin Pharmacol Ther 2013;93(2):153–8.
41. Leckband SG, Kelsoe JR, Dunnenberger HM, et al. Clinical Pharmacogenetics Implementation Consortium guidelines for HLA-B genotype and carbamazepine dosing. Clin Pharmacol Ther 2013;94(3):324–8.
42. Rubinstein WS, Maglott DR, Lee JM, et al. The NIH genetic testing registry: a new, centralized database of genetic tests to enable access to comprehensive information and improve transparency. Nucleic Acids Res 2013;41(Database issue): D925–35.
43. Sangkuhl K, Berlin DS, Altman RB, et al. PharmGKB: understanding the effects of individual genetic variants. Drug Metab Rev 2008;40(4):539–51.
44. Volpi S, Bult CJ, Chisholm RL, et al. Research directions in the clinical implementation of pharmacogenomics: an overview of US programs and projects. Clin Pharmacol Ther 2018;103(5):778–86.
45. Hicks JK, Dunnenberger HM, Gumpper KF, et al. Integrating pharmacogenomics into electronic health records with clinical decision support. Am J Health Syst Pharm 2016;73(23):1967–76.
46. Fiedorowicz JG. Depression and cardiovascular disease: an update on how course of illness may influence risk. Curr Psychiatry Rep 2014;16(10):492.

Pharmacoeconomics of Biologic Therapy

Don A. Bukstein, MD[a,b,*], Allan T. Luskin, MD[c,1]

KEYWORDS

- Severe asthma • Biologic therapy • Pharmacoeconomics • Health care resource use
- Oral corticosteroid • Personalized medicine

KEY POINTS

- Pharmacoeconomics in immune therapy with biologics involves comparing the costs of an intervention with the change in health status to establish value of an intervention.
- Accurate assessments require measuring all disease costs before and after the intervention, including direct disease costs, costs of related comorbidities, and indirect costs.
- Indirect costs include absenteeism, presenteeism, and quality of life of the patient and family/caregivers.
- Proper policy decisions demand that the cost of the intervention be compared with the cost of the lack of the intervention or alternative interventions.
- Costs of lack of the intervention or alternative therapies include both direct and indirect costs, and the direct costs should include the costs of complications of uncontrolled disease and long-term side effects medications such as corticosteroids.

The good physician treats the disease; the great physician treats the patient who has the disease.

—Sir William Osler

This article originally appeared in *Immunology and Allergy Clinics*, Volume 37, Issue 2, May 2017.

Disclosure Statement: D.A. Bukstein has served as a speaker for Merck, Genentech, Novartis Pharmaceuticals, AstraZeneca, Aerocrine, Teva Pharmaceutics, Meda Pharmaceuticals, and Circassia. He has received honoraria from AstraZeneca, Schering-Plough, Merck, Meda Pharmaceuticals, Alcon, and Aerocrine and has commercial interests in Altus Minicampus and the PBL Institute. A.T. Luskin has served as a speaker for Genentech.

[a] Allergy, Asthma & Sinus Center, Madison, WI, USA; [b] Allergy, Asthma & Sinus Center, Milwaukee, WI, USA; [c] Healthy Airways, Madison, WI, USA
[1] Present address: 10 Tower Drive, Sun Prairie, WI 53590.
* Corresponding author. 11 Glen Arbor Way, Fitchburg, WI 53711.
E-mail address: donabukstein@gmail.com

INTRODUCTION

Recent years have witnessed tremendous progress in the therapeutic approach to immune-related diseases, such as rheumatoid arthritis, psoriasis, inflammatory bowel disease, and asthma. The introduction of novel biologic agents, including antibodies and cytokine inhibitors, has allowed clinicians to achieve improved outcomes for their patients. An important factor that has affected the utilization of novel therapies is their acquisition costs, which far exceed those for older drugs. Nevertheless, these are serious chronic conditions, which can cause substantial morbidity and accelerated mortality for affected individuals. Alternative therapeutic choices often involve the use of agents such as systemic corticosteroids with potentially costly side effects. Both undertreatment with uncontrolled disease and treatment with alternative therapies have severe economic consequences to patients and their families as well as to society. Therefore, appropriate pharmacoeconomic analyses demand we take into account all relevant costs, not only of the treatments but also of the disease itself and that of alternative treatments. In this way, the value of therapies can be correctly estimated.

Previous articles have emphasized the clinical burden of severe asthma. The authors summarize the pharmacoeconomic data obtained for biologic agents in patients with inadequately controlled severe persistent allergic asthma despite high-dose inhaled corticosteroids (ICSs) plus a long-acting β-agonist (LABA) and discuss the cost-effectiveness evidence published for biologic agents in this patient population. Although there is a great deal of evidence highlighting the health, economic, and societal burden of asthma, the evidence is highly skewed toward patients with severe uncontrolled asthma, particularly when asthma is inadequately controlled. In patients who do not respond to traditional therapy but do respond to biologic therapy, the cost-effectiveness of biologics often compares well with other treatments for chronic illness in the long terms of costs.

Costs are a measure of resources consumed. By assessing costs, pharmacoeconomic studies complement studies of efficacy and safety, helping to determine the relationships of treatment and outcome. Costs are divided into 3 categories: direct costs, or costs attributable to the intervention; indirect costs, or costs resulting from reduced productivity; and intangible costs, which are incurred from pain and emotional suffering. Insurance companies, patients, doctors, and society each have different perspectives with respect to costs. The authors review different types of cost analyses and their use in studies of asthma as a model. Cost studies influence clinicians', policy makers', and third-party payers' decisions regarding the implementation of particular therapies or programs. Collection of all relevant cost data needs to be facilitated and evaluated along with clinical trials to facilitate these decisions.

This article attempts to provide a more clinically useful perspective on the pharmacoeconomics of new biologics in the treatment of immune diseases, particularly in the area of asthma. Biologics are a cornerstone of personalized medicine but are inherently costly. Therefore—especially for those with the greatest economic burden—a cost-sensitive approach to improve the health of persons who have or are at the highest risk for uncontrolled asthma and other immune disorders must be developed.

Pharmacoeconomic evaluation encompasses a collection of methods that assesses the costs and consequences of comparative health care interventions. **Table 1** summarizes types of pharmacoeconomic evaluation. Evaluating the health and economic impacts of these interventions has been a topic of long-standing interest among clinicians.[1] Such evaluation involves a variety of issues and methods and additionally has major policy implications. This review discusses the main types of

Table 1
Types of pharmacoeconomic analyses

Type	Description	Comparison (X:Y)
Cost minimization (CMA)	Compares cost in monetary terms of treatment with identical outcomes	Dollars: Outcome unit varies but equivalent in comparatory groups
Cost-effectiveness (CEA)	Compares cost in monetary terms with outcomes in natural units	Dollars: Natural units such as years, blood glucose, LDL, cholesterol
Cost utility (CUA)	Compares cost in monetary terms and outcomes in terms of years of life	Dollars: QALY quality of life-years
Cost benefit (CBA)	Compares costs and outcomes in monetary terms	Dollars: dollars

Abbreviation: LDL, low-density lipoprotein.

pharmacoeconomic evaluation used to assess the use of biologics in asthma and immune disease and will be achieved by analyzing studies to demonstrate how pharmacoeconomic evaluation has been used for asthma care strategies using biologics. Also discussed are the challenges in the practical application of pharmacoeconomic evaluation and related policy implications. This review is designed for clinicians caring for individuals with asthma and other immune diseases to assist with understanding and evaluating published economic analyses, and identifying the key costs and benefits associated with their own clinical practices.[1]

Why Should Caregivers, Insurance Companies, Payers, and Society Be Concerned About the Pharmacoeconomics of Immune Diseases?

Health care costs are increasing, and the focus of both government and private insurance on spending places demands on health care providers to reduce costs yet improve outcomes.[2] Although new medical interventions can substantially improve health outcomes, these often come at considerable cost to both the health care system and patients. In order to efficiently use limited health care resources, beyond the standard evaluations of safety and efficacy, it is necessary to also evaluate the relative cost-effectiveness of new medical technologies. First the inflammatory immune disease asthma is discussed as an example one area of medicine that is grappling with the challenge of applying biologic therapies.

ASTHMA

Asthma is considered a high-burden inflammatory disease of the lungs, affecting an estimated 17.7 million adults and 6.3 million children in the United States.[3] Approximately 1 in 2 asthma sufferers, 10.7 million people, reported having at least one asthma attack, and 3651 casualties were a result of asthma in 2014.[3] In 2010, asthma in the United States resulted in 439,435 hospitalizations, 1.8 million emergency department (ED) visits, and 14.2 million physician office visits.[3,4] Although its health implications are frightening enough, asthma's cost burden is astounding as well. Asthma is associated with an estimated $50 billion (2009 dollars) in total direct incremental costs annually.[4] Furthermore, productivity loss related to the illness accounts for an additional $3.8 billion, and productivity loss from mortality accounts for another $2.1 billion.[5]

Typically, physicians take a three-pronged approach to allergy care: minimize exposure to allergens, reduce symptoms with pharmacologic therapy, and alter the immune response with immunotherapy. For severe asthma, physicians have the option to improve control with either biologics or thermoplasty.[6] Although this 3-pronged method has been adopted by most specialty physicians for asthma treatment, to form an overall management strategy that maximizes positive patient outcomes, asthma treatment needs to be a shared decision-making process (SDM) between the patient, clinician, and payer. Each of the main stakeholders, physician, health care delivery system, employer, patient, and society as a whole, have different areas of emphasis.

Physician perspective
- How can I help these patients control asthma symptoms and prevent comorbidities and exacerbations?
- What type and mix of medical care services will achieve control, balancing benefit and risk?
- For managed-care patients:
  - How can I achieve clinical objectives of Accountable Care Organizations (ACOs), satisfy patient preference, and minimize costs?
  - How can I adhere to mandated guidelines (Pay For Performance [P4P]) and ACOs?

Health care delivery system perspective
- How can direct costs be contained? Managing insurance premiums across groups and maximizing the number of insured patients.
- How will we reduce exacerbation? Exacerbation is associated with mortality and likely higher direct costs than chronic daily symptoms.[7]
- How do we meet guidelines or regulated performance requirements, such as Healthcare Effectiveness Data and Information Set and the Affordable Care Act (ACA)?
- How can I use P4P to reduce costs?
- How do we keep plan members satisfied?
- How do we keep asthma off of our list of concerns?

Employer perspective
- How do I reduce medical costs?
- How do I maintain a productive workforce?
  - Ensure a satisfied workforce
  - Reduce workforce absenteeism
  - Reduce workforce presenteeism
  - Reduce workforce turnover

Patient Perspective
- How do I limit out-of-pocket costs?
- How do I improve my quality of life (QOL)?
- How do I prevent exacerbations and avoid going to the ED?

Societal perspective
- What are the societal costs of asthma?
- How do we control these costs in a non-Orwellian world? (ie, *a mandate such as "Get rid of the cat" or "Quit smoking" is not an option!*)
- What is the impact of the disease on family, friends, work or school, and the community?

- How do we sustain public programs?
- What is the cost-effectiveness and lifetime impact of a preventive intervention?

These various stakeholders weigh various costs differently. Health care systems place more importance on direct costs, whereas patients and employers may value indirect costs. Although all of these parties have high concerns with cost, it is vital to note that value does not equate to cost. It is important then that we define what we mean by quality value in health care and how this may outweigh any dollar costs that many fear. Value in health care is generally defined as quality/cost. More specifically, physicians have refined it to the following:

$$\frac{\text{Change in health status} + \text{Satisfaction}}{\text{Cost}}$$

The cost of a biologic intervention equates to the following:

Cost = Cost of drug − Direct Costs − Positive Change in QOL − Change in Patient Productivity

Accurate evaluation of the equation demands that all costs be measured. These costs are hidden direct costs including the costs of asthma, side effects, medications, and comorbid disease. Furthermore, comorbid disease might be favorably affected either directly by medication, such as in the case of allergic rhinitis, or indirectly by improved control, such as in the case of gastroesophageal reflux disease or obstructive sleep apnea.

Therefore, cheaper is not always less expensive when other elements are measured. As clinicians, we need to learn how to develop an understanding of the true pharmacoeconomic value of biologics, so that we can accurately convey this to health care organizations, the government, and, most importantly, patients. The evaluation depends not solely on drug acquisition costs but also on the costs of the disease itself, from short- and long-term side effects of the drug to alternative treatment costs. The most difficult cost to calculate is the change in productivity. This change in productivity is the cost generated by uncontrolled disease resulting in the loss of personal parental and spousal/family productivity. Also challenging to estimate is the long-term societal cost that is generated from the lack of education because of the effect on school performance as well as underemployment of a patient and their family. The different costs listed in the equation above will vary based on the population receiving the biologic and will depend on identifying the patients who are able to respond and those who are able to do so. The Refractory Asthma Stratification Programme in the United Kingdom (RASP-UK) points out that some patients have poorly controlled asthma simply because they are not taking their medicines correctly.[8] Identifying those patients is important, but there is another group that RASP-UK investigators hope to identify: patients with severe asthma characterized by high eosinophil or periostin levels who are taking their medicines correctly yet fail to respond to medication. Even within this group of asthma sufferers who do have the right biomarker profile, physicians may have difficulty determining which patients should receive which biologic.[8,9] The biomarkers linked to each medicine tend to go up and down together, so a patient might have a high eosinophil count in addition to high periostin levels.[9–12]

WHEN IS BIOLOGIC THERAPY COST-EFFECTIVE?

There are many ways to analyze cost data, and cost-effectiveness is a commonly used method (**Table 1**). A biologic therapy is deemed to be a cost-effective strategy when the outcome is worth the cost relative to competing alternatives. In other words, it is a cost-effective strategy when scarce resources are used to acquire the best value on the market considering all alternatives.[13]

Average cost-effectiveness is calculated as:

Cost of drug

Resulting effect = Cost per unit of effect achieved

What is the incremental cost-effectiveness of a biologic in comparison with all other treatment options?

$$\frac{\text{Cost(Option B)} - \text{Cost(Option A)}}{\text{Effect(Option B)} - \text{Effect(Option A)}} = \text{Cost to achieve one unit of effect}$$

Previous articles have discussed many of the efficacies of data variables, or what product (effect) can be consistently expected from the use of drug or health service, which was determined from clinical trials. They seek a direct relationship to morbidity and mortality such as survival/death or, as per the asthma example, asthma exacerbations avoided. These efficacy outcomes may rely on surrogate measures such as the Asthma Control Test, pulmonary function tests, fractional exhaled nitric oxide, or use of oral steroids. A randomized controlled clinical trial is the gold standard for deriving this efficacy data, but observational studies can also add insight into the real-world costs of a biologic.[14,15]

HOW AND WHAT VARIABLES SHOULD WE MEASURE?

What resources are consumed to produce one unit of the effect? There are drug product acquisition costs, drug preparation and administration costs, drug monitoring costs, treatment costs of adverse effects, and indirect institutional costs (discounting other drugs).

In order to draw the most valid conclusion about costs generated over time to achieve an effect in the future, it is necessary to consider that there is a time preference associated with money. The concept of time-value of money states that the amount of money in your hand at this moment is worth more than the same amount in the future. Therefore, future costs must be adjusted to reflect present value. For example, a $1000 cost 1 year from now requires only $930 in hand today assuming a 7% return on investment.

Sensitivity analysis (SA) is another important tool used to assess the cost-benefit ratio of biologics. Basically, by altering important variables and then recalculating the results, we can test the validity of conclusions.[14] SA becomes increasingly important because assumptions are often made without proper analysis.

For example, SA could be used for questions like:

- Would Agent A still be most cost-effective if the effect of Agent B was greater than measured in a clinical trial?
- Would Agent A still be most cost-effective if the monitoring costs of Agent B were actually lower to a much greater degree?

As an example, although oral steroids are the least costly method in terms of initial dollars for asthma treatment, they may actually be costly in the long run, due to the common health complications they cause for the patient.[16–20] Steroid complications place not only an excessive emotional burden on patients but also a financial one, because they will then be forced to pay for additional hospitalization and also potentially for more drugs for treatment. Therefore, clearly physicians need to look deeper.

THE ADOPTION OF BIOLOGICS

Since biologics were brought into the picture, oral steroid use has decreased by 5%, and clinically significant ulcer complications were reduced by 50%.[20] When questioning whether to adopt biologics, the risk of asthma attacks and exacerbations needs to be looked at. Although biologic treatment has shown to prevent these, it is also important to recognize that not all asthma patients have an equal risk of developing an exacerbation.

This then leads to several questions, including the following:

- Is paying extra for exacerbation protection justified in all patients?
- How much can the risk of asthma exacerbation be altered by using biologics?
- What value is really purchased for the extra cost?

All of these factors must be analyzed for each and every patient to determine the most effective treatment option.

What Are the Real-World Practical Applications of Pharmacoeconomics of Biologics to Shared Decision Making?

One must first collect all the data available, and that includes the true costs of medications, copays, deductibles, and prior authorizations at point of service in order to adequately partake in SDM with patients. Risk reduction for complications seen with oral steroids with biologics is unlikely to offset their increased cost in the management of average-risk patients with asthma with no or little history of exacerbations and without the TH-2 phenotype. Clinical decision making and attempts at risk reduction for other complications seen with biologics are unlikely to offset their increased cost in the management of average-risk patients with asthma-control problems with no history of frequent exacerbations and use of oral steroids.

Decreased monitoring costs of biologics and the attenuated risk of future complications with these agents do result in cost-effective care.[21] Thus, the real issue is who is at risk for steroids' adverse events currently cannot be identified, and there is no consistent method of measurement. The higher acquisition cost may then be justified.

Treating the patient on an outpatient basis creates the best value. Better outcomes are achieved at a lower overall cost: the best possible situation.[21–23] Time and money can only be spent once; choice is inevitable. Whether done unconsciously or with a consistent process, health care professionals are constantly evaluating patient care choices and acting on them.

Pharmacoeconomics and outcomes research can enhance the quality of the practice by strengthening the evaluation process and increasing the probability that better value is delivered in patient care.[22]

Will Establishing General Disease Phenotype Influence the Pharmacoeconomic Choice of a Biologic?

There are many reviews on these topics,[24–27] and in principle, it is generally accepted that therapeutic agents should be used when there is a favorable balance between their benefits and potential risks. Examples from other fields suggest that pharmacogenetic data can help predict both the benefit and the toxicity of particular drugs in individual patients.[23] The general use of disease endotypes for allergies and asthma and correct selection of the responder patient population with defined biomarkers remain essential unmet needs in the clinical settings.[24]

Whether it will be possible to define subtypes of patients with asthma who might benefit from more cost-effective, personalized management plans remains to be determined. In the area of profiling, ideally one would be able to use a limited number of reasonably inexpensive tests to predict responses to various forms of treatment rather than to rely on comprehensive analyses of the subject's response to biologics and other medications (trial of 1), waiting until exacerbation costs skyrocket, or until one can search the entire genome, metabolome, and microbiome. The same point can be made with respect to what type of testing would be needed for effectively monitoring and assessment of treatment responses.[24–27]

What Does a Decision Maker (eg, Patient, Physician, Health Maintenance Organization Pharmacy and Therapeutics Committee, Government Agency) Need to Know in Selecting the Most Cost-Effective Management Approach for a Patient?

Although the potential cost of personalized or precision medicine has been widely discussed, the costs to individual patients and health systems will vary by country, and in countries with private health care options, costs will vary further based on one's type of health insurance.[24–28] No matter who is assessing the cost-effectiveness of an intervention, they should ideally consider all of the costs and benefits of the decision, placing values on such important outcomes as long-term wellness and enhanced QOL, cost of time lost at school or work, and reductions in long-term economic productivity.

Hood[25] has emphasized the importance of involving patients, and in the case of children, their guardians, in making decisions about their health care. This participatory aspect of medicine constitutes the fourth "P" of P4 medicine, where the 4 Ps are predictive, preventive, personalized, and participatory.

It might be possible to devise approaches using biometric and other data, including data about one's genetic profile and personal environment, to identify more accurately if those patients with asthma or other immune diseases will or will not respond favorably to treatment with expensive biologics and to assess the likely effectiveness of diverse interventions. It might also be possible to define constellations of biometric and other individual characteristics that could change the trial-and-failure approach currently often used to move from first- to second- to third-line therapeutic approaches. An approach in which the caregiver, in consultation with the patient (and/ or her or his guardians), can more quickly select a treatment, which is in some cases biologic, will likely result in a higher probability of success for that person. Such precision care approaches not only will permit health care resources to be used in a more cost-effective manner, but more importantly, would result in improved satisfaction of patients and their families with their management and treatment, along with producing favorable social and economic effects by improving attendance and performance in school or at work. If we can overcome the significant impediments to establishing such new approaches, then we will be able to offer a much brighter future to those subjects at risk of allergic diseases and to those patients who already have them.[24] This is the basis for the process of initiating patient activation, and possibly improved adherence to biologic therapy.[29–31]

We cannot remain stuck in the past. Even if a study done in 2010 says a biologic is not very cost-effective, the criteria available then do not mean in the near future with improved phenotyping and patient selection, that biologic will not be extremely cost-effective in 2017.[24]

Which of the Potential Biologic Agents Will Be the Most Pharmacoecomonically Realistic and Valuable Choice? In Asthma? What Do We Use?

The past decade has been marked by the introduction and expanding use of biologic therapies for the induction and maintenance of response in patients with asthma and other immune diseases. Traditional cost analyses had shown that biologics and medication costs contributed minimally toward the overall costs associated with the disease; however, these studies were all conducted before the introduction of biologic therapies. At that time, a small minority of patients accounted for a disproportionately large percentage of the overall costs.[17,32,33] This suggested that cost savings could be realized if interventions decreased the utilization of health care resources and associated costs. More recent studies have been heterogeneous in their design and findings. Some have suggested that cost savings realized, due to a decrease in the utilization of health care services, may partially offset the higher costs of biologic agents. Incorporation of data on indirect cost savings and QOL improvements into ongoing and future analyses is required to allow for more accurate analyses of overall costs and cost savings.

Uncontrolled diseases, like asthma, are costlier than controlled diseases, regardless of severity. To appropriately stratify the uncontrolled population, we need not only additional medications but also an improved guide to SDM to make sure the specific biologic is appropriate for the underlying phenotype. Without stratification of uncontrolled asthma for anticipated clinical and economic benefit, the pharmacoeconomics of specific biologics are unclear. Data are conflicting regarding the cost-effectiveness of omalizumab, despite the drug being used on patients for over a decade.[34,35] It has been proposed that omalizumab is a cost-saving option only if given to patients who are predicted to be hospitalized 5 or more times, or 20 days, per year, despite maximal medical management.[35] However, these studies evaluated patients only on severity of disease, not the patients most likely to respond, and thus are fatally flawed.

One commonly used approach in cost-effectiveness analyses is to calculate the incremental cost-effectiveness ratio (ICER), in the form of cost per quality-adjusted life-years (QALY). QALY is an index of survival that is weighted or adjusted by the patient's QOL during the survival period.[36] QALY is particularly useful because it allows for comparisons between interventions and across different conditions. For example, the cost-effectiveness of a therapy for asthma can be compared with one for rheumatoid arthritis.[37,38]

In order to provide estimates of ICER, economic modeling is often necessary. Although general methodological guidelines exist offering helpful modeling principles, evaluating treatments for autoimmune disorders remains challenging.[37,38]

What About Gains in Quality-Adjusted Life-Years with the Use of Biologics?

A recent model suggests that omalizumab may cost as much as $117,000 per QALY, compared with standard therapy with ICS/LABA at a much lower cost of $15,000 per QALY.[39,40] Of course, failure of ICS/LABA therapy administered according to Global Initiative for Asthma guidelines is the criterium used to define the patient who might benefit from biologics used in asthma therapy. There are almost no data at this time on the 2 other biologics mepolizumab and reslizumab, and the price for 1 year of mepolizumab is estimated to be more than $32,500.[41] Although often of minimal importance to the patient, these costs certainly put into question the long-term sustainability of these high costs on the health care system. Omalizumab has recently been reviewed by the National Institute for Health and Care Excellence and is recommended as an option for treating severe persistent allergic asthma as an add-on to optimized standard therapy in patients who need continuous or frequent courses of oral corticosteroids (OCSs).[42]

Points to consider:

- How long must a patient stay on this biologic therapy before they are considered a treatment failure[43]?
- What is the timeframe until we see efficacy and the plateau of that efficacy?
- Before initiating and continuing biologic therapy, SDM needs to take place on these issues, but without studies, this is difficult to quantify.
- Rational use in consideration of the underlying phenotype and with real assessment of costs, risks, and benefits, both long and short term, is the basis for rational decision making on biologic use in asthma rather than experimenting until something appears to work.
- Is there a better way of predicting exacerbations[44]?

The significant progress in asthma therapy with the arrival of omalizumab and use of the new biological drugs has increased the focus on the economic aspects because of the very large price tag related to those treatments. Several more recent economic evaluations suggest that current expensive biologics as compared with pharmacotherapy might be cost-effective for asthma therapy in patients who remain uncontrolled per asthma guidelines. To date, the cost-effectiveness of biologics for comorbid allergic problems has not been investigated.[39–56]

Because of the short amount of time mepolizumab has been on the market, there are limited data on its costs. Early reports estimate a cost per year of treatment from $10,000 to $15,000 per patient.[46] After US Food and Drug Administration approval, the real cost is $32,500 per year per patient and approximately $2700 for a single 4-week injection.[46] To the authors' knowledge, the only real cost-effectiveness analysis was recently conducted and published by the Institute for Clinical and Economic Review Group, which was based on a simulation model of asthma outcomes and costs in a representative population of suitable patients to mepolizumab therapy.[41] The investigators evaluated the incremental cost-effectiveness of mepolizumab, applying drug costs obtained from current prices and estimates of reductions in asthma exacerbations and OCS use from available clinical literature data. In a scenario analysis, it was determined that the price of mepolizumab that would produce cost-effectiveness results at willingness-to-pay thresholds of $50,000 per QALY, $100,000 per QALY, and $150,000 per QALY, respectively. At the moment, based on current purchase prices, the cost-effectiveness estimates are not affordable. To obtain a value correlated with the clinical benefit, a discount of two-thirds to three-quarters from the current acquisition costs of mepolizumab would be necessary. According to the authors of this report, mepolizumab should have a value-based cost between $7800 and $12,000 per year, whereas the full list price per patient in the United States is $32,500 per year. Other doubts arise from the lack of clinical trials evaluating benefits in the long term.

Another group of researchers[47] conducted a study with the aim to evaluate the cost-effectiveness of the newest strategies for the treatment of severe refractory asthma, such as biologic drugs (omalizumab and mepolizumab), as well as bronchial thermoplasty. The investigators used a theoretic model based on the US health care perspective, with a cohort of 10,000 adult patients affected by refractory asthma in an annual cycle and 10-year time horizon. The addition of bronchial thermoplasty to biologic treatment in responder patients was found to not be cost-effective. However, in biologic nonresponders, bronchial thermoplasty remained a cost-effective option as an add-on treatment. Mepolizumab without bronchial thermoplasty was the most cost-effective option for biologic responders, with a 10-year per-patient cost of $116,776 and 5.46 QALYs gained (Institute for Clinical and Economic Review: $21,388). Bronchial thermoplasty is a cost-effective treatment option only in the nonresponders group to biologic treatment ($33,161 per QALY).

A recent draft guidance of the National Institute for Health and Care Excellence does not recommend mepolizumab as an add-on therapy for severe refractory eosinophilic asthma. This is most certainly due to the fact that the costs of mepolizumab compared with usual asthma treatments are above the range usually considered to be a cost-effective use of National Health Service resources.[47]

In the authors' opinion, because it occurred in the past for omalizumab, the increase in the number of eligible patients evaluated in clinical trials may dispel doubts about the real cost-effectiveness ratio of mepolizumab in clinical practice. Cost-effectiveness and pharmacoeconomics of the currently available, extremely expensive biologics approved for use in uncontrolled severe asthma (mepolizumab, reslizumab, and benralizumab) are not well-established figures. Studies in the future should be aimed at defining real-life usefulness of these drugs, and establishing their correct position in treatment guidelines. Pharmacoeconomic studies carried out so far are controversial, but it is likely that they will be necessary to work toward a reduction of purchase costs to extend the availability of these promising therapeutic options.

If Biologics Are Used for Asthma, What Is Their Duration of Benefit?

With respect to clinical benefits, economic evaluations of biologics as compared with pharmacotherapy have indicated that the cost-effectiveness of biologics primarily depends on the duration of the clinical benefit of biologics following treatment cessation.[48] For instance, one study showed that a reduction in the time horizon of the analysis had a negative impact on the cost-effectiveness of the biologic therapy omalizumab.[52] Data on the duration of the clinical benefit of biologics used in economic evaluations were derived from clinical trials, observational studies, expert opinion literature, or authors' assumptions. Although assumptions were informed by clinical trials, the quality of the clinical evidence can be questioned, and uncertainty surrounds the quantitative estimate of the duration of clinical benefit following cessation of biologics.[57–59] Data from the XPORT trial suggest that almost 50% of patients can be successfully withdrawn from omalizumab after 5 years of therapy. Factoring this into the pharmacoeconomic models would make omalizamab appear a much more favorable therapy.[57–59]

What Is the Cost Benefit of Biologics Compared with Pharmacotherapy in Asthma Treatment?

With respect to costs, the cost-effectiveness of biologics as compared with pharmacotherapy depends on the break-even point of cumulative costs between treatment alternatives (ie, the point in time when cumulative costs of biologics equal cumulative costs of pharmacotherapy). Biologics (plus drugs as needed) tend to be more expensive during the first years of treatment, but cumulative costs of pharmacotherapy start to exceed those associated with biologics (if pharmacotherapy is able to be decreased or stopped altogether) at a later stage when biologics has stopped, but its clinical benefit is maintained. Although steps down in therapy after control is maintained is suggested, it is rarely practiced. The break-even point tends to differ between economic evaluations and cannot be transferred given that, for instance, cost estimates reported in economic evaluations are specific to the study setting, and is unlikely to be generalizable.[60]

No economic evaluation has involved a direct comparison of biologics with the combination of biologics with subcutaneous immunotherapy[61–64] except for one study that did not give a conclusive answer because of methodological limitations.[64] Therefore, the question of the cost-effectiveness of biologics versus biologics plus immunotherapy has not been resolved to date. The literature does suggest that any future economic evaluation needs to consider such aspects as safety profile, compliance rate, and administrative costs, which may affect the cost-effectiveness of sublingual versus subcutaneous immunotherapy.[64] Also, where the biologic is given—intravenously or subcutaneously in a medical facility or subcutaneously at home—needs to be considered.

The literature on the cost-effectiveness of biologics consists of studies conducted in Europe and in the United States. The results of these studies should be interpreted with care when assessing their generalizability to another country because the patient population and the specific biologics and administrative costs used are likely to vary between countries, as well as the funding, organization, regulation, and real-life practices governing biologic use in asthma.

Existing economic evaluations have used a variety of outcome measures, such as the peak expiratory flow rate, symptom scores, the number of symptom-free days, the number of patients free from symptoms, and the number of exacerbations. This makes it difficult to compare cost-effectiveness results between studies. Existing economic evaluations of respiratory allergy have shown that improvement in these outcome measures resulting from biologics translate into better QOL.[65] However, there is a need for additional economic evaluations that consider QOL by means of instruments such as the EQ-5D (QOIL scale used in europe Don).[66] This instrument can be used to calculate QALYs and to express the cost-effectiveness of immunotherapy in terms of the additional costs per QALY gained as compared with the alternative. Comparing it with the threshold value set by the health care industry, the payer can then assess the cost-effectiveness of asthma biologics. For instance, the National Institute for Health and Clinical Excellence in England and Wales uses a threshold value of £20,000–£30,000 per QALY[42] that determines which health technologies will be recommended for use by the National Health Service. Economic evaluations of biologics like immunotherapy for asthma should be carried out with real world clinical studies. Thus, cost-effectiveness can be based on randomized controlled trials to provide a degree of internal validity, whereas analyses based on observational studies reflect real-life practice. Alternatively, the use of modeling techniques that critically depend on the study design and the quality of data that are extracted from the literature or other sources are used as input in the cost-effectiveness model.[65]

Some economic evaluations included direct health care costs from the perspective of the third-party payer or the health care system. As a result, these studies focused on the costs of biologics and examined the cost impact of biologics on the use of medicines, physician consultations and hospitalization, ED visits, and exacerbations.[65] The central outcome of exacerbations and use of OCSs most often determines biologic use in asthma. OCS use is the way most physicians determine the number of exacerbations in a patient. This exacerbation history is most often not based on pharmacy data of oral steroid use but on patient history. However, data suggest that relying on patient history could miss as many as 58% of patients who have had 3 or more exacerbations in the past year.[44] Identifying these patients can result in additional interventions that would further reduce their risk for future exacerbations, so a review of pharmacy refill data for OCS bursts, rather than patient history alone, should become a routine component of comprehensive care for asthma patients. Also, although OCS may help control asthma and manage exacerbations, it must be considered that OCS side effects may result in additional health care resource use and costs, highlighting the need for OCS-sparing asthma therapies.[19,20]

A central and extremely important issue is that biologic use is predicated on the number of asthma exacerbations, which for most physicians involves asking the patient how many bursts of OCS they have been on in the past year. The issue is that this is often not a reliable number and may underestimate OCS use.[44] Although OCS are economical from a drug-cost and acquisition perspective, OCS have been associated with dose- and duration-dependent debilitating adverse events, including bone fractures, diabetes mellitus, infections, hypertension, and cataracts. Thus, evidence related to the economic costs attributable to OCS-related side effects has the potential to inform health care insurance company about the tradeoffs of OCS use versus trial of biologic for improved asthma control. Thus, it is high-OCS users with possible OCS-related side effects that are more likely to use health care services than those without such side effects.[65]

EMBRACING QUALITY HEALTH CARE IN THE UNITED STATES

There is pressure on medical providers to embrace payment reform models that give incentives to provide the right care, to the right patient, at the right venue, at the right time, and at the right cost. The United States is at the core of multiple experiments aimed to shift care delivery from a volume-based to a value-based system. On April 16, 2015, President Obama signed into law H.R. 2, the Medicare Access and CHIP Reauthorization Act, a bill that ushers in a new era in physician payment for Medicare. Under either the Merit-based Incentive Payment System (MIPS) or alternative payment models, health care providers will assume some level of financial risk for their clinical decisions. On April 27, Centers for Medicare and Medicaid Services published proposed rules on MIPS implementation and the process and requirements Alternative Payment Models must meet in order to be classified as Advanced Alternative Payment Models. Although fee-for-service is all about volume and reinforces work in silos with little incentive to integrate, the new emphasis for physician reimbursement is on value, with the triple aim of improving quality, enhancing the patient consumer experience, and most importantly, constraining cost growth.

There are huge problems with the current pharmacoeconomic analysis of the costs of biologics in asthma and other immune diseases. Because of fragmented, inefficient, and unorganized delivery of care, extreme variability in treatment practices without apparent benefits, misalignment of incentives, lack of transparency in pricing and costs, and inadequate pharmacoeconomic data to assess value (ie, interaction of quality, cost and patient satisfaction, and experience), biologics and asthma treatment costs are on an unsustainable course. Until some of these issues are addressed and repaired, cost-effective utilization of biologics may remain a mystery.

So What Can Insurance Companies, Society, and Caregivers Do to Move the Study of Pharmacoeconomics of Biologics in the Right Direction? Furthermore, How Can Pharmacoeconomics Enhance the Physicians' and Patients' Outcomes and Reduce Direct Costs, Indirect Costs, and Long-Term Complication Costs?

Improvements in the study of pharmacoeconomics are an aid to decision making with strong potential to:

- Mitigate the influence of marketing
- Help put physicians in the driver's seat
- Enhance the position of allergists from payer's perspective
- Help set practice priorities

- Affect Medicare plans to decrease payout to stem the tide of budget deficits
- Help private payers actively develop quality report cards

POTENTIAL PROBLEMS INTERPRETING PHARMACOECONOMIC DATA

1. The cost of uncontrolled asthma and immune disease is significant and increasing.
2. The cost of an intervention is only partly reflected in drug acquisition costs, and a great deal of the accuracy of pharmacoeconomic evaluations depends on ability to measure change in total disease costs.
3. The pharmacoeconomic equation changes based on the variation in importance of the various costs to user of the data. The individual and family will place more importance on sleep and cough, the employer and perhaps society on productivity, and the ACO on direct costs only without full appreciation for QOL or presenteeism.
4. Drug acquisition data have often been obtained from studies of all comers, completely contrary to personalized medicine, and if personalized therapy is the goal, the pharmacoeconomic data of relevance are the cost-benefits in that population. For example, what are the pharmacoeconomic data for anti–IL-5 biologic therapies in all patients versus patients with blood eosinophil levels of 150, 300, and 400 cells per microliter? The equations will look quite different.
5. Only models that look at responders, with discontinuation of drug in nonresponders, is appropriate. Models looking at 5- or 10-year costs with a drug continued is clinically irrelevant.
6. Models must account for all costs. Hidden direct costs are often overlooked. Indirect costs are difficult to measure and typically ignored but are extremely important to many users of pharmacoeconomic data.
7. Most importantly, pharmcoeconomic data are most appropriately evaluated not using drug versus no drug, but drug versus alternative therapy.
8. That leads to the importance of evaluating all costs of alternative therapy, including the costs of side effects. Because alternative therapy is typically OCSs, it is critical to better understand the costs of side effects of OCSs, both medical and psychiatric.
9. The hidden direct costs and indirect costs, including the ability to put a cost on QOL, are critical for evaluating omalizumab for hives and dupilumab for atopic dermatitis, in which direct costs may not be as great as with respiratory disease.
10. The omilizamab pediatric indication and upcoming dupilumab atopic dermatitis approval make it even more important to understand the costs of disease on parents and caregivers. This is almost invariably overlooked.

SUMMARY

Poorly controlled, therapy-resistant asthma negatively impacts QOL and health care costs. Medication adherence, socioeconomics, and other factors complicate asthma biologic treatments. Cost-effective models of biologic use commonly evaluate the benefit of treatments using QALYs that incorporate both the quantity and the quality of life. Cost-effectiveness information on biologic use can thus assist decision makers in evaluating the overall value of a new treatment or new technology. Long-term savings to the health care system do not always result in short-term patient or payer savings. Pharmacoeconomics and outcomes research can enhance the quality of the practice by strengthening the evaluation process and increasing the probability that better value in patient care is delivered. More of the costs in biologics will be borne by the patients in the future because these patients already have high indirect costs. The international literature suggests that biologics may be cost-effective as compared with pharmacotherapy for certain asthma phenotypes. One economic evaluation has suggested that biologics as compared with pharmacotherapy is unlikely to be cost-effective for asthma. The reader should note that this evidence originated from a limited number of economic evaluations that suffered from several methodological shortcomings. The question of the cost-effectiveness of biologics versus pharmaco-therapy has not been resolved to date. No economic evaluation has examined the cost-effectiveness of biologics in asthma taking into account the comorbidities that the biologic also improves. Time and money can only be spent once, so choice is inev-itable. Whether done unconsciously or with a consistent process, health care profes-sionals are constantly evaluating care choices and acting on them.

REFERENCES

1. Eisenberg JM. Clinical economics: a guide to the economic analysis of clinical practices. JAMA 1989;262:2879–86.
2. Trueman P, Drummond M, Hutton J. Developing guidance for budget impact analysis. Pharmacoeconomics 2001;19:609–21.
3. Centers for Disease Control and Prevention. Most recent asthma data. In: CDC website. 2016. Available at: http://www.cdc.gov/asthma/most_recent_data.htm. Accessed June 30, 2016.
4. Centers for Disease Control and Prevention. Asthma facts: CDC's National Asthma Control Program Grantees. In: CDC website. 2013. Available at: http://www.cdc. gov/asthma/pdfs/asthma_facts_program_grantees.pdf. Accessed November 18, 2015.
5. Bahadori K, Doyle-Waters MM, Marra C, et al. Economic burden of asthma: a sys-tematic review. BMC Pulm Med 2009;9:24.
6. Reddel HK, Bateman ED, Becker A, et al. A summary of the new GINA strategy: a roadmap to asthma control. Eur Respir J 2015;46:622–39.
7. Healthcare Cost and Utilization Project (HCUP). Chronic Condition Indicator (CCI) for ICD-9-CM. In: HCUP website. 2016. Available at: http://www.hcup-us. ahrq.gov/toolssoftware/chronic/chronic.jsp. Accessed July 8, 2016.
8. Heaney LG, Djukanovic R, Woodcock A, et al. Research in progress: medical research council United Kingdom refractory asthma stratification programme (RASP-UK). Thorax 2016;71(2):187–9.
9. Nair P, Pizzichini MM, Kjarsgaard M, et al. Mepolizumab for prednisone-dependent asthma with sputum eosinophilia. N Engl J Med 2009;360:985–93.
10. Haldar P, Brightling CE, Hargadon BN, et al. Mepolizumab and exacerbations of refractory eosinophilic asthma. N Engl J Med 2009;360:973–84.
11. Ortega HG, Liu MC, Pavord ID, et al. Mepolizumab treatment in patients with se-vere eosinophilic asthma. N Engl J Med 2014;371:1198–207.
12. Bel EH, Wenzel SE, Thompson PJ, et al. Oral glucocorticoid-sparing effect of me-polizumab in eosinophilic asthma. N Engl J Med 2014;371:1189–97.
13. Cangelosi MJ, Ortendahl JD, Meckley LM, et al. Cost-effectiveness of bronchial thermoplasty in commercially insured patients with poorly controlled, severe, persistent asthma. Expert Rev Pharmacoecon Outcomes Res 2015;15(2):1–8.
14. Einarson TR, Bereza BG, Nielsen TA, et al. Systematic review of models used in economic analyses in moderate-to-severe asthma and COPD. J Med Econ 2016; 19(4):319–55.

15. Antonova E, Trzaskoma B, Omachi TA, et al. Poor asthma control is associated with overall daily activity impairment: 3-year data from the EXCELS study of omalizumab. J Allergy Clin Immunol 2016;137(2 Suppl 1):AB14.

16. Morishima T, Ikai H, Imanaka Y. Cost-effectiveness analysis of omalizumab for the treatment of severe asthma in Japan and the value of responder prediction methods based on a multinational trial. Value Health Reg Issues 2013;2:29–36.

17. Barnett SBL, Nurmagambetov TA. Costs of asthma in the United States: 2002–2007. J Allergy Clin Immunol 2011;127(1):145–52.

18. Rowe B, Spooner C, Ducharme F, et al. Corticosteroids for preventing relapse following acute exacerbations in asthma. Cochrane Database Syst Rev 2007;(3):CD000195.

19. Liu D, Ahmet A, Ward L, et al. A practical guide to the monitoring and management of the complications of systemic corticosteroid therapy. Allergy Asthma Clin Immunol 2013;9(1):30.

20. Luskin AT, Antonova E, Broder MS, et al. Healthcare resource use and costs associated with possible side effects of high oral corticosteroid use in asthma: a claims-based analysis. Presented at: Academy of Managed Pharmacy NEXUS 2015. Orlando (FL), October 26–28, 2015.

21. Dominguez-Ortega J, Phillips-Angles E, Barranco P, et al. Cost-effectiveness of asthma therapy: a comprehensive review. J Asthma 2015;52:529–37.

22. Zelger RS, Schatz M, Dalal AA, et al. Utilization and costs of severe uncontrolled asthma in a managed-care setting. J Allergy Clin Immunol Pract 2016;4:120–9.

23. Diaz RA, Charles Z, George E, et al. NICE guidance on omalizumab for severe asthma. Lancet Respir Med 2013;1:189–90.

24. Galli SJ. Toward precision medicine and health: opportunities and challenges in allergic diseases. J Allergy Clin Immunol 2016;137:1289–98.

25. Hood L. Systems biology and P4 medicine: past, present, and future. Rambam Maimonides Med J 2013;4(2):e0012.

26. Ferkol T, Quinton P. Precision medicine: at what price? Am J Respir Crit Care Med 2015;192:658–9.

27. Joyner MJ, Paneth N. Seven questions for personalized medicine. JAMA 2015;314:999–1000.

28. Akdis CA, Akdis M. Advances in allergen immunotherapy: aiming for complete tolerance to allergens. Sci Transl Med 2015;7:280ps6.

29. Marcum ZA, Sevick MA, Handler SM. Medication nonadherence: a diagnosable and treatable medical condition. JAMA 2013;309(20):2105–6.

30. Goldberg EL, Dekoven M, Schabert VF, et al. Patient medication adherence: the forgotten aspect of biologics. Biotechnol Healthc 2009;6(2):39–42, 44.

31. Bender BG. Overcoming barriers to nonadherence in asthma treatment. J Allergy Clin Immunol 2002;109(6 Suppl):S554–9.

32. Cisternas MA, Blanc PD, Yen IH, et al. A comprehensive study of direct and indirect costs of adult asthma. J Allergy Clin Immunol 2003;111:1212–8.

33. Colice GJ, Wu EQ, Birnbaum H, et al. Healthcare and workloss costs associated with patients with persistent asthma in a privately insured population. Occup Environ Med 2006;48:794–802.

34. Norman G, Faria R, Paton F, et al. Omalizumab for the treatment of severe persistent allergic asthma: a systematic review and economic evaluation. Health Technol Assess 2013;17(52):1–342.

35. Humbert M, Beasley R, Ayres J, et al. Benefits of omalizumab as add-on therapy in patients with severe persistent asthma who are inadequately controlled despite

best available therapy (GINA 2002 step 4 treatment): INNOVATE. Allergy 2005; 60(3):309–16.

36. Drummond MF, Jefferson TO. Guidelines for authors and peer reviewers of economic submissions to the BMJ. The BMJ Economic Evaluation Working Party. BMJ 1996;313:275–83.

37. Maetzel A, Tugwell P, Boers M, et al. Economic evaluation of programs or interventions in the management of rheumatoid arthritis: defining a consensus-based reference case. J Rheumatol 2003;30:891–6.

38. Economics Working Group report. a proposal for a reference case for economic evaluation in rheumatoid arthritis. J Rheumatol 2003;30:886–90.

39. Oba Y, Salzman G. Cost-effectiveness analysis of omalizumab in adults and adolescents with moderate-to-severe allergic asthma. J Allergy Clin Immunol 2004; 114:265–9.

40. Zafari Z, Sadatsafavi M, Marra CA, et al. Cost-effectiveness of bronchial thermoplasty, omalizumab, and standard therapy for moderate-to-severe allergic asthma. PLoS One 2016;11(1):e0146003.

41. Tice JA, Ollendorf D, Campbell JD, et al. Mepolizumab (Nucala, GlaxoSmithKline plc.) for the treatment of severe asthma with eosinophilia: effectiveness, value and value-based benchmarks: final report. Boston: Institute for Clinical and Economic Review; 2016.

42. National Institute for Health and Care Excellence (NICE). Omalizumab for treating severe persistent allergic asthma. In: NICE website. 2013. Available at: https://www.nice.org.uk/guidance/ta278. Accessed July 10, 2016.

43. Rodrigo GJ, Neffen H, Castro-Rodriguez JA. Efficacy and safety of subcutaneous omalizumab vs placebo as add-on therapy to corticosteroids for children and adults with asthma: a systemic review. Chest 2011;139:28–35.

44. Bukstein D, Steven G, Luskin A. Pharmacy data more reliable at predicting asthma exacerbations. Presented at: American College of Allergy, Asthma and Immunology (ACAAI) annual meeting. Baltimore (MD), November 7–11, 2015. [abstract: 72].

45. UK Medicines Information. New drugs online report for mepolizumab. In: UK Medicines Information website. Available at: http://www.ukmi.nhs.uk/applications/ndo/record_view_open.asp?newDrugID4675. Accessed March 6, 2016.

46. Institute for Clinical and Economic Review (ICER). ICER draft reports on Nucala® (mepolizumab) for asthma and Tresiba® (insulin degludec) for diabetes posted for public comment edit. In: ICER website. 2015. Available at: http://www.icer-review.org/icer-draft-reports-on-nucala-mepolizumab-for-asthma-and-tresiba-insulin-degludec-for-diabetes-posted-for-public-comment. Accessed March 5, 2016.

47. Bogart M, Roberts A, Wheeler S. Cost-effectiveness of refractory asthma treatment strategies: a decision tree analysis. Value Health 2015;18:A174.

48. Kuprys-Lipinska I, Piotr Kuna P. Loss of asthma control after cessation of omalizumab treatment: real life data. Postepy Dermatol Alergol 2014;31(1):1–5.

49. Molimard M, Mala L, Bourdeix I, et al. Observational study in severe asthmatic patients after discontinuation of omalizumab for good asthma control. Respir Med 2014;108(4):571–6.

50. Nopp A, Johansson SG, Adedoyin J, et al. After 6 years with Xolair: a 3-year withdrawal follow-up. Allergy 2010;65:56–60.

51. Bonifazi F, Jutel M, Bilo BM, et al. EAACI Interest Group on Insect Venom Hypersensitivity. Prevention and treatment of hymenoptera venom allergy: guidelines for clinical practice. Allergy 2005;60:1459–70.

52. Turner SJ, Nazareth T, Raimundo K, et al. Impact of omalizumab on all-cause and asthma-related healthcare resource utilization in patients with moderate or severe persistent asthma. Am J Respir Crit Care Med 2014;189:A6580.

53. Bégin P, Dominguez T, Wilson SP, et al. Phase 1 results of safety and tolerability in a rush oral immunotherapy protocol to multiple foods using Omalizumab. Allergy Asthma Clin Immunol 2014;10(1):7.

54. Schneider LC, Rachid R, LeBovidge J, et al. A pilot study of omalizumab to facilitate rapid oral desensitization in high-risk peanut-allergic patients. J Allergy Clin Immunol 2013;132:1368–74.

55. Pauwels B, Jonstam K, Bachert C. Emerging biologics for the treatment of chronic rhinosinutis. Expert Rev Clin Immunol 2015;11(3):349–61.

56. Umetsu DT. Targeting IgE to facilitate oral immunotherapy for food allergy: a potential new role for anti-IgE therapy? Expert Rev Clin Immunol 2014;10(9):1125–8.

57. Busse WW, Trzaskoma B, Omachi TA, et al. Evaluating omalizumab persistency of response after long-term therapy (XPORT). Presented at the Annual Meeting of the American Thoracic Society (ATS). San Diego (CA), May 16–21, 2014. [abstract: A31].

58. Busse W, Trzaskoma B, Omachi TA, et al. Evaluating omalizumab persistency of response after long-term therapy (XPORT). Presented at the Annual Meeting of the European Respiratory Society (ERS). Munich (Germany), September 6–10, 2014. Eur Respir J 2014;44(Suppl 58):P3485.

59. Antonova J, Trzaskoma B, Raimundo K, et al. Longitudinal change in asthma symptom control in patients who continued vs discontinued omalizumab: results from the XPORT study. Presented at the 71st American College of Allergy, Asthma & Immunology (ACAAI) annual scientific meeting. Atlanta (GA), November 8–11, 2014.

60. Campbell JD, McQueen RB, Briggs A. The "e" in cost-effectiveness analyses: a case study of omalizumab efficacy and effectiveness for cost-effectiveness analysis evidence. Ann Am Thorac Soc 2014;11(Suppl 2):S105–11.

61. Larenas-Linnemann D, Wahn U, Kopp M. Use of omalizumab to improve desensitization safety in allergen immunotherapy. J Allergy Clin Immunol 2014;133(3):937–937.e2.

62. Kamin W, Kopp MV, Erdnuess F, et al. Safety of anti-IgE treatment with omalizumab in children with seasonal allergic rhinitis undergoing specific immunotherapy simultaneously. Pediatr Allergy Immunol 2010;21(1 Pt 2):e160–5.

63. Casale TB, Stokes JR. Future forms of immunotherapy. J Allergy Clin Immunol 2011;127:8–15.

64. Casale TB, Busse WW, Kline JN, et al. Omalizumab pretreatment decreases acute reactions after rush immunotherapy for ragweed-induced seasonal allergic rhinitis. J Allergy Clin Immunol 2006;117:134–40.

65. Sullivan PW, Campbell JD, Ghushchyan VH, et al. Characterizing the severe asthma population in the United States: claims-based analysis of three treatment cohorts in the year prior to treatment escalation. J Allergy Clin Immunol 2014;133(Suppl 2):AB41.

66. Pickard AS, Wilke C, Jung E, et al. Use of a preference-based measure of health (EQ-5D) in COPD and asthma. Respir Med 2008;102(4):519–36.

The Role of PET/MR Imaging in Precision Medicine

Eugene Huo, MD[a], David M. Wilson, MD[a],
Laura Eisenmenger, MD[a], Thomas A. Hope, MD[a,b],*

KEYWORDS

• PET/CT • PET/MR imaging • Precision medicine • Molecular imaging

KEY POINTS

- The superior capabilities of MR imaging to characterize soft tissue offers an advantage compared with computed tomography in the diagnosis of malignancy.
- PET tracers targeting specific pathologic processes can be more accurate and sensitive for primary and metastatic disease when compared with conventional contrast agents and nontargeted radiotracers.
- Precision PET tracers combined with MR imaging can provide diagnostic options unavailable with any other modality.
- PET tracers can be combined with radioactive sources to act as not just diagnostic agents but also radiotherapeutics.

INTRODUCTION

PET/computed tomography (CT) has become commonplace in the diagnosis and evaluation of malignancy; however, PET/MR imaging is emerging as a strong competitor with current and potential applications in precision medicine. Precision medicine is loosely defined as an approach to disease treatment and prevention that takes into account individual variability in the patient's tumor. As therapies have become more disease specific, diagnostic imaging must continue to advance with tailored disease-specific agents.

PET imaging has always provided valuable functional information about physiologic processes beyond simple evaluation of anatomy or lesion size. Using various combinations of radioisotopes and tracers, PET has advanced past identification of glucose metabolism and can now precisely identify specific disease processes, clusters of

This article originally appeared in *PET Clinics*, Volume 12, Issue 4, October 2017.

Disclosure Statement: T.A. Hope receives research support from GE Healthcare.

[a] Department of Radiology and Biomedical Imaging, University of California San Francisco, 505 Parnassus Avenue, San Francisco, CA 94143, USA; [b] Department of Radiology, San Francisco VA Health Care System, 4150 Clement Street, San Francisco, CA 94121, USA

* Corresponding author. 505 Parnassus Avenue, M-391, San Francisco, CA 94143.

E-mail address: thomas.hope@ucsf.edu

Clinics Collections 8 (2020) 83–100

https://doi.org/10.1016/j.ccol.2020.07.007

2352-7986/20/Published by Elsevier Inc.

malignant cells, or mutations.[1] Through the development of new targeted molecular imaging methods, PET is better able to assay in vivo biological processes noninvasively and quantitatively, with the potential to identify patients with specific tumors or genotypes of disease.

Early studies have shown combining the use of these targeted precision medicine PET agents with MR imaging has some definite advantages compared with PET/CT. Unlike the low intrinsic soft tissue contrast of CT,[2] the superior soft tissue contrast of MR imaging allows for the improved assessment of fine anatomic detail[3–5] and can provide additional information on tissue composition and function not possible with CT. In allowing for more precise evaluation of disease-specific markers in combination with excellent anatomic detail, PET/MR imaging offers a way not only to identify those patients who may benefit from targeted treatment but also a better method of evaluating disease response. This article reviews both the current and future directions of PET/MR imaging in precision medicine.

PET/MR IMAGING VERSUS PET/COMPUTED TOMOGRAPHY

PET/MR imaging as a modality is still in its fledgling stages but has shown much promise, with the unique information that can be obtained from both modalities. The current literature has begun to show that PET and MR imaging can be complementary in evaluating primary tumor, as well as assessing metastatic or recurrent disease.[6,7] There are 2 primary advantages of PET/MR imaging compared with PET/CT. First, with the advent of hybrid PET/MR imaging scanners that acquire and fuse metabolic information from PET with anatomic and functional data from MR imaging, it is now possible for complete spatial and temporal matching of PET and MR imaging data.[3,8] This is advantageous compared with the sequential nature of data acquisition inherent to PET/CT, reducing misregistration and allowing for easier transition of PET/MR imaging into the clinical setting.

The second major advantage is the superior soft tissue information provided by MR imaging. PET/CT may detect small foci of radionuclide uptake; however, due to the low soft tissue contrast of CT and the sequential data acquisition of PET/CT, lesion localization may suffer in some circumstances and anatomic correlates for small PET findings may be overlooked. The superior soft tissue contrast of MR imaging allows for the improved assessment of fine anatomic detail, including clear depiction of lesion margins, local tumor infiltration, and the relationship of lesions to adjacent structures.[3–5] MR imaging contrast agents can also provide specific imaging information regarding soft tissues, such as macrophage infiltration with the use of ferumoxytol and hepatobiliary imaging with gadoxetate disodium. With this fine anatomic detail and specialized contrast agents, PET/MR imaging will often help in detection of small lesions that may be difficult for either modality to demonstrate alone.

In addition to the anatomic detail and contrast enhancement, MR imaging is capable of providing functional information with diffusion-weighted imaging (DWI), perfusion imaging, and spectroscopy not possible with CT and without the use of ionizing radiation. DWI has proven particularly valuable in the assessment of lesion cellularity, and may be used as a whole-body screening technique for the detection of neoplastic lesions, including small lesions less than 10 mm in diameter.[9,10] Magnetic resonance spectroscopy's ability to detect metabolites can also help to differentiate normal versus abnormal tissue and distinguish proliferation versus necrosis in masses.[11] Dynamic contrast-enhanced MR imaging can be used to evaluate lesion perfusion, with certain malignant lesions demonstrating characteristic perfusion patterns.[12] This functional information can further assist in diagnosis and evaluation of disease response.

Even though there are many potential advantages, PET/MR imaging does have some disadvantages. Because MR imaging cannot directly measure density, alternative methods of attenuation-correction must be used.[13] The cost of a combined PET/MR imaging scanner is greater than the combined cost of a separate PET and MR imaging scanner, while decreasing the flexibility in utilization. Specific body regions are known to have decreased imaging sensitivity on PET/MR imaging compared with PET/CT, including evaluation of bowel-based tumors due to peristaltic motion and in the evaluation for pulmonary nodules.[14] Despite these limitations, the combination of PET and MR imaging has already proven to be helpful with the use of ^{18}F-fluorodeoxyglucose (FDG), and may have increased utility when applied to precision medicine.

Issues related to attenuation correction with PET/MR imaging cannot be overlooked when considering precision medicine. Accurate quantification of uptake is critical for tumor characterization and inclusion of imaging modalities in clinical trials. Quantitative accuracy in PET relies on 2 main processes: attenuation correction and PET reconstruction parameters. In PET/CT, measurement of attenuation maps is straightforward because the CT component measures density directly. Therefore, phantoms used in PET/CT disregard attenuation as a source of error and methods to evaluate quantitative accuracy focus on PET reconstruction parameters. Using PET/CT phantoms, one can create protocols that deliver reproducible PET quantification.[15,16] These same phantoms cannot be used in PET/MR imaging because the phantoms cannot reproduce the MR imaging and density characteristics that would be required to evaluate the accuracy of the attenuation map produced in PET/MR imaging. Additionally, these phantoms create significant artifacts when imaged using MR imaging due to the materials they are made of.[17,18] Currently, when one measures activity in a phantom in PET/MR imaging, a predetermined density map is used for attenuation rather than one acquired directly from the phantom at the time of imaging. In particular, this is relevant for the pelvis, where bone is not included in the attenuation map in the currently commercially available systems, which can result in a 20% error in quantitative accuracy.[19,20] It is imperative that radiologists develop phantoms and reconstruction parameters specific to PET/MR imaging to delineate the quantitative error in PET/MR imaging. This will allow PET/MR imaging to be included in multicenter clinical trials and verify that the measured uptake is accurate and valid, thereby making it appropriate for use in precision medicine applications.

PRECISION MEDICINE

Many malignancies in the past have been treated by surgery, radiation, or generalized chemotherapies, but more and more frequently treatments are more targeted.[21–24] Although not all patients respond to targeted therapies, those patients who harbor specific mutations can be given therapy directed specifically to the tumor genotype. The tumor molecular profile can also be used to predict prognosis and response to therapy.[1] Some of these some principles can and are being applied to PET/MR imaging.

PET imaging can take 2 major forms: nontargeted imaging and targeted molecular imaging. Nontargeted molecular imaging typically images cellular processes, such as glucose metabolism and cell proliferation. Because this method focuses on general cellular processes, it often does not characterize individual patient's tumors. For targeted molecular imaging, probes directly image specific molecular targets, such as transporters or enzymes. Both nontargeted molecular imaging and targeted molecular imaging can be useful in disease diagnosis and monitoring (see later discussion).

POTENTIAL OF HYPERPOLARIZED MR IMAGING

One aspect of MR imaging that has not yet been used in the setting of PET/MR imaging is hyperpolarized MR imaging. New MR imaging–compatible molecular imaging techniques have the potential to identify cancer and other diseases, providing metabolic information that has traditionally been the domain of high-sensitivity methods like PET.[25,26] Specifically, hyperpolarized ^{13}C MR imaging uses a recently developed technique, solution dynamic nuclear polarization (DNP), to dramatically increase the signal of ^{13}C-enriched metabolic agents. The resulting increase in sensitivity (up to 10^6) allows real-time observation of metabolism in living systems, based on the conversion of an introduced ^{13}C substrate into its metabolic products. Metabolism is observed by new resonances in the hyperpolarized ^{13}C spectrum, reflecting the subtle frequency shift between different ^{13}C small molecules in vivo.

One important target has been pyruvate, a 3-carbon molecule that sits at the crossroads of human metabolism. In cancer, pyruvate is converted primarily to lactate, reflecting the glycolytic phenotype observed in many human neoplasms. This conversion can typically be observed within the first few seconds of introducing hyperpolarized ^{13}C pyruvate into human cancers, including those of the prostate, brain, and liver.[27] Although hyperpolarized ^{13}C MR imaging is a relatively new technology (solution DNP was first reported in 2003), a wealth of data has been generated in cell and animal models relevant to human cancer.[28] Furthermore, the method is not limited to ^{13}C pyruvate, with numerous newer probes applied to study in vivo perfusion, reduction and oxidation (redox), pH, necrosis, and glutaminolysis.

A successful in vivo hyperpolarized ^{13}C MR imaging experiment requires expertise in chemistry, biochemistry, engineering, pulse sequence design, pharmaceutical sciences, and data processing. Not surprisingly, successful use in humans has been challenging, with the potential of the method recently met in a first-in-human clinical trial in subjects with prostate cancer.[29] This study demonstrated the safety of ^{13}C pyruvate in a series of subjects with cancer, and showed that both hyperpolarized ^{13}C pyruvate and its metabolic product ^{13}C lactate could be detected in the human prostate. Future work will extend this method to other human cancers, including those of the brain (glioblastoma multiforme) and liver (metastatic breast cancer). To extend this technology into widespread clinical practice, there are ongoing efforts to improve coil design and data acquisition, as well as to engineer robust solution DNP systems. Furthermore, combined modality imaging such as PET/MR imaging highlights the potential of using multiple metabolic techniques in tandem to better diagnose and treat the metabolic disturbances in patients with cancer. PET is typically limited to 1 targeted probe; however, the combination of hyperpolarized MR imaging and PET allows for the simultaneous imaging of multiple targets and pathways.

NONTARGETED MOLECULAR PROBES

Currently, PET/MR imaging is primarily used with less specific nontargeted molecular imaging agents. Through the imaging of cell processes, nontargeted molecular imaging can be used to identify abnormal cell physiology and monitor cellular changes over time. Nontargeted molecular probes are radiolabeled versions of compounds used or retained in higher amounts within a targeted pathologic process when compared with normal physiologic ones. The most common cellular processes imaged by nontargeted molecular imaging and PET/MR imaging are glucose metabolism (^{18}F-FDG), lipogenesis (^{11}C-choline, ^{11}C-acetate), cellular proliferation or DNA synthesis (^{18}F-fluorothymidine, ^{18}F-FMAU), and cellular hypoxia (^{18}F-fluoromisonidazole, nitroimidazole compounds).

The most commonly used nontargeted agent is FDG PET (**Fig. 1**). Because glucose metabolism is not specific to tumors, areas of naturally high or increased metabolism also demonstrate increased uptake, such as the brain, heart, or bowel, in addition to inflammatory or infectious processes. Despite the limitations of [18]FDG, the information from a PET scan when combined with the soft-tissue resolution of MR imaging has

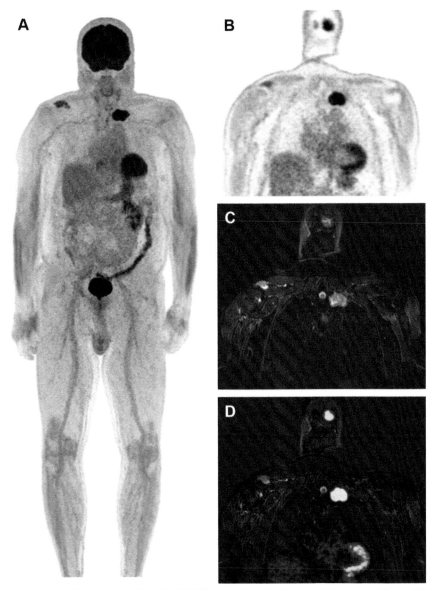

Fig. 1. Fluorodeoxyglucose (FDG) PET/MR imaging. A 79-year-old man with multiple myeloma after radiation, stem cell transplant, and thalidomide. (*A*) MIP and (*B*) coronal PET images demonstrations uptake within the left lung apex and right shoulder, corresponding to active disease. Corresponding (*C*) short tau inversion recovery and (*D*) fused PET/MR imaging images.

resulted in an examination that can affect treatment decisions. Rectal cancer is among the diseases that have the potential to benefit from the combination of modalities.

Treatment of rectal cancer changes greatly based on both the presence of distant metastatic disease and local T-staging. MR imaging is the best current imaging modality for identifying depth of invasion, which is the key prognostic factor in determining T-stage. Preoperative radiation therapy has a high morbidity when given in T1, T2, and early T3 disease but offers a reduction in recurrence rate postresection when given in advanced T3 or greater disease. However, detection of nodal and metastatic disease is extremely variable, depending on the reader, and requires a significant amount of expertise.[30] Metastatic disease is most commonly found in the liver and lymph nodes, and although distant disease changes the treatment algorithm, resection is still possible. PET has been shown to significantly improve the detection of disease compared with CT alone, revealing unknown disease in 19% of patients, and changing the therapeutic approach 17% of patients.[31] PET also has a role in the evaluation of rectal cancer after resection, successfully differentiating recurrent or residual rectal cancer from scar.[32]

[18]F-choline is a nontargeted molecular probe that demonstrates increased uptake in prostate and parathyroid cancers due to increased choline kinase activity and increased choline transport.[33,34] PET/MR imaging with ^{18}F-choline has been shown to improve the detection rate of prostate cancer in targeted biopsies compared with MR imaging alone.[35] ^{18}F-choline agents have shown better detection of both androgen-dependent and independent prostate cancers in vitro.[36] A few studies have noted the discovery of incidental parathyroid adenomas on[18]F-choline PET/MR imaging studies for prostate cancer staging[37–39] (**Fig. 2**). One pilot study demonstrated an 89% sensitivity and 100% specificity for identification of histologically confirmed adenomas in patients with prior inconclusive ultrasound and [99]mTc-sestamibi scintigraphy. PET/MR imaging not only located the responsible adenomas but also was able to provide detailed anatomic information to the surgeons.[40] Because the sensitivity of conventional dual-tracer subtraction scintigraphy using [99]mTc-tetrofosmin and ^{123}I coupled with ultrasonography drops to as low as 30% if multiple parathyroid glands are involved,[41–44] dynamic contrast-enhanced CT and ^{18}F-choline PET/CT have emerged as imaging modalities that can identify these subtle parathyroid adenomas.[37,45–49]

TARGETED MOLECULAR IMAGING

Targeted molecular imaging images specific molecular targets such as transporters or enzymes, which have the potential to be earlier and more sensitive biomarkers of therapeutic efficacy. In addition, many preclinical and clinical studies suggest that targeted molecular imaging provides useful methods for monitoring targeted therapy in PET/MR imaging. The targeted molecular imaging probes in common use can be divided by different targeted ligands, monoclonal antibodies or their fragments, natural peptide ligands or their analogues, tyrosine kinase inhibitors or their analogues, and high-affinity peptides. Precision medicine PET/MR imaging with targeted molecular imaging is being applied in a few disease processes currently, most commonly in prostate and neuroendocrine tumor (NET).

Prostate Carcinoma

For the evaluation of prostate cancer, MR imaging is known to be superior to CT,[50] gaining acceptance in American Urological Association guidelines.[51] CT has not been shown to have a role in prostate cancer evaluation except for the identification

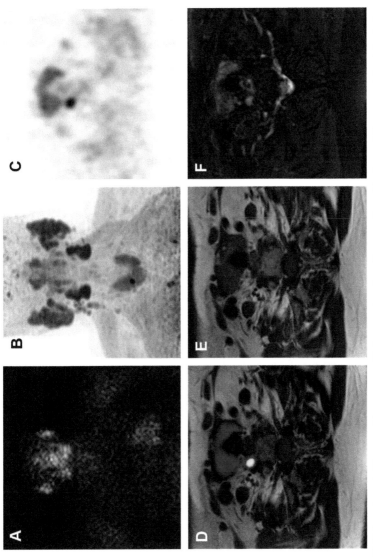

Fig. 2. Choline PET/MR imaging. A 65-year-old woman with hypercalcemia, after parathyroidectomy. Isthmus nodule detected on ultrasound with a benign biopsy and (A) negative sestamibi scan. A focus of uptake on choline PET/MR imaging (B) MIP and (C) axial images was identified posterior to the right thyroid lobe. (D) Fused PET/MR imaging images demonstrate the right paraesophageal adenoma with (E) T1 hypointensity and (F) T2 hyperintensity.

of nodal disease and evaluation of sclerotic osseous metastases.[50] For evaluation of the primary tumor, multiparametric MR imaging (mpMR imaging) combines anatomic and functional MR imaging, including T2-weighted, DWI, and dynamic-contrast enhanced MR imaging.[52] The diffusion component of mpMR imaging is the strongest predictive factor of cancer in the peripheral zone,[53] which is reflected in the weight given to it in the Prostate Imaging Reporting and Data System (PIRADS) version 2 reporting system.[52] Newer studies have shown that DWI can also predict tumor grading[54,55] in the peripheral zone and may have a role as a predictive biomarker for biochemical recurrence.[56]

There have been several new developments over the past 5 years in the imaging of prostate cancer, including probes-targeting bombesin[57] and prostate-specific membrane antigen (PSMA). PMSA is a transmembrane protein expressed in high levels in more than 90% of prostate carcinomas.[58] The expression of PMSA correlates with unfavorable prognostic factors, such as a high Gleason score, infiltrative growth, metastasis, and hormone independence.[58] 68-gallium (^{68}Ga)-PSMA has demonstrated a high sensitivity and specificity for prostate cancer, allowing for detection of even small amounts of tumor, both local and metastatic.[59–61] The most commonly used PSMA-targeted probe is ^{68}Ga-PSMA N,N'-bis [2-hydroxy-5-(carboxyethyl) benzyl] ethylenediamine-N,N'- diacetic acid (HBED-CC or PSMA-11).[62]

The 4 main applications of imaging in prostate cancer are in patients with low-risk disease, evaluation of high-risk preprostatectomy patients, post-treatment biochemical recurrence, and CRPC.

Active surveillance describes the observation of patients with lower grade biopsies (Gleason score <6) who may not benefit from definitive therapy. In this approach, immediate radical prostatectomy or radiation therapy is deferred in favor of continuous surveillance.[63] To date, there has been no evaluation of patients under active surveillance, although there is the belief that the combination of MR imaging and PET could detect clinically significant cancers. Currently, there is a clinical trial evaluating a PSMA targeted compound in active surveillance patients but without MR imaging for comparison (NCT02615067).[64] This is a large unmet need and the combination of hyperpolarized MR imaging with PET may have better imaging characteristics than MR imaging alone.[27] Eiber and colleagues[65] compared PET/MR imaging with the already established mpMR imaging, as well as the PET, and found that ^{68}Ga-PSMA-11 PET/MR imaging had a higher diagnostic accuracy than either mpMR imaging or PET alone for the evaluation of the primary tumor (**Fig. 3**). This study was in subjects with intermediate to high-grade tumors in which detection of the primary tumor is not as critical; however, it does suggest that this approach may be applicable in the active surveillance population.

The most common classification schema for risk stratification of patients with prostate cancer is the D'Amico criteria.[66] Approximately 15% of patients diagnosed with prostate cancer fit into this category. With a diagnosis of high-risk prostate cancer, 22% have osseous metastases and 33% have pelvic nodal disease.[67] With the high specificities in detecting nodal and osseous metastatic disease, PET/MR imaging can be useful in the evaluation of these patients before definitive therapy. Initial studies have been performed evaluating PSMA PET for nodal staging of high-risk patients[68] but comparisons between PET/CT and PET/MR imaging have not yet been performed.

Biochemical recurrence is defined as an elevation in prostate-specific antigen (PSA) of greater than 0.2 ng/mL after treatment, confirmed by a second test.[69] Up to 32% of patients after radical-prostatectomy and 41% of patients postradiation therapy will have recurrence.[70,71] Afshar-Oromieh and colleagues[72] used ^{68}Ga-PSMA-11 to demonstrate the superiority of PET/MR imaging to PET/CT in prostate cancer

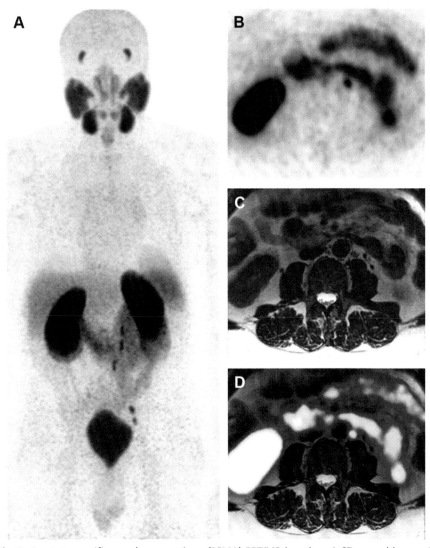

Fig. 3. Prostate-specific membrane antigen (PSMA) PET/MR imaging. A 67-year-old man after radical prostatectomy and external beam radiation treatment, now with biochemical recurrence, prostate-specific antigen = 6.1. (*A*) PSMA maximum intensity projection (MIP) and (*B*) axial images demonstrate uptake in multiple retroperitoneal lymph nodes also seen on T2 MR imaging (*C*) but are more readily identified on (*D*) fused PET/MR imaging images. Based on the imaging findings, management was changed from planned pelvic salvage radiation to monotherapy with androgen deprivation therapy.

evaluation. This study noted that the higher lesion contrast and higher imaging resolution of MR imaging enabled a subjectively easier evaluation, in addition to classifying unclear findings on PET/CT as characteristic of prostate cancer metastases on PET/MR imaging. Freitag and colleagues[73] also demonstrated the additional value of using mpMR imaging in a PET/MR imaging protocol. In this study, the ^{68}Ga-PSMA-11 PET-component of either PET/MR imaging or PET/CT found at least 1 pathologic lesion in

93 out of 119 subjects with an additional 18 out of 119 subjects (15.1%) diagnosed with a local recurrence in multiparametric portion of the PET/MR imaging. This demonstrated the additional value of hybrid ^{68}Ga-PSMA-11 PET/MR imaging by gaining complementary diagnostic information from mpMR imaging compared with the capabilities of PET/CT.

Castrate-resistant prostate cancer (CRPC) describes patients with persistent elevation of their PSA despite a low level of testosterone, typically while being treated with androgen-deprivation therapy. CRPC still responds to secondary hormonal treatments that target the androgen receptor. CRPC also demonstrates increased PSMA expression,[74] which enables PSMA-labeled radiopharmaceuticals to be used for imaging and therapy of CRPC. Early attempts with PSMA-directed radiolabeled ligands with antibodies were limited by the slow clearance and toxicity.[40] PSMA radioligand therapy with ^{177}Lu-PSMA showed at least a partial response in 56% of subjects,[75] with less overall toxicity than the PSMA antibody treatments [177]LU-DOTA (1,4,7,10-tetraazacyclododecane-1,4,7,10-tetraacetic acid)-J591.[76] Median progression-free survival was at least comparable to other treatments for CRPC. Although the role of PSMA peptide receptor radionuclide therapy (PRRT) has yet to be determined, PET/MR imaging may play a role for patient selection and evaluation of disease response in these patients.

NEUROENDOCRINE TUMORS

Another area that has been under investigation for the utility of precision medicine in PET/MR imaging is NETs. NETs include a variety of tumor types; however, well-differentiated NETs express somatostatin receptors (SSTRs), particularly type 2 receptors.[77] NETs are generally slow-growing and clinically indolent. Accurate localization and evaluation of the full extent of NET disease burden is important to determine treatment options. Up to 13% of patients present with metastatic disease, and 75% of small bowel NET and up to 85% of pancreatic NET patients are discovered to have hepatic metastatic disease during the course of their disease.[78] In many of these patients, detection and possibly treatment with PRRT may offer their only chance in changing the course of disease.[79]

In the last 15 years, ^{68}Ga-labeled peptides targeting SSTRs have been developed, demonstrating increased sensitivity compared with octreotide for the evaluation of NETs.[80,81] These agents include DOTA-D-Phe1-Tyr3-octreotide (DOTA-TOC), DOTA-1-Nal3-octreotide (DOTA-NOC), and DOTA-DPhe1-Tyr3-octreotate (DOTA-TATE).[80,81] In addition to the improvement in sensitivity and spatial resolution, ^{68}Ga-labeled peptides can be used in both PET/CT and PET/MR imaging and also provide patients with shorter examinations and less radiation exposure than Octreoscan examinations.[82]

Gaertner and colleagues[83] conducted one of the first studies to demonstrate that anatomic correlates to ^{68}Ga-DOTA-TOC PET were significantly better delineated on MR imaging compared with CT images, and that there was better coregistration of functional and morphologic data on PET/MR imaging. This study proved at least equivalence of ^{68}Ga-DOTA-TOC PET/MR imaging and PET/CT. Other early investigations have suggested that PET/MR imaging has some advantages compared with PET/CT that can improve detection of NET metastatic disease.[84] MR imaging has higher sensitivity for hepatic lesion detection compared with CT due to DWI and the hepatobiliary agent gadoxetate disodium (Eovist, Bayer Healthcare, Wayne, NJ, USA)[85–88] (**Figs. 4** and **5**). For example, hepatobiliary phase MR imaging detected 99% of hepatic metastasis compared with 46% for CT and 64% for PET

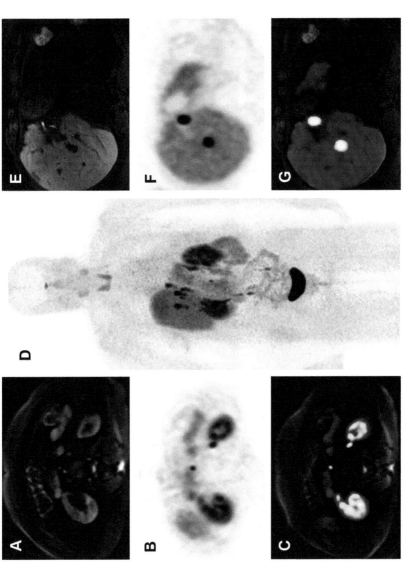

Fig. 4. DOTA-TOC PET/MR imaging. A 71-year-old woman with pancreatic neuroendocrine tumor after left hepatectomy and pancreatectomy. Multiple hepatic metastatic lesions previously treated with bland embolization. Retroperitoneal lymph nodes are noted on (A) diffusion-weighted imaging (DWI) b = 600 imaging but only 1 has increased (B, C) DOTA-TOC uptake. PET (D) MIP also demonstrates multiple hepatic imaging seen on axial (E) hepatobiliary phase, (F) PET, and (G) fusion images.

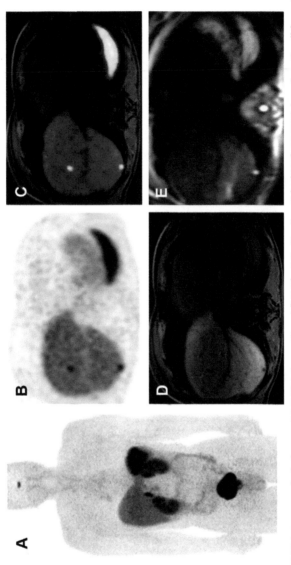

Fig. 5. DOTA (1,4,7,10-tetraazacyclododecane-1,4,7,10-tetraacetic acid)-D-Phe1-Tyr3-octreotide (TOC) PET/MR imaging. Small bowel NET status after partial hepatectomy for metastatic disease. PET (A) MIP, (B) axial, and (C) fused PET/MR imaging images demonstrate 2 small lesions with DOTA-TOC uptake. On (D) hepatobiliary phase and (E) diffusion-weighted imaging, only the posterior lesion is visible.

$(P<.001).$[84,89] Additionally, the anatomic detail provided by the MR imaging component of PET/MR imaging is useful in compensating for the decreased uptake in poorly differentiated NETs from decreased SSTR expression.[90]

Targeted agents selective for SSTRs have also been developed for therapeutic uses. Tumors with high expression of SSTRs detected by diagnostic imaging agents are also excellent targets for PRRT. ^{90}Y-DOTA-TOC and ^{177}Lu-DOTA-TATE have been used for therapy, especially useful in patients who have failed treatments with first-line somatostatin analogues. A recently concluded trial compared 229 subjects with metastatic midgut NETs treated with ^{177}Lu-DOTA-TATE or high-dose octreotide-long-acting release; there was a 79% lower risk of progression or death in the ^{177}Lu-DOTA-TATE group.[79] The role of imaging for patient selection and treatment response has yet to be determined but, given that less than 20% of subjects demonstrated a radiographic response in the trial, PET/MR imaging may play a role in determining how patients have responded to therapy.

SUMMARY

With the development of more targeted therapies for the treatment of malignancy, earlier and more accurate identification of treatment response could prove essential in improving patient outcomes. Although clinical studies have suggested that targeted molecular imaging can provide a useful method for monitoring targeted therapy in PET/MR imaging, there are currently several barriers limiting the research and clinical use of PET/MR imaging precision medicine.

Major barriers include the relatively small numbers of PET agents approved by the US Food and Drug Administration, accessibility to PET/MR imaging scanners, and relative lack of data supporting the use of PET/MR imaging compared with PET/CT using these tracers. Despite this, progress is being made in demonstrating the superiority of PET/MR imaging compared with PET/CT, including applications in targeted evaluation of prostate cancer, NETs, and parathyroid disease. It is hoped that these studies and larger clinical trials will lay the groundwork for determining clinical indications and standardizing PET/MR imaging protocols. With current and continued development in both PET and MR technology, PET/MR imaging will be a large contributor in precision medicine now and in the future.

REFERENCES

1. Teng FF, Meng X, Sun XD, et al. New strategy for monitoring targeted therapy: molecular imaging. Int J Nanomedicine 2013;8:3703–13.
2. Catalano OA, Masch WR, Catana C, et al. An overview of PET/MR, focused on clinical applications. Abdom Radiol (NY) 2017;42(2):631–44.
3. Delso G, Furst S, Jakoby B, et al. Performance measurements of the Siemens mMR integrated whole-body PET/MR scanner. J Nucl Med 2011;52(12):1914–22.
4. Torigian DA, Zaidi H, Kwee TC, et al. PET/MR imaging: technical aspects and potential clinical applications. Radiology 2013;267(1):26–44.
5. von Schulthess GK, Schlemmer HP. A look ahead: PET/MR versus PET/CT. Eur J Nucl Med Mol Imaging 2009;36(Suppl 1):S3–9.
6. Drzezga A, Souvatzoglou M, Eiber M, et al. First clinical experience with integrated whole-body PET/MR: comparison to PET/CT in patients with oncologic diagnoses. J Nucl Med 2012;53(6):845–55.
7. Al-Nabhani KZ, Syed R, Michopoulou S, et al. Qualitative and quantitative comparison of PET/CT and PET/MR imaging in clinical practice. J Nucl Med 2014; 55(1):88–94.

8. Zaidi H, Ojha N, Morich M, et al. Design and performance evaluation of a whole-body Ingenuity TF PET-MRI system. Phys Med Biol 2011;56(10):3091–106.

9. Nasu K, Kuroki Y, Nawano S, et al. Hepatic metastases: diffusion-weighted sensitivity-encoding versus SPIO-enhanced MR imaging. Radiology 2006;239(1): 122–30.

10. Padhani AR, Koh DM, Collins DJ. Whole-body diffusion-weighted MR imaging in cancer: current status and research directions. Radiology 2011;261(3):700–18.

11. Nguyen ML, Willows B, Khan R, et al. The potential role of magnetic resonance spectroscopy in image-guided radiotherapy. Front Oncol 2014;4:91.

12. Fusco R, Sansone M, Filice S, et al. Pattern recognition approaches for breast cancer DCE-MRI classification: a systematic review. J Med Biol Eng 2016; 36(4):449–59.

13. Delso G, ter Voert E, de Galiza Barbosa F, et al. Pitfalls and limitations in simultaneous PET/MRI. Semin Nucl Med 2015;45(6):552–9.

14. Chandarana H, Heacock L, Rakheja R, et al. Pulmonary nodules in patients with primary malignancy: comparison of hybrid PET/MR and PET/CT imaging. Radiology 2013;268(3):874–81.

15. Sunderland JJ, Christian PE. Quantitative PET/CT scanner performance characterization based upon the society of nuclear medicine and molecular imaging clinical trials network oncology clinical simulator phantom. J Nucl Med 2015; 56(1):145–52.

16. Fahey FH, Kinahan PE, Doot RK, et al. Variability in PET quantitation within a multicenter consortium. Med Phys 2010;37(7):3660–6.

17. Tropp J. Image brightening in samples of high dielectric constant. J Magn Reson 2004;167(1):12–24.

18. Ziegler S, Braun H, Ritt P, et al. Systematic evaluation of phantom fluids for simultaneous PET/MR hybrid imaging. J Nucl Med 2013;54(8):1464–71.

19. Samarin A, Burger C, Wollenweber SD, et al. PET/MR imaging of bone lesions–implications for PET quantification from imperfect attenuation correction. Eur J Nucl Med Mol Imaging 2012;39(7):1154–60.

20. Leynes AP, Yang J, Shanbhag DD, et al. Hybrid ZTE/Dixon MR-based attenuation correction for quantitative uptake estimation of pelvic lesions in PET/MRI. Med Phys 2017;44(3):902–13.

21. Ou SH. Crizotinib: a novel and first-in-class multitargeted tyrosine kinase inhibitor for the treatment of anaplastic lymphoma kinase rearranged non-small cell lung cancer and beyond. Drug Des Devel Ther 2011;5:471–85.

22. Moon YW, Park S, Sohn JH, et al. Clinical significance of progesterone receptor and HER2 status in estrogen receptor-positive, operable breast cancer with adjuvant tamoxifen. J Cancer Res Clin Oncol 2011;137(7):1123–30.

23. Scartozzi M, Bearzi I, Berardi R, et al. Epidermal growth factor receptor (EGFR) status in primary colorectal tumors does not correlate with EGFR expression in related metastatic sites: implications for treatment with EGFR-targeted monoclonal antibodies. J Clin Oncol 2004;22(23):4772–8.

24. Zidan J, Dashkovsky I, Stayerman C, et al. Comparison of HER-2 overexpression in primary breast cancer and metastatic sites and its effect on biological targeting therapy of metastatic disease. Br J Cancer 2005;93(5):552–6.

25. Di Gialleonardo V, Wilson DM, Keshari KR. The potential of metabolic imaging. Semin Nucl Med 2016;46(1):28–39.

26. Kurhanewicz J, Bok R, Nelson SJ, et al. Current and potential applications of clinical 13C MR spectroscopy. J Nucl Med 2008;49(3):341–4.

27. Wilson DM, Kurhanewicz J. Hyperpolarized 13C MR for molecular imaging of prostate cancer. J Nucl Med 2014;55(10):1567–72.
28. Keshari KR, Wilson DM. Chemistry and biochemistry of 13C hyperpolarized magnetic resonance using dynamic nuclear polarization. Chem Soc Rev 2014;43(5): 1627–59.
29. Nelson SJ, Kurhanewicz J, Vigneron DB, et al. Metabolic imaging of patients with prostate cancer using hyperpolarized [1-(1)(3)C]pyruvate. Sci Transl Med 2013; 5(198):198ra108.
30. Kaur H, Choi H, You YN, et al. MR imaging for preoperative evaluation of primary rectal cancer: practical considerations. Radiographics 2012;32(2):389–409.
31. Shin SS, Jeong YY, Min JJ, et al. Preoperative staging of colorectal cancer: CT vs. integrated FDG PET/CT. Abdom Imaging 2008;33(3):270–7.
32. Ito K, Kato T, Tadokoro M, et al. Recurrent rectal cancer and scar: differentiation with PET and MR imaging. Radiology 1992;182(2):549–52.
33. Ramirez de Molina A, Rodriguez-Gonzalez A, Gutierrez R, et al. Overexpression of choline kinase is a frequent feature in human tumor-derived cell lines and in lung, prostate, and colorectal human cancers. Biochem Biophys Res Commun 2002;296(3):580–3.
34. Awwad HM, Geisel J, Obeid R. The role of choline in prostate cancer. Clin Biochem 2012;45(18):1548–53.
35. Piert M, Montgomery J, Kunju LP, et al. 18F-Choline PET/MRI: the additional value of PET for MRI-guided transrectal prostate biopsies. J Nucl Med 2016;57(7): 1065–70.
36. Price DT, Coleman RE, Liao RP, et al. Comparison of [18F]Fluorocholine and [18F] Fluorodeoxyglucose for positron emission tomography of androgen dependent and androgen independent prostate cancer. J Urol 2002;168(1):273–80.
37. Cazaentre T, Clivaz F, Triponez F. False-positive result in 18F-fluorocholine PET/ CT due to incidental and ectopic parathyroid hyperplasia. Clin Nucl Med 2014; 39(6):e328–30.
38. Mapelli P, Busnardo E, Magnani P, et al. Incidental finding of parathyroid adenoma with 11C-choline PET/CT. Clin Nucl Med 2012;37(6):593–5.
39. Hodolic M, Huchet V, Balogova S, et al. Incidental uptake of (18)F-fluorocholine (FCH) in the head or in the neck of patients with prostate cancer. Radiol Oncol 2014;48(3):228–34.
40. Bouchelouche K, Turkbey B, Choyke PL. PSMA PET and radionuclide therapy in prostate cancer. Semin Nucl Med 2016;46(6):522–35.
41. Borley NR, Collins RE, O'Doherty M, et al. Technetium-99m sestamibi parathyroid localization is accurate enough for scan-directed unilateral neck exploration. Br J Surg 1996;83(7):989–91.
42. Hindie E, Melliere D, Jeanguillaume C, et al. Unilateral surgery for primary hyperparathyroidism on the basis of technetium Tc 99m sestamibi and iodine 123 subtraction scanning. Arch Surg 2000;135(12):1461–8.
43. Johnston LB, Carroll MJ, Britton KE, et al. The accuracy of parathyroid gland localization in primary hyperparathyroidism using sestamibi radionuclide imaging. J Clin Endocrinol Metab 1996;81(1):346–52.
44. Rubello D, Pelizzo MR, Casara D. Nuclear medicine and minimally invasive surgery of parathyroid adenomas: a fair marriage. Eur J Nucl Med Mol Imaging 2003;30(2):189–92.
45. Hoang JK, Sung WK, Bahl M, et al. How to perform parathyroid 4D CT: tips and traps for technique and interpretation. Radiology 2014;270(1):15–24.

46. Bahl M, Muzaffar M, Vij G, et al. Prevalence of the polar vessel sign in parathyroid adenomas on the arterial phase of 4D CT. AJNR Am J Neuroradiol 2014;35(3): 578–81.

47. Orevi M, Freedman N, Mishani E, et al. Localization of parathyroid adenoma by (1)(1)C-choline PET/CT: preliminary results. Clin Nucl Med 2014;39(12):1033–8.

48. van Raalte DH, Vlot MC, Zwijnenburg A, et al. F18-Choline PET/CT: a novel tool to localize parathyroid adenoma? Clin Endocrinol (Oxf) 2015;82(6):910–2.

49. Lezaic L, Rep S, Sever MJ, et al. (1)(8)F-Fluorocholine PET/CT for localization of hyperfunctioning parathyroid tissue in primary hyperparathyroidism: a pilot study. Eur J Nucl Med Mol Imaging 2014;41(11):2083–9.

50. Hricak H, Choyke PL, Eberhardt SC, et al. Imaging prostate cancer: a multidisciplinary perspective. Radiology 2007;243(1):28–53.

51. Rosenkrantz AB, Verma S, Choyke P, et al. Prostate magnetic resonance imaging and magnetic resonance imaging targeted biopsy in patients with a prior negative biopsy: a consensus statement by AUA and SAR. J Urol 2016;196(6):1613–8.

52. Weinreb JC, Barentsz JO, Choyke PL, et al. PI-RADS prostate imaging - reporting and data system: 2015, version 2. Eur Urol 2016;69(1):16–40.

53. Westphalen AC, Rosenkrantz AB. Prostate imaging reporting and data system (PI-RADS): reflections on early experience with a standardized interpretation scheme for multiparametric prostate MRI. AJR Am J Roentgenol 2014;202(1): 121–3.

54. NiMhurchu E, O'Kelly F, Murphy IG, et al. Predictive value of PI-RADS classification in MRI-directed transrectal ultrasound guided prostate biopsy. Clin Radiol 2016;71(4):375–80.

55. Kim TH, Kim CK, Park BK, et al. Relationship between Gleason score and apparent diffusion coefficients of diffusion-weighted magnetic resonance imaging in prostate cancer patients. Can Urol Assoc J 2016;10(11–12):E377–82.

56. Park SY, Kim CK, Park BK, et al. Prediction of biochemical recurrence following radical prostatectomy in men with prostate cancer by diffusion-weighted magnetic resonance imaging: initial results. Eur Radiol 2011;21(5):1111–8.

57. Mansi R, Minamimoto R, Macke H, et al. Bombesin-targeted PET of prostate cancer. J Nucl Med 2016;57(Suppl 3):67s–72s.

58. Kratochwil C, Afshar-Oromieh A, Kopka K, et al. Current status of prostate-specific membrane antigen targeting in nuclear medicine: clinical translation of chelator containing prostate-specific membrane antigen ligands into diagnostics and therapy for prostate cancer. Semin Nucl Med 2016;46(5):405–18.

59. Eiber M, Maurer T, Souvatzoglou M, et al. Evaluation of Hybrid (6)(8)Ga-PSMA Ligand PET/CT in 248 patients with biochemical recurrence after radical prostatectomy. J Nucl Med 2015;56(5):668–74.

60. Perera M, Papa N, Christidis D, et al. Sensitivity, specificity, and predictors of positive 68Ga-Prostate-specific membrane antigen positron emission tomography in advanced prostate cancer: a systematic review and meta-analysis. Eur Urol 2016;70(6):926–37.

61. Freitag MT, Radtke JP, Hadaschik BA, et al. Comparison of hybrid (68)Ga-PSMA PET/MRI and (68)Ga-PSMA PET/CT in the evaluation of lymph node and bone metastases of prostate cancer. Eur J Nucl Med Mol Imaging 2016;43(1):70–83.

62. Afshar-Oromieh A, Malcher A, Eder M, et al. PET imaging with a [68Ga]gallium-labelled PSMA ligand for the diagnosis of prostate cancer: biodistribution in humans and first evaluation of tumour lesions. Eur J Nucl Med Mol Imaging 2013; 40(4):486–95.

63. Chen RC, Rumble RB, Loblaw DA, et al. Active surveillance for the management of localized prostate cancer (Cancer Care Ontario Guideline): American Society of Clinical Oncology Clinical Practice Guideline Endorsement. J Clin Oncol 2016; 34(18):2182–90.

64. Molecular Insight Pharmaceuticals I. Study to evaluate 99mTc-MIP-1404 SPECT/CT imaging in men with biopsy proven low-grade prostate cancer. 2015. Available at: https://ClinicalTrials.gov/show/NCT02615067.

65. Eiber M, Weirich G, Holzapfel K, et al. Simultaneous 68Ga-PSMA HBED-CC PET/MRI improves the localization of primary prostate cancer. Eur Urol 2016;70(5): 829–36.

66. D'Amico AV, Whittington R, Malkowicz SB, et al. Biochemical outcome after radical prostatectomy, external beam radiation therapy, or interstitial radiation therapy for clinically localized prostate cancer. JAMA 1998;280(11):969–74.

67. Miller DC, Hafez KS, Stewart A, et al. Prostate carcinoma presentation, diagnosis, and staging. Cancer 2003;98(6):1169–78.

68. Maurer T, Gschwend JE, Rauscher I, et al. Diagnostic efficacy of (68)Gallium-PSMA positron emission tomography compared to conventional imaging for lymph node staging of 130 consecutive patients with intermediate to high risk prostate cancer. J Urol 2016;195(5):1436–43.

69. Cookson MS, Aus G, Burnett AL, et al. Variation in the definition of biochemical recurrence in patients treated for localized prostate cancer: the American Urological Association Prostate Guidelines for Localized Prostate Cancer Update Panel report and recommendations for a standard in the reporting of surgical outcomes. J Urol 2007;177(2):540–5.

70. Kwon O, Kim KB, Lee YI, et al. Salvage radiotherapy after radical prostatectomy: prediction of biochemical outcomes. PLoS One 2014;9(7):e103574.

71. Roehl KA, Han M, Ramos CG, et al. Cancer progression and survival rates following anatomical radical retropubic prostatectomy in 3,478 consecutive patients: long-term results. J Urol 2004;172(3):910–4.

72. Afshar-Oromieh A, Haberkorn U, Schlemmer HP, et al. Comparison of PET/CT and PET/MRI hybrid systems using a 68Ga-labelled PSMA ligand for the diagnosis of recurrent prostate cancer: initial experience. Eur J Nucl Med Mol Imaging 2014; 41(5):887–97.

73. Freitag MT, Radtke JP, Afshar-Oromieh A, et al. Local recurrence of prostate cancer after radical prostatectomy is at risk to be missed in 68Ga-PSMA-11-PET of PET/CT and PET/MRI: comparison with mpMRI integrated in simultaneous PET/MRI. Eur J Nucl Med Mol Imaging 2017;44(5):776–87.

74. Wright GL Jr, Grob BM, Haley C, et al. Upregulation of prostate-specific membrane antigen after androgen-deprivation therapy. Urology 1996;48(2):326–34.

75. Baum RP, Kulkarni HR, Schuchardt C, et al. 177Lu-labeled prostate-specific membrane antigen radioligand therapy of metastatic castration-resistant prostate cancer: safety and efficacy. J Nucl Med 2016;57(7):1006–13.

76. Vallabhajosula S, Goldsmith SJ, Hamacher KA, et al. Prediction of myelotoxicity based on bone marrow radiation-absorbed dose: radioimmunotherapy studies using 90Y- and 177Lu-labeled J591 antibodies specific for prostate-specific membrane antigen. J Nucl Med 2005;46(5):850–8.

77. Hassan MM, Phan A, Li D, et al. Risk factors associated with neuroendocrine tumors: a U.S.-based case-control study. Int J Cancer 2008;123(4):867–73.

78. Frilling A, Sotiropoulos GC, Li J, et al. Multimodal management of neuroendocrine liver metastases. HPB (Oxford) 2010;12(6):361–79.

79. Strosberg J, El-Haddad G, Wolin E, et al. Phase 3 trial of 177Lu-Dotatate for Midgut neuroendocrine tumors. N Engl J Med 2017;376(2):125–35.

80. Yang J, Kan Y, Ge BH, et al. Diagnostic role of Gallium-68 DOTATOC and Gallium-68 DOTATATE PET in patients with neuroendocrine tumors: a meta-analysis. Acta Radiol 2014;55(4):389–98.

81. Buchmann I, Henze M, Engelbrecht S, et al. Comparison of 68Ga-DOTATOC PET and 111In-DTPAOC (Octreoscan) SPECT in patients with neuroendocrine tumours. Eur J Nucl Med Mol Imaging 2007;34(10):1617–26.

82. Hope TA, Pampaloni MH, Flavell RR, et al. Somatostatin receptor PET/MRI for the evaluation of neuroendocrine tumors. Clin Transl Imaging 2017;5:63.

83. Gaertner FC, Beer AJ, Souvatzoglou M, et al. Evaluation of feasibility and image quality of 68Ga-DOTATOC positron emission tomography/magnetic resonance in comparison with positron emission tomography/computed tomography in patients with neuroendocrine tumors. Invest Radiol 2013;48(5):263–72.

84. Hope TA, Pampaloni MH, Nakakura E, et al. Simultaneous (68)Ga-DOTA-TOC PET/MRI with gadoxetate disodium in patients with neuroendocrine tumor. Abdom Imaging 2015;40(6):1432–40.

85. Sankowski AJ, Cwikla JB, Nowicki ML, et al. The clinical value of MRI using single-shot echoplanar DWI to identify liver involvement in patients with advanced gastroenteropancreatic-neuroendocrine tumors (GEP-NETs), compared to FSE T2 and FFE T1 weighted image after i.v. Gd-EOB-DTPA contrast enhancement. Med Sci Monit 2012;18(5):MT33–40.

86. Mayerhoefer ME, Ba-Ssalamah A, Weber M, et al. Gadoxetate-enhanced versus diffusion-weighted MRI for fused Ga-68-DOTANOC PET/MRI in patients with neuroendocrine tumours of the upper abdomen. Eur Radiol 2013;23(7):1978–85.

87. Giesel FL, Kratochwil C, Mehndiratta A, et al. Comparison of neuroendocrine tumor detection and characterization using DOTATOC-PET in correlation with contrast enhanced CT and delayed contrast enhanced MRI. Eur J Radiol 2012;81(10):2820–5.

88. Schreiter NF, Nogami M, Steffen I, et al. Evaluation of the potential of PET-MRI fusion for detection of liver metastases in patients with neuroendocrine tumours. Eur Radiol 2012;22(2):458–67.

89. Flechsig P, Zechmann CM, Schreiweis J, et al. Qualitative and quantitative image analysis of CT and MR imaging in patients with neuroendocrine liver metastases in comparison to (68)Ga-DOTATOC PET. Eur J Radiol 2015;84(8):1593–600.

90. Hofman MS, Lau WF, Hicks RJ. Somatostatin receptor imaging with 68Ga DOTA-TATE PET/CT: clinical utility, normal patterns, pearls, and pitfalls in interpretation. Radiographics 2015;35(2):500–16.

Genomic Approaches to Hypertension

Sheriff N. Dodoo, MD[a], Ivor J. Benjamin, MD[b,c],*

KEYWORDS

- Hypertension • Blood pressure • Genomic approaches

KEY POINTS

- Genomic insights and analyses of Mendelian hypertension (HTN) syndromes and Genome-Wide Association study (GWAS) on essential HTN have contributed to the depth of understanding of the genetics origins of hypertension.
- Mendelian syndromes are important for the field, since such knowledge leads to specific insights about disease pathogenesis and the potential for precision medicine.
- The clinical impact of findings of GWAS on essential HTN is continuously evolving, and the accrued insights will refine efforts to combat the societal impact of hypertension.
- Comprehensive identification of all genomic variants of hypertension, along with their individual associated mechanisms, is paving the way forward in the era of personalized medicine.
- The overriding challenge for care providers is to reduce health inequities through improved compliance and, perhaps, new paradigms for implementation science that incorporates genomic medicine.

INTRODUCTION

Hypertension is the leading cause of cardiovascular morbidity and mortality worldwide,[1–3] affecting more than a third of the US adult population[4,5] with a disproportionate burden in underrepresented and ethnic minorities including African Americans.[6] In both personal and societal terms, blood pressure control has emerged as an important health indicator in the US population and for 1 billion people

---

This article originally appeared in *Cardiology Clinics*, Volume 35, Issue 2, May 2017.

Disclosure statement: The authors have no financial or commercial conflicts of interest to declare.

[a] Department of Internal Medicine, Meharry Medical College, 1005 Dr DB Todd Jr Boulevard, Nashville, TN 37208, USA; [b] Cardiovascular Center, Department of Medicine, Medical College of Wisconsin, 8701 Watertown Plank Road, Milwaukee, WI 53226, USA; [c] Division of Cardiology, Department of Medicine, Medical College of Wisconsin, 8701 Watertown Plank Road, Milwaukee, WI 53226, USA

* Corresponding author. Cardiovascular Center, Medical College of Wisconsin, 8701 Watertown Plank Road, Milwaukee, WI 53226.

E-mail address: ibenjamin@mcw.edu

Clinics Collections 8 (2020) 101–115

https://doi.org/10.1016/j.ccol.2020.07.008

worldwide. To attain the American Heart Association Strategy Impact Goals to improve cardiovascular health of all Americans by 2020 and beyond, an ideal blood pressure target (<120/80 mm Hg) ranks among the 7 ideal health indicators[7] being directly targeted in populations. Although an in-depth review of the clinical manifestations, diagnostic evaluation, and treatment options of asymptomatic and symptomatic hypertension are covered elsewhere, this article reviews the genetic causes and provides a conceptual framework by which genomic analyses have propelled novel insights into the mechanisms of systemic and arterial hypertension.

Hypertension remains a significant public health problem with far-reaching impact on disease burden globally from stroke, heart failure, aortic dissection, atrial fibrillation, myocardial infarction[8] and end-stage kidney disease. In fact, a recent publication by Lawes and colleagues[8] concluded that 13.5% of premature deaths, 54% of strokes and 47% of ischemic heart disease worldwide are attributable to uncontrolled hypertension. Among the most easily recognizable and reversible risk factors, these authors further concluded that about 80% of the attributable burden occurred in low-income and middle-income economies. In spite of evidence of medical therapeutics and access to advanced systems of medical care, fewer than 50% of Americans treated for hypertension reach the target blood pressure goals. To achieve effective gains, both highly motivated and educated individuals affected with hypertension along with knowledgeable medical providers are prerequisites for proper blood pressure control and management.

Although the etiology of essential hypertension is unknown, both genetic and environmental factors play important roles in the pathophysiologic mechanisms in modern societies.[9] In epidemiologic studies among members of the Luo tribe in Kenya, for example, Poulter and colleagues[10] have highlighted lower blood pressure in their traditional rural environment compared with the urban center of Nairobi where urinary sodium and potassium concentrations was higher and lower, respectively. Because the renin-angiotensin- aldosterone system (RAS) has features for adaptation in sodium conservation, it has been hypothesized that a sodium-deprived environment favors sodium conservation as the default phenotype, underscoring the importance of salt reabsorption in the pathogenesis of hypertension in societies with high dietary salt intake.[11] In recent decades, substantial progress has been made to elucidate the mechanisms underlying the physiologic pathways and molecular targets of genes causally linked to rare Mendelian forms of hypertension in people.

GENOMIC VARIATION AND HUMAN INHERITABLE DISEASES

Thanks to the Human Genome Project, the promise to identify the consequence of germ line mutations (ie, single-nucleotide variants [SNV] and copy-number variants [CNV]) has yielded almost 3000 protein-coding genes linked to disease-associated mutations in people.[12] Innovations of genome sequencing coupled with technologies that dramatically reduce the amount of DNA required for coverage of coding regions have revolutionized the identification of rare variants and disease-causing mutations. Genomic approaches such as whole exome capture and sequencing technologies for increased sensitivity and specificity have provided an important means to investigate inheritability factors of hypertension. Indeed, proof of concept for whole-exome sequencing has been validated as a clinical diagnostic tool for the evaluation of patients with previously undiagnosed genetic disease.[13]

For Mendelian diseases, the discovery of the genetic basis is central to establishing causality between genotype and phenotype and the foundation for genetic screening and diagnosis in affected populations. Studies from family and twin research suggest that blood pressure is moderately heritable (30%–50%).[14] However, the extent to which the percentage of inheritability influences the development of hypertension has been previously challenged.[15] When single-gene mutations result in the large effects on the phenotype, then applications of next-generation sequencing have identified rare variants with moderate-to-large effects, especially in populations of phenotypic extremes.

Along with traditional cardiovascular risks factors, 2 broad groups of genomic variants have been proposed to influence the development of hypertension. These are the effects of genomic variants on the development of rare familial syndromes that lead to monogenic hypertension (HTN) and the genetic variants underlying common essential HTN. These rare familial genome variants with monogenic hypertension have large effects, potentially triggering hypertensive crises with severe cardiovascular morbidity and mortality. However, the many genetic variants with small effects likely underlie the polygenic trait of common essential HTN in people. Thus, familial hypertensive syndromes are rarely caused by monogenetic variants that significantly influence an increase in blood pressure with variable effect size. In these hypertensive syndromes, patients develop HTN at an early age (**Table 1**) and have effect sizes as much as 10 mm Hg in systolic blood pressure.

THE GENOMIC VARIANTS IN BLOOD PRESSURE REGULATION CAUSING RARE FAMILIAL HYPERTENSIVE SYNDROMES

Because large fractions of interindividual variability can be attributed to genetic determinants, the pursuit of rare disease-causing mutations using genetic approaches has successfully yielded substantial insights into the pathophysiology of hypertension while simultaneously affording new opportunities for tailored therapies in the era of precision medicine. Several monogenic variants have established Mendelian modes of inheritance.[33,34] Twelve genes have been identified, modulating and influencing the development of 8 distinct rare familial hypertensive syndromes, all of which are inherited in a Mendelian fashion. **Table 1** summarizes these genetic variants including key features of each clinical syndrome. Recently, 2 of the 4 genes known to cause Gordon syndrome were identified.[22,24] Other Mendelian HTN syndromes have been mapped to genomic regions, although their specific defects are yet to be demonstrated. These conditions remain an active area of exploration and intense research.

KEY FEATURES OF MONOGENIC HYPERTENSION

The monogenic hypertension genes that follow the rules of classical Mendelian may be inherited as autosomal-dominant and recessive disorders. An autosomal-dominant pattern of inheritance refers to an affected individual who has 1 copy of a mutant gene and 1 normal gene on a pair of autosomal chromosomes. An autosomal-recessive pattern of inheritance has both copies of the mutant gene on a pair of autosomal chromosomes. A polygenic trait is one whose phenotype is influenced by more than 1 gene. Complex traits such as hypertension are polygenic and display a continuous distribution, such as height or skin color. Phenotypic features of renal salt homeostasis, electrolyte, and hormonal disturbance are contributing factors to familial monogenic hypertensive syndromes.[34,35] More precise phenotypic analysis by biochemical analysis is required for measurements of aldosterone, renin, and additional hormones. Furthermore, 7 out of the 12 genes presented as loss-of-function mutations. These syndromes (see **Table 1**) often lead to severe hypertensive crises in one of 2 ways, either a reduction of an inhibitory effect on blood pressure or a positive feedback loop that leads to an increase in blood pressure. The identification of

Table 1
Genes associated with monogenic hypertension

Gene(s)	Chr	Disease Name	Key Features of Clinical Syndrome	Mode of Inheritance and Genetic Mechanism	% HTN (N)—% Early Onset HTN (N)c	Estimated Frequency; Occurrence in the General Population
CYP11B1 (11-beta hydroxylase gene)[16]	8q	(MIM: 202010) CAH type IV (congenital adrenal hyperplasia, caused by 11-beta-hydroxylase deficiency)	HTN, hypokalemia, virilization (variable); 2 of 3 patients have severe, classic form with HTN in the first years of life; otherwise HTN is usually mild to moderate in intensity; accounts for 5%–8% of all CAH cases	AR; LOF	63% (38)—NA[17]	~1/100,000 births ~1/5–7000 in Jewish families of North African origin (Morocco, Tunisia)
CYP11B2 (aldosterone synthase gene)[18]	8p	(MIM: 103900) Glucocorticoid remediable aldosteronism: familial hyperaldosteronism type I: glucocorticoid suppressible hyperaldosteronism	HTN, low plasma renin, increased aldosterone, response to dexamethasone; high genetic heterogeneity and potassium level often normal; high prevalence of intracranial aneurysms	AD; GOF gene expressed under ACTH control (fusion of the promoter region of the gene for CYP11B1 and the coding sequences of CYP11B2)	88% (8)–41% (12)[19]	Rare defect

Gene	Locus	Syndrome	Clinical features	Inheritance; mechanism	Frequency	Notes
WNK1, WNK4 (lysine-deficient protein kinase 1 and 4 genes)[20]	12p	Pseudohypoaldosteronism type 2 (PHA2): Gordon syndrome WNK1: PHA2C (MIM: 614492) WNK4: PHA2B (MIM: 614491) KLHL3: PHA2D (MIM: 614495) CUL3: PHA2E (MIM: 614496)	HTN, hyperkalemia, response to thiazides	WNK1: AR; GOF WNK4: AR; LOF; ↑ expression of the thiazide-sensitive Na-Cl co-transporter SLC12A3 (NCCT) KLHL3: AD or AR; LOF (inhibition of KLHL3 increases the activity of SLC12A3) CUL3: AD; LOF	WNK1: 84% (12)–13%[21,22] WNK4: 50% (18)–10%[22,23] KLHL3 dominant: 27% (15)–17%[24] KLHL3 recessive: 100% (5)–14%[24] CUL3: NA—94%[22]	Rare defect
KLHL3 (kelch-like 3 gene)[22,24]	5q					
CUL3 (cullin 3 gene)[22]	2q					
SCNN1B, SCNN1G (amiloride-sensitive sodium channel, beta and gamma subunit gene encoding 2 subunits of the ENaC sodium channel)[25,26]	16p	(MIM: 177200) Liddle's syndrome: pseudoaldosteronism[27,28]	HTN, hypokalemia, metabolic alkalosis, low plasma renin, low aldosterone, respond to amiloride	AD; GOF	SCNN1B: 100% (18)[27] SCNN1G: 100% (6)–50% (6)[26]	Rare defect
CYP17A1- (steroid 17-hydroxylase/17 ,20 lyase gene)[29]	10q	(MIM: 202110) Congenital adrenal hyperplasia, caused by 17-alpha-hydroxylase deficiency: CAH type V	HTN, hypokalemia, hypogonadism/ androgen deficiency	AR; LOF	NA[30]	Very rare defect

(continued on next page)

Table 1
(continued)

Gene(s)	Chr	Disease Name	Key Features of Clinical Syndrome	Mode of Inheritance and Genetic Mechanism	% HTN (N)—% Early Onset HTN (N)c	Estimated Frequency; Occurrence in the General Population
HSD11B2(11-beta-hydroxy steroid dehydrogenase 2 gene)[31]	16q	(MIM: 218030) Cortisol 11-beta-ketoreductase deficiency; syndrome of apparent mineralocorticoid excess	HTN, hypokalemia, low plasma renin, responsiveness to spironolactone; severe HTN	AR; LOF	100% (9) to >89% (9)[31]	Very rare defect
NR3C2 (mineralocorticoid receptor gene)[51]	4q	(MIM: 605115) Early-onset autosomal dominant HTN with exacerbation in pregnancy	HTN, severe HTN in pregnancy	AD; GOF	100%(8)–100% (8)d[51]	One large pedigree reported
KCNJ5 (potassium inwardly rectifying channel gene, subfamily J, member 5)[32]	11q	(MIM: 613677) Familial hyperaldosteronism type III	HTN, hypokalemia, high aldosterone, high 18-oxocortisol and 18-hydroxycortisol	AD; LOF	100% (3)–100% (3)[32]	One pedigree reported

The percentage of patients with HTN and with early-onset HTN (≤18 years of age) is indicated in this review.

The age limit for early-onset HTN was less than 20 years.

Abbreviations: AD, autosomal dominant; AR, autosomal recessive; GOF, gain of function; LOF, loss of function; NA, not available.

From Ehret GB, Caulfield MJ. Genes for blood pressure: an opportunity to understand hypertension. Eur Heart J 2013;34(13):953–4; with permission.

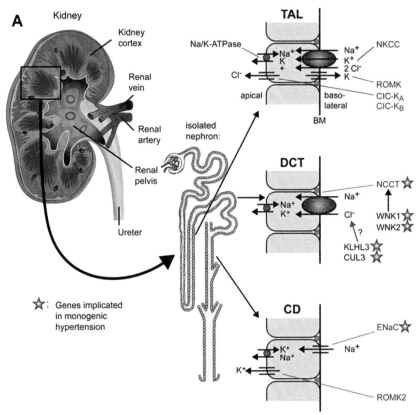

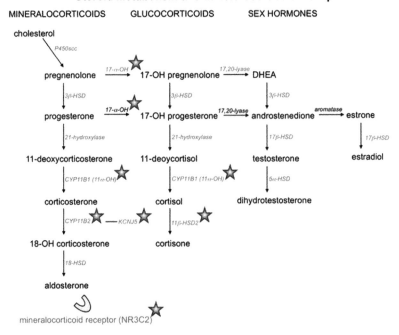

the genetic basis of these hypertensive disease states may be important in our request for therapeutic approaches to these rare disease entities. Such patients with suspected monogenic HTN syndromes should be referred to advanced specialized centers.

MECHANISTIC PATHWAYS OF THE MONOGENIC HYPERTENSIVE SYNDROMES

Mutations linked to genes affecting mineralocorticoid metabolism have provided the earliest evidence for genetic determinants of hypertension in people. Recent efforts have now well-established 12 genes covering 2 general pathways in the pathogenesis of monogenic hypertension: namely, renal sodium homeostasis and steroid hormone metabolism linked to mineralocorticoid receptor activity as illustrated in **Fig. 1**.

The epithelial sodium channel ($E_{NA}C$) functions in the final common pathway for sodium reabsorption in the distal nephron. The gain-of-function mutation of $E_{NA}C$ results in the salt-dependent hypertension or Liddle Syndrome. Pseudohypoaldosteronism Type II (PHAII) is a rare Mendelian syndrome characterized by hypertension, metabolic acidosis, and hyperkalemia, and it is caused by mutations encoding the *Klech-like 3* and *Cullen 3* genes (16). The renal physiology has features underscored by salt reabsorption and both K^+ and H^+ excretion. Maximum salt reabsorption appears to be orchestrated due to elevated aldosterone by increased levels of angiotensin II (16). In certain instances, hypertension contributes to inheritable forms of the metabolic syndrome when clustered with comorbidities and risk factors of early onset coronary artery disease, central obesity, and diabetes.[36]

Other known monogenic defects include Peroxisome-proliferator-activated-receptor (PPAR) gamma mutations in the pathogenesis of diabetes and HTN21 or RET gene mutations underlying the manifestation of pheochromocytoma, HTN, and other malignancies. The finding that genetic defects in HTN syndromes localize to proteins of the kidney and to steroid hormone activity suggested that similar mechanisms also contribute to the genetic origin of essential HTN. Of note, there is also the partial overlap between the pathways of monogenic HTN and commonly used antihypertensive drugs used to treat essential HTN (eg, thiazide diuretics, aldosterone receptor antagonists).

GENOME-WIDE ASSOCIATION STUDIES AND HYPERTENSION

For human genetic studies, linkage analysis has been a valuable tool used to identify genomic loci of high penetrance. The first large-scale attempt to validate HTN variants by GWAS was carried out by the Welcome Trust Case Control Consortium in in a British population, identifying genome-wide significant variants among 7 common diseases using 2000 cases and 3000 controls.[37] Since then, several consortia and individual trials have published 43 variants that could be replicated in independent samples (**Table 2**) using GWAS or similar methods. Most investigations have been carried out using samples of European origin, including CHARGE (Cohorts for Heart and

---

Fig. 1. Disease-causing pathways affected in monogenic hypertension. Genes encoding the mutated gene products are shown to be located in the context of physiologic pathways associated with salt reabsorption homeostasis. Two groups of pathways are affected, pathways affecting the kidney (*A*) and pathways affecting steroid metabolism and the mineralocorticoid receptor (*B*). A selection of important structures (eg, ion channels) or enzymes is labeled in gray. Proteins mutated in monogenic HTN syndromes are marked by a red star. CD, collecting duct; DCT, distal-convoluted tubule; TAL, thick ascending limb of the loop of Henle. (*From* Ehret GB, Caulfield MJ. Genes for blood pressure: an opportunity to understand hypertension. Eur Heart J 2013;34(13):955; with permission.)

Table 2
Summary of genetic variants associated with alterations of blood pressure

Locus Name	Sentinel SNP	chr	Position (hg19)	CA	SBP Beta	SBP P-Value	DBP Beta	DBP P-Value	HTN Beta	HTN P-Value	Ethnicity	Max N
CASZ1[38,39]	rs880315	1	10,796,866	C	0.61	5.20×10^9	NA	NA	NA	NA	EU, AS	52,155
MTHFR (3′)-NPPB[44]	rs4846049	1	11,850,365	T	NA	NA	−0.34	3.00×10^{10}	NA	NA	EU	84,467
MTHFR (5′)-NPPB[40–43]	rs17367504	1	11,862,778	G	−0.90	8.72×10^{22}	−0.55	3.55×10^{19}	−0.10	2.34×10^{10}	EU	125,000
ST7L-CAPZA1[47]	rs17030613	1	113,190,807	C	0.49	8.40×10^8	0.38	1.20×10^8	NA	NA	AS	49,952
MOV1[40]	rs2932538	1	113,216,543	G	0.39	1.17×10^9	0.24	9.88×10^{10}	0.05	2.89×10^7	EU, AS	195,000
AGT[44–46]	rs2004776	1	230,848,702	T	0.42	3.80×10^6	0.32	5.00×10^8	0.08	3.70×10^7	EU, AS	86,588
FIGN_GRB14[47,48]	rs16849225	2	164,906,820	C	0.75	3.50×10^{10}	0.29	2.70×10^5	NA	NA	AS, EU	49,511
SLC4A7[40]	rs13082711	3	27,537,909	T	−0.32	1.51×10^6	−0.24	3.77×10^9	−0.03	3.56×10^4	EU	198,000
ULK4[40,49]	rs3774372	3	41,877,414	T	−0.07	3.95×10^1	−0.37	9.02×10^{14}	−0.02	1.81×10^1	EU	162,000
MAP4[48]	rs319690	3	47,927,484	T	−0.423	4.74×10^8	−0.265	6.88×10^9	NA	NA	EU	93,496
MECOM[40]	rs419076	3	169,100,886	T	0.41	1.78×10^{13}	0.24	2.12×10^{12}	0.03	3.06×10^4	EU	194,000
FGF5[40,41,46,47,52]	rs1458038	4	81,164,723	T	0.71	1.47×10^{23}	0.46	8.46×10^{25}	0.07	1.85×10^7	EU, AS	140,000
SLC39A8[40]	rs13107325	4	103,188,709	T	−0.98	3.27×10^{14}	−0.68	2.28×10^{17}	−0.10	4.89×10^7	EU	151,000
ENPEP[47]	rs6825911	4	111,381,638	C	0.6	7.30×10^8	0.39	9.00×10^9	NA	NA	AS	49,515
GUCY1A3-1B3[40]	rs13139571	4	156,645,513	C	0.32	1.16×10^6	0.26	2.17×10^{10}	0.04	2.49×10^5	EU	185,000
NPR3-C5orf23[40,47]	rs1173771	5	32,815,028	G	0.50	1.79×10^{16}	0.26	9.11×10^{12}	0.06	3.23×10^{10}	EU, AS	159,000
EBF1[40]	rs11953630	5	157,845,402	T	−0.41	3.02×10^{11}	−0.28	3.81×10^{13}	−0.05	1.68×10^7	EU	161,000
HFE[40]	rs1799945	6	26,091,179	G	0.63	7.69×10^{12}	0.46	1.45×10^{15}	0.09	1.76×10^{10}	EU	144,000
BAT2-BAT5[40]	rs805303	6	31,616,366	G	0.38	1.49×10^{11}	0.23	2.98×10^{11}	0.05	1.12×10^{10}	EU	202,000
PIK3CG[48]	rs17477177	7	106,411,858	T	−0.552	5.67×10^{11}	−0.081	1.40×10^1	NA	NA	EU	112,996
NOS3[45,50]	rs3918226	7	150,690,176	T	NA	NA	0.78	2.20×10^9	NA	NA	EU	84,467
BLK-GATA4[38]	rs2898290	8	11,433,909	C	−0.53	3.40×10^9	NA	NA	NA	NA	EU	52,155
CYP11B2[46]	rs1799998	8	143,999,600	T	0.91	1.50×10^5	0.53	1.80×10^5	NA	NA	AS	19,426

(continued on next page)

Table 2
(continued)

Locus Name	Sentinel SNP	chr	Position (hg19)	CA	SBP Beta	SBP P-Value	DBP Beta	DBP P-Value	HTN Beta	HTN P-Value	Ethnicity	Max N
CACNB2(5')[40]	rs4373814	10	18,419,972	G	−0.37	4.81×10^{11}	−0.22	4.36×10^{10}	−0.05	8.53×10^{8}	EU	188,000
CACNB2(3')[40,49,53]	rs1813353	10	18,707,448	T	0.57	2.56×10^{12}	0.41	2.30×10^{15}	0.08	6.24×10^{10}	EU, AS	102,000
C10orf107[40,43]	rs4590817	10	63,467,553	G	0.65	3.97×10^{12}	0.42	1.29×10^{12}	0.10	9.82×10^{9}	EU	111,000
PLCE1[40]	rs932764	10	95,895,940	G	0.48	7.10×10^{16}	0.18	8.06×10^{7}	0.06	9.35×10^{9}	EU	161,000
CYP17A1-NT5C2[46,47,49,51-54]	rs11191548	10	104,846,178	T	1.10	6.90×10^{26}	0.46	9.44×10^{13}	0.10	1.40×10^{5}	EU, AS	162,000
ADRB1[45]	rs1801253	10	115,805,056	G	−0.57	4.70×10^{10}	−0.36	9.50×10^{10}	−0.06	3.30×10^{4}	EU	86,588
ADM[40]	rs7129220	11	10,350,538	G	−0.62	2.97×10^{12}	−0.30	6.44×10^{8}	−0.04	1.11×10^{3}	EU	183,000
PLEKHA7[40,49,54]	rs381815	11	16,902,268	T	0.57	5.27×10^{11}	0.35	5.34×10^{10}	0.06	3.41×10^{6}	EU, AS	97,000
FLJ32810-TMEM1[40,55]	rs633185	11	100,593,538	G	−0.56	1.21×10^{17}	−0.33	1.95×10^{15}	−0.07	5.41×10^{11}	EU, AS	160,000
ATP2B1[39,40,49,52,54,56,57]	rs17249754	12	90,060,586	G	0.93	1.82×10^{18}	0.52	1.16×10^{14}	0.13	1.13×10^{14}	EU, AS	96,000
SH2B3[40,41,48,58]	rs3184504	12	111,884,608	T	0.60	3.83×10^{18}	0.45	3.59×10^{25}	0.06	2.62×10^{6}	EU, AF	121,000
ALDH2[47]	rs11066280	12	112,817,783	T	1.56	7.90×10^{31}	1.01	1.30×10^{35}	NA	NA	AS	46,957
TBX5-TBX3[40,47,49,58]	rs10850411	12	115,387,796	T	0.35	5.38×10^{8}	0.25	5.43×10^{10}	0.05	5.18×10^{6}	EU, AS	161,000
CYP1A1-ULK3[40,41,49,57,58]	rs1378942	15	75,077,367	C	0.61	5.69×10^{23}	0.42	2.69×10^{26}	0.07	1.04×10^{8}	EU, AS, AF	163,000
FURIN-FES[40]	rs2521501	15	91,437,388	T	0.65	5.20×10^{19}	0.36	1.89×10^{15}	0.06	7.02×10^{7}	EU, AS, AF	127,000
UMOD[59]	rs13333226	16	20,365,654	G	−0.49	2.60×10^{5}	−0.3	1.50×10^{5}	NA	1.50×10^{13}	EU	79,133
GOSR2[40]	rs17608766	17	45,013,271	T	−0.56	1.13×10^{10}	−0.13	1.66×10^{2}	−0.02	7.99×10^{2}	EU	152,000
ZNF652[40,43]	rs12940887	17	47,402,807	T	0.36	1.79×10^{10}	0.27	2.29×10^{14}	0.05	1.20×10^{7}	EU	188,000
JAG1[40]	rs1327235	20	10,969,030	G	0.34	1.87×10^{8}	0.30	1.41×10^{15}	0.03	4.57×10^{4}	EU, AS	158,000
GNAS-EDN3[40]	rs6015450	20	57,751,117	G	0.90	3.87×10^{23}	0.56	5.63×10^{23}	0.11	4.18×10^{14}	EU, AS	159,000

The table includes loci associated with SBP, DBP, HTN that were replicated in independent samples. Only data from unbiased experiments as the GWAS and similar experiments are included, and only single marker analyses were considered. Only SNPs discovered using an additive model were included, and the maximal r2 between 2 pairs of SNPs was set to be 0.3. The locus name is the name of the nearest gene or a composite of the flanking genes if several genes are near.38

Abbreviations: AF, individuals of African-American or African origin; AS, individuals of Asian origin; CA, coded allele; DBP, diastolic blood pressure; EU, individuals of European ancestry; NA, not available; SBP, systolic blood pressure.

From Ehret GB, Caulfield MJ. Genes for blood pressure: an opportunity to understand hypertension. Eur Heart J 2013;34(13):958-9; with permission.

Aging Research in Genomic Epidemiology) consortium, the Global BP Gen (Global BP Genetics) consortium, and the ICBP (International Consortium for BP GWAS). Notable Non-European samples particularly involve cohorts of Asian origin and include studies of the Korea Association Resource consortium and the Asian Genetic Epidemiology Network. The study using participants of African origin is the CARe (Candidate-gene Association Resource) consortium.

To date, the largest contribution to the total number of genomic loci discovered for systolic blood pressure (SBP), diastolic blood pressure (DBP), and HTN is by the International Consortium for Blood pressure (ICBP) GWAS,[40] although many other studies have contributed additional variants. The ICBP study included total discovery GWAS data involving 69,395 individuals and further replication genotyping/look-ups in up to 133,661 subjects. The experiment replicated 13 genomic loci discovered in several other overlapping studies[41,49] and demonstrated 29 SNPs with genome-wide significance, all of which have been independently validated to increase the risk of HTN.

PERSPECTIVES FROM THE DISCOVERY OF 43 VARIANTS FOR ESSENTIAL HYPERTENSION BY GWAS

From 3 decades of research on the genetics of essential HTN, what lessons have emerged from variants identified by the GWAS and other similar linkage analyses thus far? The overall BP effect sizes of individual genetic variant are small, typically 1 mm Hg for SBP and 0.5 mm Hg for DBP (see **Table 2** - subset of SNPs). Collectively, all 29 variants tested in 1 experiment account for only 1% to 2% of SBP and DBP variance.[40] One repeatedly tested hypothesis is that only a small subset of all blood pressure-associated SNPs has been identified. Hence the heritability of blood pressure is about 25 times larger than the difference currently explained by SNPs identified through GWAS. In addition, only a portion of the total heritability of hypertension can currently be explained by the GWAS contributing to the term missing heritability.[60] The expectation is that many more loci yet to be discovered will include variants in the rare allele spectrum with larger effect sizes. For SNPs with effect sizes similar to those in **Table 2** the total number of variants denoting blood pressure variation has been extrapolated to be about 116.[40] In 1 well-designed experiment, a risk score of the combined effects of the 29 SNPs has been clearly associated with blood pressure and HTN in multiple populations.[40] This partially explains the overall phenotypic variance of HTN and hence may not be useful in HTN risk prediction. Of the 43 variants significantly associated with SBP, DBP, and HTN outlined in **Table 2**, only a few are near a gene that has been established to be related to blood pressure. The remaining variants are localized in genomic loci that were previously thought not to be associated with blood pressure. It is hoped that other GWAS consortia could identify over-represented biological pathways in analyses using GWAS SNPs,[61] but efforts in this direction have not been successful for blood pressure thus far. Confounding factors may be attributed to the intrinsic properties of the phenotype or to the small number of variants identified so far. Many variants identified may not be peculiar to individuals of European decent, but also found in cohorts of Asian and African origin. This evidence suggests that, although, genomic analysis in multiple ethnicities is far from complete, many of these variants identified may have significant impact across ethnicities. Such hypotheses are clearly the focus of further studies.

SUMMARY

Genomic insights and analyses of Mendelian HTN syndromes and GWAS on essential HTN have contributed to the depth of current understanding of the genetics origins of hypertension. These rare monogenic hypertensive syndromes are likely to be encountered by practitioners at specialized centers, and warrant attention to the heterogeneous category of essential hypertension encountered on a regular basis.

Mendelian syndromes are important for the field, since such knowledge leads to specific insights about disease pathogenesis and the potential for precision medicine. Furthermore, the clinical impact of findings of GWAS on essential HTN is continuously evolving, and the accrued insights accrued will refine efforts to combat the societal impact of hypertension. Comprehensive identification of all genomic variants of hypertension, along with their individual associated mechanisms, is paving the way forward in the era of personalized medicine. Notwithstanding, the overriding challenge for care providers is to reduce health inequities through improved compliance and, perhaps, new paradigms for implementation science incorporating genomic medicine.

ACKNOWLEDGMENTS

The authors thank Abigail Stein for her editorial assistance. An NIH Director's Pioneer Award Grant HL17650 and the Advancing a Healthier Wisconsin Endowment at the Medical College of Wisconsin, Cardiovascular Center Grant 5520311 for I.J.B, supported this work.

REFERENCES

1. Hsu CY, McCulloch CE, Darbinian J, et al. Elevated blood pressure and risk of end-stage renal disease in subjects without baseline kidney disease. Arch Intern Med 2005;165:923–8.
2. Lawes CM, Vander Hoorn S, Rodgers A. Global burden of blood pressure-related disease, 2001. Lancet 2008;371:1513–8.
3. Lewington S, Clarke R, Qizilbash N, et al. Age-specific relevance of usual blood pressure to vascular mortality: a meta-analysis of individual data for one million adults in 61 prospective studies. Lancet 2002;360:1903–13.
4. Burt VL, Whelton P, Roccella EJ, et al. Prevalence of hypertension in the US adult population. Results from the third national health and Nutrition Examination Survey, 1988–1991. Hypertension 1995;25:305–13.
5. Go AS, Mozaffarian D, Roger VL, et al. Executive summary: heart disease and stroke statistics—2013 update: a report from the American Heart Association. Circulation 2013;127:143–52.
6. Hajjar I, Kotchen TA. Trends in prevalence, awareness, treatment, and control of hypertension in the United States, 1988–2000. JAMA 2003;290:199–206.
7. Lloyd-Jones DM, Hong Y, Labarthe D, et al. Defining and setting national goals for cardiovascular health promotion and disease reduction: the American Heart Association's strategic Impact Goal through 2020 and beyond. Circulation 2010;121:586–613.
8. Lawes CM, Vander HS, Rodgers A. Global burden of blood-pressure-related disease, 2001. Lancet 2008;371:1513–8.
9. Munroe GB, Rice PB, Bochud KM, et al. Genetic variants in novel pathways influence blood pressure and cardiovascular disease risk. Nature 2011;478:103–9.
10. Poulter N, Khaw KT, Hopwood BE, et al. Blood pressure and its correlates in an African tribe in urban and rural environments. J Epidemiol Community Health 1984;38:181–5.
11. Brunner HR, Gavras H. Is the renin system necessary? Am J Med 1980;69:739–45.

12. Chong JX, Buckingham KJ, Jhangiani SN, et al. The genetic basis of mendelian phenotypes: discoveries, challenges, and opportunities. Am J Human Genetics 2015;97:199–215.

13. Choi M, Scholl UI, Ji W, et al. Genetic diagnosis by whole exome capture and massively parallel DNA sequencing. Proc Natl Acad Sci USA 2009;106:19062.

14. Miall WE, Oldham PD. The hereditary factor in arterial blood-pressure. Br Med J 1963;1:75–80.

15. Levy D, DeStefano AL, Larson MG, et al. Evidence for a gene influencing blood pressure on chromosome 17. Genome scan linkage results for longitudinal blood pressure phenotypes in subjects from the Framingham heart study. Hypertension 2000;36:477–83.

16. White PC, Dupont J, New MI, et al. A mutation in CYP11B1 (Arg-448—His) associated with steroid 11 beta-hydroxylase deficiency in Jews of Moroccan origin. J Clin Invest 1991;87:1664–7.

17. Rosler A, White PC. Mutations in human 11 beta-hydroxylase genes: 11 betahydroxylase deficiency in Jews of Morocco and corticosterone methyl-oxidase II deficiency in Jews of Iran. J Steroid Biochem Mol Biol 1993;45:99–106.

18. Lifton RP, Dluhy RG, Powers M, et al. A chimaeric 11 beta-hydroxylase/aldosterone synthase gene causes glucocorticoidremediable aldosteronism and human hypertension. Nature 1992;355:262–5.

19. Rich GM, Ulick S, Cook S, et al. Glucocorticoid-remediable aldosteronism in a large kindred: clinical spectrum and diagnosis using a characteristic biochemical phenotype. Ann Intern Med 1992;116:813–20.

20. Wilson FH, Disse-Nicodeme S, Choate KA, et al. Human hypertension caused by mutations in WNK kinases. Science 2001;293:1107–12.

21. Disse-Nicodeme S, Achard JM, Desitter I, et al. A newlocus on chromosome 12p13.3 for pseudohypoaldosteronism type II, an autosomal dominant form of hypertension. Am J Hum Genet 2000;67:302–10.

22. Boyden LM, Choi M, Choate KA, et al. Mutations in kelch-like 3 and cullin 3 cause hypertension and electrolyte abnormalities. Nature 2012;482:98–102.

23. Mayan H, Munter G, Shaharabany M, et al. Hypercalciuria in familial hyperkalemia and hypertension accompanies hyperkalemia and precedes hypertension: description of a large family with the Q565E WNK4 mutation. J Clin Endocrinol Metab 2004;89:4025–30.

24. Louis-Dit-Picard H, Barc J, Trujillano D, et al. KLHL3 mutations cause familial hyperkalemic hypertension by impairing ion transport in the distal nephron. Nat Genet 2012;44:456–60. S1–3.

25. Shimkets RA, Warnock DG, Bositis CM, et al. Liddle's syndrome: heritable human hypertension caused by mutations in the beta subunit of the epithelial sodium channel. Cell 1994;79:407–14.

26. Hansson JH, Nelson-Williams C, Suzuki H, et al. Hypertension caused by a truncated epithelial sodium channel gamma subunit: genetic heterogeneity of Liddle syndrome. Nat Genet 1995;11:76–82.

27. Botero-Velez M, Curtis JJ, Warnock DG. Brief report: Liddle's syndrome revisited–a disorder of sodium reabsorption in the distal tubule. N Engl J Med 1994;330:178–81.

28. Liddle GW, Island DP, Ney RL, et al. Nonpituitary neoplasms and Cushing's syndrome. Ectopic 'adrenocorticotropin' produced by nonpituitary neoplasms as a cause of Cushing's syndrome. Arch Intern Med 1963;111:471–5.

29. Goldsmith O, Solomon DH, Horton R. Hypogonadism and mineralocorticoid excess. The 17-hydroxylase deficiency syndrome. N Engl J Med 1967;277: 673–7.
30. Imai T, Yanase T, Waterman MR, et al. Canadian Mennonites and individuals residing in the Friesland region of The Netherlands share the same molecular basis of 17 alpha-hydroxylase deficiency. Hum Genet 1992;89:95–6.
31. Mune T, Rogerson FM, Nikkila H, et al. Human hypertension caused by mutations in the kidney isozyme of 11 beta-hydroxysteroid dehydrogenase. Nat Genet 1995;10:394–9.
32. Choi M, Scholl UI, Yue P, et al. K+ channel mutations in adrenal aldosterone-producing adenomas and hereditary hypertension. Science 2011;331:768–72.
33. Lifton RP. Molecular genetics of human blood pressure variation. Science 1996; 272:676–80.
34. Lifton RP, Gharavi AG, Geller DS. Molecular mechanisms of human hypertension. Cell 2001;104:545–56.
35. Lifton RP. Genetic dissection of human blood pressure variation: common pathways from rare phenotypes. Harvey Lect 2004;100:71–101.
36. Keramati AR, Fathzadeh M, Go GW, et al. A form of the metabolic syndrome associated with mutations in DYRK1B. N Engl J Med 2014;370:1909–19.
37. Wellcome Trust Case Control Consortium. Genome-wide association study of 14,000 cases of seven common diseases and 3,000 shared controls. Nature 2007;447:661–78.
38. Ho JE, Levy D, Rose L, et al. Discovery and replication of novel blood pressure genetic loci in the Women's Genome Health Study. J Hypertens 2011;29:62–9.
39. Takeuchi F, Isono M, Katsuya T, et al. Blood pressure and hypertension are associated with 7 loci in the Japanese population. Circulation 2010;121:2302–9.
40. Ehret GB, Munroe PB, Rice KM, et al. Genetic variants in novel pathways influence blood pressure and cardiovascular disease risk. Nature 2011;478:103–9.
41. Newton-Cheh C, Johnson T, Gateva V, et al. Genome-wide association study identifies eight loci associated with blood pressure. Nat Genet 2009;41:666–76.
42. Tomaszewski M, Debiec R, Braund PS, et al. Genetic architecture of ambulatory blood pressure in the general population: insights from cardiovascular gene-centric array. Hypertension 2010;56:1069–76.
43. Newton-Cheh C, Larson MG, Vasan RS, et al. Association of common variants in NPPA and NPPB with circulating natriuretic peptides and blood pressure. Nat Genet 2009;41:348–53.
44. Johnson T, Gaunt TR, Newhouse SJ, et al. Blood pressure loci identified with a gene-centric array. Am J Hum Genet 2011;89:688–700.
45. Johnson AD, Newton-Cheh C, Chasman DI, et al. Association of hypertension drug target genes with blood pressure and hypertension in 86,588 individuals. Hypertension 2011;57:903–10.
46. Takeuchi F, Yamamoto K, Katsuya T, et al. Reevaluation of the association of seven candidate genes with blood pressure and hypertension: a replication study and meta-analysis with a larger sample size. Hypertens Res 2012;35(8):825–31.
47. Kato N, Takeuchi F, Tabara Y, et al. Meta-analysis of genome-wide association studies identifies common variants associated with blood pressure variation in east Asians. Nat Genet 2011;43:531–8.
48. Wain LV, Verwoert GC, O'Reilly PF, et al. Genome-wide association study identifies six new loci influencing pulse pressure and mean arterial pressure. Nat Genet 2011;43:1005–11.

49. Levy D, Ehret GB, Rice K, et al. Genome-wide association study of blood pressure and hypertension. Nat Genet 2009;41:677–87.
50. Salvi E, Kutalik Z, Glorioso N, et al. Genomewide association study using a high-density single nucleotide polymorphism array and case-control design identifies a novel essential hypertension susceptibility locus in the promoter region of endothelial NO synthase. Hypertension 2012;59:248–55.
51. Geller DS, Farhi A, Pinkerton N, et al. Activating mineralocorticoid receptor mutation in hypertension exacerbated by pregnancy. Science 2000;289:119–23.
52. Tabara Y, Kohara K, Kita Y, et al. Common variants in the ATP2B1 gene are associated with susceptibility to hypertension: the Japanese Millennium Genome Project. Hypertension 2010;56:973–80.
53. Lin Y, Lai X, Chen B, et al. Genetic variations in CYP17A1, CACNB2 and PLEKHA7 are associated with blood pressure and/or hypertension in She ethnic minority of China. Atherosclerosis 2011;219:709–14.
54. Hong KW, Jin HS, Lim JE, et al. Recapitulation of two genomewide association studies on blood pressure and essential hypertension in the Korean population. J Hum Genet 2010;55:336–41.
55. Ehret GB, O'Connor AA, Weder A, et al. Follow-up of a major linkage peak on chromosome 1 reveals suggestive QTLs associated with essential hypertension: GenNet study. Eur J Hum Genet 2009;17:1650–7.
56. Cho YS, Go MJ, Kim YJ, et al. A large-scale genome-wide association study of Asian populations uncovers genetic factors influencing eight quantitative traits. Nat Genet 2009;41:527–34.
57. Hong KW, Go MJ, Jin HS, et al. Genetic variations in ATP2B1, CSK, ARSG and CSMD1 loci are related to blood pressure and/or hypertension in two Korean cohorts. J Hum Hypertens 2010;24:367–72.
58. Fox ER, Young JH, Li Y, et al. Association of genetic variation with systolic and diastolic blood pressure among African Americans: the Candidate Gene Association Resource study. Hum Mol Genet 2011;20:2273–84.
59. Padmanabhan S, Melander O, Johnson T, et al. Genome-wide association study of blood pressure extremes identifies variant near UMOD associated with hypertension. PLoS Genet 2010;6:e1001177.
60. Manolio TA, Collins FS, Cox NJ, et al. Finding the missing heritability of complex diseases. Nature 2009;461:747–53.
61. Lango Allen H, Estrada K, Lettre G, et al. Hundreds of variants clustered in genomic loci and biological pathways affect human height. Nature 2010;467:832–8.

Precision Medicine and PET/Computed Tomography in Cardiovascular Disorders

Elizabeth H. Dibble, MD*, Don C. Yoo, MD

KEYWORDS

- PET/CT • Cardiovascular disease • Myocardial perfusion imaging • Cardiac viability
- Cardiac sarcoidosis • Cardiac amyloidosis • Infection • Vasculitis

KEY POINTS

- PET myocardial perfusion imaging effectively evaluates coronary vasculature.
- PET/computed tomography (CT) can evaluate for hibernating myocardium in patients who are potential candidates for revascularization procedures.
- PET/CT can evaluate the metabolic and anatomic involvement of a variety of inflammatory, infectious, and malignant cardiovascular disorders.
- PET/CT can identify cardiac involvement in sarcoidosis and amyloidosis.
- Novel targeted radiopharmaceutical agents and novel use of established techniques show promise in diagnosing and monitoring cardiovascular diseases.

INTRODUCTION

Despite advances in prevention, diagnosis, treatment, and understanding of cardiovascular disease, it remains the number 1 cause of death for both men and women in the United States.[1] In addition to heart disease and stroke, which are the leading causes of morbidity and mortality related to cardiovascular disease, inflammatory disorders, amyloidosis, infection, and malignancy can also affect the cardiovascular system.

Advances in imaging have allowed improved noninvasive evaluation of cardiovascular disease. Ultrasonography, MR imaging, and nuclear medicine play critical roles in its evaluation. Over the past 2 decades, single-photon emission computed tomography (SPECT) has been the primary nuclear cardiac imaging technology; use of PET was limited by availability and cost. The past decade has seen increased availability of

This article originally appeared in *PET Clinics*, Volume 12, Issue 4, October 2017.

Disclosures: E.H. Dibble has nothing to disclose; D.C. Yoo is a consultant for Endocyte.

Department of Diagnostic Imaging, The Warren Alpert Medical School of Brown University, Rhode Island Hospital, 593 Eddy Street, Providence, RI 02903, USA

* Corresponding author.

E-mail address: edibble@lifespan.org

PET/computed tomography (CT) scanners, primarily used in cancer imaging, which can evaluate metabolic and anatomic involvement of a variety of inflammatory, infectious, and malignant cardiovascular disorders. PET/CT is useful in evaluating coronary vasculature, hibernating myocardium, cardiac sarcoidosis, cardiac amyloidosis, cerebrovascular disease, acute aortic syndromes, cardiac and vascular neoplasms, cardiac and vascular infections, and vasculitis. Novel targeted radiopharmaceutical agents and novel use of established techniques show promise in diagnosing and monitoring cardiovascular diseases.

NORMAL ANATOMY AND IMAGING TECHNIQUE
Normal Cardiac Anatomy

The normal heart consists of endocardium, myocardium, epicardium, and pericardium. The right atrium receives venous drainage from the body, and the right ventricle pumps that blood to the lungs for oxygenation. Oxygenated blood returns to the left atrium and is pumped through the body by the left ventricle. The vascular supply to the heart comes from the right coronary artery (RCA) and the left main coronary artery (LM); the LM branches into the left anterior descending artery (LAD) and left circumflex artery. The RCA supplies blood to the inferior left ventricle, the LAD supplies blood to the anterior left ventricle and septum, and the left circumflex artery supplies blood to the lateral and posterior left ventricle.

Cardiac Imaging Techniques

Myocardial perfusion imaging is indicated for patients with known or suspected coronary artery disease. The 2 most commonly used radiopharmaceuticals for PET cardiac perfusion imaging are 82-Rb and 13-N-ammonia. 82-Rb does not require an on-site cyclotron, which is a distinct advantage compared with 13-N-ammonia, which requires an on-site cyclotron. PET myocardial perfusion imaging is faster than SPECT myocardial imaging, has superior attenuation correction, and has higher spatial and temporal resolution. Exercise stress is challenging to perform with PET perfusion radiopharmaceuticals primarily because of the short half-lives. 18F-based tracers have longer half-lives and allow for exercise stress; initial studies have shown promise, but 18F tracers are not yet routinely used.[2] Pharmacologic stress can be performed with adenosine, dipyridamole, regadenoson, or dobutamine.

Cardiac viability imaging is indicated to determine the extent of hibernating myocardium in patients who are potential candidates for revascularization procedures. Viability studies can be performed with 18F fluorodeoxyglucose (FDG) and thallium-201 but FDG is preferred because of its higher spatial resolution and accuracy. Patients are administered a glucose load so that glucose receptors are stimulated to take up FDG. If there is viable tissue in an area of perfusion defect on prior SPECT or PET myocardial perfusion study (ie, hibernating myocardium), it takes up FDG in the corresponding area on viability scan.

Normal Vascular Anatomy (Noncoronary)

The left ventricle pumps blood to the body via the aorta, which branches into progressively smaller arteries, eventually perfusing the body at the level of the capillaries then returning to the heart via the venous system. Arteries are composed of 3 layers: the intima (inner), media (middle), and adventitia (outer). Atherosclerosis affects the intimal layer; other cardiovascular diseases can affect other layers.

Vascular Imaging Techniques

The coronary vasculature can be evaluated by PET perfusion imaging as previously described. In addition, FDG-PET/CT can be used to evaluate for infectious, inflammatory, or neoplastic processes involving the vasculature.

IMAGING PROTOCOLS
Myocardial Perfusion

Myocardial perfusion imaging is indicated for patients with known or suspected coronary artery disease. As previously described, the most common radiopharmaceuticals used for myocardial perfusion imaging are 82-Rb and 13-N-ammonia. Patient preparation includes overnight fasting and avoidance of caffeine and caffeine-containing foods for 24 hours and theophylline-containing medications for 48 hours. Rest images are usually acquired first. Rest and stress images can be acquired on different days; for 2-day studies, stress images are usually acquired first. Scout images are acquired to confirm adequate field of view to cover the heart (standard field of view includes the top of the lung apices to the base of heart). A rest dose of radiopharmaceutical (eg, 30–40 mCi Rb-82) should be administered over 20 to 30 seconds (or the lowest radiation dose necessary to acquire a diagnostic-quality image for the individual PET/CT scanner). An emission scan (typically around 5 minutes) should be obtained for a single bed position. Once a 12-lead electrocardiogram (ECG) is in place and intravenous (IV) access established, the pharmacologic stress agent can be administered (eg, dipyridamole 0.56 mg/kg over 4 minutes). Patients should have ECG, blood pressure, and heart rate monitored. At stress target, a second dose of radiopharmaceutical should be injected (eg, 30–40 mCi Rb-82) followed by an emission scan.

Cardiac Viability

Cardiac viability imaging is indicated for patients who are potential candidates for revascularization procedures and in whom there is suspicion of hibernating myocardium. Studies are performed with a glucose load to push FDG into the myocardium. Contraindications include recent ingestion of food, significant exercise within the prior 24 hours, and increased blood glucose level. Nondiabetic patients should fast for 6 hours before the examination. Patients with diabetes controlled with oral medications should avoid breakfast on the morning of the examination and take regularly scheduled medications. Patients with diabetes who are on insulin should continue their usual diets and medications. On arrival, blood glucose level should be checked with a fingertip stick. If less than 150 mg/dL, 50 g of oral glucose should be administered and FDG can be injected. If blood glucose level is 150 to 200 mg/dL, 25 g of oral glucose should be administered and 2 units of regular insulin should be administered via IV; if blood glucose level is greater than 200 mg/dL, regular insulin should be given via IV. Glucose should be checked again 30 to 40 minutes after glucose or insulin administration and, if it is less than 150 mg/dL, FDG can be administered. The FDG dose should be weight based (typically 0.1–0.15 mCi/kg of FDG depending on the individual PET/CT scanner), should be the lowest dose necessary to acquire a diagnostic-quality image, and it should be administered 60 to 75 minutes before imaging. Parameters for CT acquisition vary by scanner, but scans should be performed at low dose for attenuation correction. Gating can also be performed. CT should cover the cardiac region from the top of the lung apices to the base of heart at a single bed position. Camera setup, patient position, acquisitions, processing, and display for interpretation vary by scanner and software; in our institution, once images have been acquired, they must be reconstructed to provide short axis, horizontal long axis, and vertical long axis views.

Cardiac Sarcoidosis

Cardiac sarcoidosis imaging is indicated for patients with suspected cardiac sarcoidosis. Patient preparation includes fasting (except for water) for at least 6 hours, and preferably 12 hours, to downregulate glucose receptors. Preferred diet before fasting is high fat, high protein, low carbohydrate to maximize free fatty acid metabolism. Nondiabetic patients can take all medications; insulin-dependent diabetic patients should take half of their usual dose on the morning of the test; non–insulin-dependent patients should not take oral diabetes medications on the day of the scan. On arrival, blood glucose level should be checked with a fingertip stick. If less than 70 mg/dL or greater than 200 mg/dL, the physician should be alerted. If glucose level is acceptable and an IV is established, 10 mCi FDG (or the lowest dose necessary to acquire a diagnostic-quality image) should be administered. After 60 minutes, the patient should be scanned from the top of the lung apices to the base of heart for 10 minutes at a single bed position. This field of view also provides information about nodal status in the chest. If a whole-body sarcoid scan is desired, then the patient can be scanned from the skull to the thighs. A recent study examined the feasibility of using somatostatin receptor–based PET/CT in a small number of patients with suspected cardiac sarcoidosis with promising results, although larger studies are warranted.[3]

Cardiac Amyloidosis

Three radiopharmaceuticals have been approved by the United States Food and Drug Administration (FDA) for imaging amyloid plaques: 18F-florbetapir (Eli Lilly); 18F-flutemetamol (GE Healthcare); and 18F-florbetaben (Piramal Pharma).[4] Although these tracers are typically used for imaging amyloid plaques in the brain in the setting of known or suspected Alzheimer disease, these radiopharmaceuticals (along with 18F-NaF PET/CT) have also been used to image cardiac amyloidosis.[5–9] Because these radiopharmaceuticals are not glucose analogs, fasting is not necessary. The lowest dose necessary to acquire a diagnostic-quality image should be administered; optimal timing of PET image acquisition has not yet been established for amyloid agents[7] and may be shorter for 18F-NaF.[9] The patient should be scanned from the top of the lung apices to the base of heart at a single bed position.

Cardiovascular Infection, Inflammation, and Neoplasm

Whole-body and skull-to-thigh FDG-PET are most commonly used to evaluate malignancy but is also useful in evaluating infection and inflammation. As with other PET imaging, patient preparation includes fasting, avoidance of significant exercise within the prior 24 hours, and having normal blood glucose levels (<200 mg/dL; higher than this level prompts consultation with the attending physician). The radiopharmaceutical dose should be weight based and as low as reasonable to achieve diagnostic-quality imaging. At our institution, we use 0.14 mCi/kg. We use low-dose CT for attenuation correction; as mentioned earlier, specific parameters vary by scanner and radiologist preference. At our institution, all patients are scanned at 120 kV, 5 mm × 5 mm helical acquisition, 0.5-second rotation, and dose modulation. Scan length and tube current vary based on patient size. Patients are scanned approximately 75 minutes after radiopharmaceutical injection; at 65 to 70 minutes after injections, patients should empty their bladders. Once positioned on the table, a CT scout and localizer scan is performed, and the PET scan is performed of the corresponding anatomy (skull to thighs [eg, most staging or restaging malignancy scans] versus whole body [eg, melanoma, cutaneous lymphoma, fever of unknown origin]).

Table 1 summarizes PET/CT cardiovascular imaging protocols.

IMAGING FINDINGS/PATHOLOGY
Cardiac/Pericardiac Imaging

Perfusion
Normal myocardial perfusion rest images should show radiopharmaceutical uptake throughout the myocardium. A defect on rest imaging could be caused by a fixed defect from prior myocardial infarction or artifact. Stress images are acquired after patients are injected with radiopharmaceutical at the designated target time (adenosine, dipyridamole, or regadenoson) or target heart rate (dobutamine). Normal stress images without perfusion defects imply no hemodynamically significant narrowing of the coronary arteries. A perfusion defect of the inferior wall implies RCA narrowing; a perfusion defect of the anterior wall, septum, and/or apex implies LAD narrowing; and a perfusion defect of the anterolateral or inferolateral wall implies left circumflex narrowing.

Viability
Areas of hibernating myocardium, or viable tissue, take up FDG on a viability scan in areas of fixed defect seen on prior perfusion imaging. In contrast, areas of scar/infarct (ie, nonviable tissue) do not take up FDG on viability scan in areas of fixed defect on perfusion imaging (**Fig. 1**).

Nonischemic cardiomyopathies and inflammatory disorders
Sarcoidosis Sarcoidosis is characterized by accumulation of noncaseating granulomas caused by an inciting pathogen or environmental agent[10] that can affect multiple organ systems. Cardiac sarcoidosis can manifest as cardiomyopathy or arrhythmias and is difficult to diagnose on biopsy. Twenty-five percent of patients with sarcoidosis have cardiac involvement on autopsy, although approximately 80% is clinically occult.[11] It can involve the pericardium, myocardium, and endocardium of atria or ventricles; the lateral left ventricular wall at the heart base is affected most commonly followed by the basal septum, with a tendency to involve the conducting system; however, myocardial involvement is usually patchy, which likely contributes to the low diagnostic yield on biopsy.[10] Inflammation from granulomas can eventually lead to scarring. PET/CT can detect early myocardial inflammation before myocardial impairment occurs[12]; it can also show involvement of lung parenchyma and mediastinal lymph nodes. Sarcoid imaging evaluates whether defects on resting perfusion scans are caused by infarct or inflammation; areas of defect on rest perfusion imaging with corresponding uptake on sarcoid imaging suggest inflammation caused by myocardial sarcoidosis (**Fig. 2**). PET also shows promise in detecting sarcoidosis treatment response.[13,14]

Nonischemic inflammatory cardiomyopathies PET/CT has shown other nonischemic inflammatory cardiomyopathies, including inflammatory myocarditis[15] and stress myocardial stunning, or Takotsubo cardiomyopathy. The mechanism of Takotsubo cardiomyopathy is unknown but is likely related to increased catecholamine levels and stress-related neuropeptides, which may cause vascular spasm or myocyte injury.[16]

Amyloidosis Amyloidosis is caused by abnormal folding of extracellular proteins that form pathologic deposits of amyloid plaques.[17] As discussed earlier, 3

Table 1
Imaging protocols

Imaging Technique	Indications	Patient Preparation	Radiopharmaceutical	Wait Time Before Scan	Scan Protocol
Myocardial perfusion	Suspected coronary artery disease	Overnight fast, avoidance of caffeine and caffeine-containing foods for 24 h and theophylline-containing medications for 48 h	82-Rb 13-N-ammonia	None	Scout, inject, scan, stress, inject, scan
Cardiac viability	Planned revascularization with suspected hibernating myocardium	Short fast, oral glucose administration	18F-FDG	60 min	Inject, scout, scan
Cardiac sarcoidosis	Sarcoidosis with suspected cardiac involvement	Prolonged fast, high fat, high protein, low carb	18F-FDG	60 min	Inject, scout, scan
Cardiac Amyloidosis	Amyloidosis with suspected cardiac involvement	None with amyloid agents, prolonged fast with NaF	18F-florbetapir 18F-flutemetamol 18F-florbetaben 18F-NaF	30–60 min	Inject, scout, scan
Whole-body PET/CT	Malignancy, inflammation including atherosclerosis, infection	Prolonged fast to evaluate suspected cardiac malignancy	18F-FDG	60 min	Inject, scout, scan

Abbreviation: carb, carbohydrate.

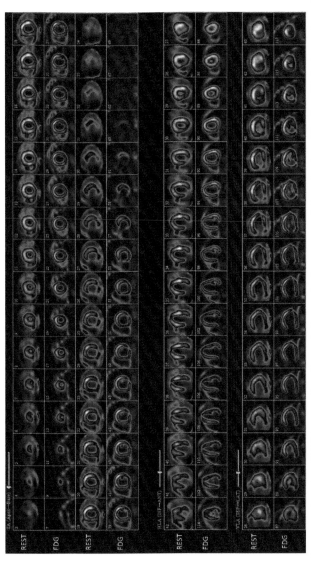

Fig. 1. Rest images from a technetium (Tc)-99m tetrofosmin perfusion study show severe defects in the mid to basal inferior wall. FDG-PET images show predominantly matched defects with only minimal mismatch in the basal inferoseptal wall indicating that most of the defects are nonviable myocardium and the patient will not benefit from revascularization.

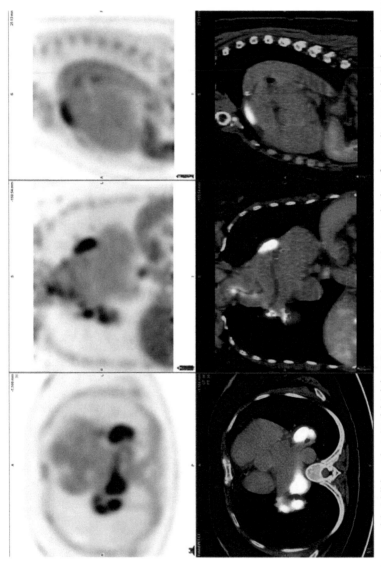

Fig. 2. Axial (*left*), coronal (*middle*), and sagittal (*right*) FDG-PET images in a patient worked up for cardiac sarcoidosis show intense uptake in mediastinal and hilar adenopathy consistent with known sarcoidosis. There is no increased uptake in the left ventricular wall greater than background cardiac blood pool activity to indicate cardiac involvement with sarcoidosis. Rest images from a Tc-99m tetrofosmin perfusion study were normal (not shown).

radiopharmaceuticals have been approved by the FDA for imaging amyloid plaques in the setting of known or suspected Alzheimer disease, but they (along with 18F-NaF PET/CT) have also been used to image cardiac amyloidosis, which can cause restrictive cardiomyopathy and heart failure.[5–9] Targeted agents may be able to differentiate myocardial thickening caused by amyloidosis from that caused by hypertensive heart disease,[7] and 18F-NaF PET may be able to differentiate transthyretin-related cardiac amyloidosis from the light-chain cardiac amyloidosis,[9] which is typically associated with poorer outcomes.[18] Imaging findings are specific cardiac uptake with amyloid agents or uptake over mediastinal background with NaF PET/CT.

Neoplasm
The most common primary cardiac neoplasm is the myxoma, and the most common primary cardiac malignancy is sarcoma; however, secondary cardiac malignancies are approximately 40 times more common than primary cardiac malignancies[15] (**Fig. 3**). FDG-avid primary and metastatic cardiac malignancies show focal FDG uptake in the heart, and the heart must be windowed appropriately to minimize background myocardial uptake. Longer fasting and a low-carbohydrate, high-fat, high-protein diet may be helpful in minimizing myocardial uptake.[19] Pericardial metastatic disease shows focal FDG activity within the pericardium. Lack of FDG uptake in an intracardiac mass seen on CT may suggest thrombus.[20]

Infection
Although the ability to diagnose endocarditis in native valves is limited by low sensitivity,[21] recent studies have shown promise in the ability of PET to diagnose prosthetic valve infection and infections of implanted electronic devices.[21–23] PET has also shown endocarditis caused by infected atrial septal defect surgical patch closure.[24] Extracardiac embolic infections can be identified in the setting of endocarditis; one study with 72 patients showed clinically important new findings (not identified by standard work-up) in 1 out of 7 patients imaged with PET/CT.[25] PET has also shown infectious myocarditis, typically in patients with cancer.[15]

Vascular Imaging

Atherosclerosis
Although myocardial perfusion imaging can show altered myocardial metabolism caused by altered coronary blood flow, PET/CT can also directly show atherosclerotic plaque by assessing arterial FDG uptake related to inflammation[26–28] from activated intimal macrophages[29] (symptomatic, unstable plaques show increased uptake compared with asymptomatic plaques[30]) or molecular cardiovascular calcification with 18F NaF PET/CT.[31–33] Inflammation and calcification may represent distinct pathophysiologic processes in the development of atherosclerosis,[34,35] and PET can assess both processes. Protocol alterations to minimize background cardiac uptake may improve visualization of coronary arterial atherosclerotic plaque.[36,37] Recent research has shown the potential of novel PET tracers to target the vascular cell adhesion molecule (VCAM)-1, a molecule implicated in atherosclerosis, by labeling anti–VCAM-1 nanobody (cAbVCAM-1-5) with 18F.[38]

PET may be useful in monitoring response to intervention for atherosclerosis and has shown decreased FDG uptake by atherosclerotic plaques in patients treated with simvastatin compared with diet modification alone.[39]

Aneurysm
Aortic aneurysms can show FDG uptake related to inflammation and macrophage accumulation; FDG uptake may suggest an unstable aneurysm at risk of causing

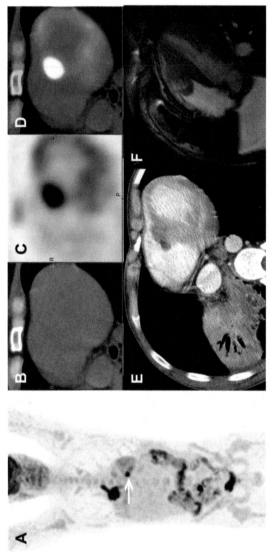

Fig. 3. Maximum intensity projection image (A) after IV administration of FDG shows an intensely hypermetabolic focus in the right lung representing the patient's known lung cancer and linear intense uptake in the right hilum/right aspect of the mediastinum. There is a discrete focus of intense activity in the heart (white arrow). Axial PET (C) and PET/CT (D) images centered at the focally increased activity show an intense focus of increased uptake in the interventricular septum without corresponding abnormality on CT (B). Contrast-enhanced CT (E) shows subtle hypodensity in the interventricular septum. MR imaging (F) confirms a mass arising from the interventricular septum. This mass was biopsied and confirmed to represent metastasis.

pain, expanding, and/or rupturing versus a stable aneurysm without FDG uptake, which may have a more benign course.[29,40]

Dissection and intramural hematoma

Similarly, there is more uptake in acute versus chronic aortic dissection.[41] FDG uptake in the aortic wall also can be seen in intramural hematoma; platelets adhere to leukocytes, which accumulate FDG.[29] Intramural hematoma has been identified incidentally on PET performed for malignancy, allowing earlier diagnosis and treatment.[29,42] Lack of uptake may suggest that the hematoma is chronic (**Fig. 4**).

Vasculitis

Aortic vasculitis results from accumulation of inflammatory cells in the media (giant cell arteritis and Takayasu arteritis) or periaorta (inflammatory abdominal aortic aneurysms).[29] PET can show active inflammation related to large vessel inflammatory arthritides and may be helpful in monitoring disease activity[43] (**Fig. 5**). Increased vascular activity also can be seen in the setting of systemic inflammatory conditions, including psoriasis and rheumatoid arthritis, even when adjusting for cardiovascular risk factors.[44–46]

Cerebrovascular disease

Using 15-O and 11-C radiopharmaceuticals, PET can image cerebral circulation and metabolism in the setting of stroke and can provide information about ischemic penumbra for intervention planning,[47] although the need for an on-site cyclotron and advances in MR imaging have limited its use. PET is also useful in distinguishing vascular dementia from other neurodegenerative disorders[47] based on the distribution of altered metabolism. Cerebrovascular disease is characterized by decreased uptake with distinct margins in 1 or more vascular territorial distributions or multifocal areas of hypometabolism caused by small infarcts or small vessel disease. PET can also show altered metabolism and/or altered blood flow in the setting of intracerebral hemorrhage.[47]

Infection

PET/CT can identify vascular graft infections; the most suspicious findings are focal and intense FDG uptake, particularly in the setting of fluid collection or abscess formation.[48] PET/CT can also monitor response of graft infections to therapy[49] and complications, for example, fistula to bone causing osteomyelitis.[50] PET/CT has also been used to help diagnose involvement of abdominal aortic aneurysms and aortoiliac reconstructions in patients with *Coxiella burnetii*.[51]

Neoplasm

Although primary vascular tumors are rare, PET/CT has been helpful in the diagnosing and staging sarcomas of the great vessels.[52,53] 68Ga-DOTANOC (68Ga-labelled [1,4,7,10-tetraazacyclododecane-1,4,7,10-tetraacetic acid]-1-Nal3-octreotide) PET/CT has shown mesenteric vascular thrombosis with a pancreatic neuroendocrine carcinoma.[54]

Diagnostic Criteria

Atherosclerosis

In the setting of suspected atherosclerosis with cardiac risk factors, diagnosis of atherosclerosis on myocardial perfusion imaging requires a perfusion defect in a vascular territory on stress imaging that is not present on rest imaging. Atherosclerosis can also show increased activity in the wall of a blood vessel caused by inflammation or the presence of targeted molecules related to atherosclerosis.

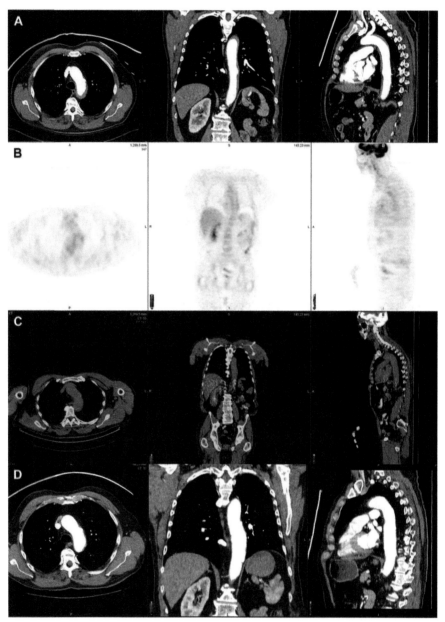

Fig. 4. (*A*) Axial (*left*), coronal (*middle*), and sagittal (*right*) contrast-enhanced CT images show a type B intramural hematoma. PET/CT was performed because there was clinical concern that the patient could have a vasculitis. (*B, C*) FDG-PET images show only minimal activity within the aortic wall consistent with intramural hematoma and not a vasculitis. (*D*) Follow-up contrast-enhanced CT images 4 months after the PET/CT scan show resolution of the intramural hematoma.

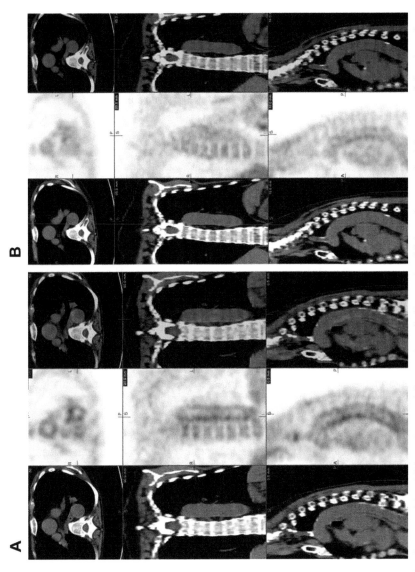

Fig. 5. (A) Axial (*top*), coronal (*middle*), and sagittal (*bottom*) CT (*left*), PET (*middle*), and PET/CT (*right*) images of the chest show intense circumferential activity throughout the wall of the thoracic aorta with only minimal atherosclerotic disease seen in the thoracic aorta. (B) After treatment with corticosteroids, the circumferential activity in the wall of the thoracic aorta is no longer seen on the PET images.

Hibernating myocardium

In the setting of suspected hibernating myocardium in patients who are potential candidates for revascularization procedures, criteria to diagnose hibernating myocardium or viable tissue on imaging include uptake of FDG on viability scan in areas that did not show uptake in comparable SPECT or PET perfusion imaging. Lack of uptake on viability scan suggests myocardial scar or infarct rather than hibernating myocardium.

Cardiac sarcoidosis

In the setting of known or suspected sarcoidosis, myocardial involvement by sarcoidosis can be diagnosed when patchy increased activity is identified, most commonly involving the left ventricle or septum.

Cardiac amyloidosis

Diagnostic criteria include specific cardiac uptake with amyloid agents or uptake over mediastinal background with NaF.

Cerebrovascular disease

Cerebrovascular disease can be diagnosed when PET shows decreased uptake with distinct margins in 1 or more vascular territorial distributions or multifocal areas of decreased uptake, presumably caused by small infarcts/small vessel disease.

Acute aortic syndromes

Increased activity involving an aortic aneurysm, dissection, or intramural hematoma may suggest acuity of findings; lack of uptake suggests a more benign course.

Cardiac or vascular neoplasm

Focal increased activity in the heart, particularly in the setting of known metastatic primary cancer, suggests cardiac metastasis. Focal increased activity associated with a mass in the heart or vasculature without a known malignancy suggests a primary neoplasm.

Cardiac or vascular infection

In the setting of suspected infection (eg, fever, bacteremia), prosthetic valve or implanted electronic device infections show increased activity in the affected area. Vascular graft infection shows focal and intense FDG uptake and is particularly suspicious in the setting of fluid collection or abscess formation.

Vasculitis

Linear or circumferential uptake along blood vessel walls, typically more diffuse than that seen in atherosclerosis, can suggest inflammatory vasculitis and can delineate the extent and distribution of involvement. Findings are particularly suggestive in the setting of a known inflammatory syndrome.

Diagnostic criteria are summarized in **Table 2.**

Differential Diagnosis

Atherosclerosis

On myocardial perfusion imaging, cardiac metastatic lesions can mimic perfusion defects[55] and motion artifact and errors in attenuation correction can mimic defects.

On whole-body PET/CT imaging, uptake caused by vasculitis can mimic atherosclerosis.

Hibernating myocardium

If proper diet preparation is not heeded, hibernating myocardium may be mistaken for myocardial infarction.

Table 2
Diagnostic criteria

Diagnosis	Diagnostic Criteria
Atherosclerosis	Perfusion defect in a vascular territory on stress imaging but not on rest imaging; linear uptake along blood vessel wall
Hibernating myocardium	Radiopharmaceutical uptake in areas without corresponding uptake on perfusion imaging
Cardiac sarcoidosis	Patchy increased myocardial uptake, typically involving the left ventricle or septum
Cardiac amyloidosis	Specific cardiac uptake with amyloid agents or uptake over mediastinal background with NaF
Cerebrovascular disease	Decreased uptake with distinct margins in 1 or more vascular territorial distributions or multifocal areas of hypometabolism caused by small infarcts or small vessel disease
Acute aortic syndromes	Increased uptake involving an aortic aneurysm, dissection, or intramural hematoma may suggest acuity of findings; lack of uptake suggests a more benign course
Cardiac or vascular neoplasm	Focal increased uptake in the heart in the setting of known metastatic disease; focal increased uptake associated with a mass in the heart or vasculature
Cardiac or vascular infection	Focal intense uptake particularly when associated with prosthetic valve, implanted electronic device, or vascular graft in the appropriate clinical setting
Vasculitis	Linear or circumferential uptake along blood vessel walls

Cardiac sarcoidosis
Cardiac tumor can mimic the patchy myocardial involvement of sarcoidosis. Late-stage sarcoidosis may have uptake that is similar or decreased compared with normal myocardium, thus appearing falsely negative on PET imaging.

Cardiac amyloidosis
Targeted amyloid PET imaging agents are specific for identification of amyloid plaques. Further studies are needed to differentiate subtypes of amyloidosis and confirm that imaging findings correlate histologically with plaque burden and ultimately with clinical significance.

Cerebrovascular disease
Multifocal decreased uptake can be seen in the setting of prior insult (eg, hemorrhage, trauma, encephalitis), metastatic disease, or errors in attenuation correction.

Acute aortic syndromes
Uptake in aortic aneurysm, dissection, or intramural hematoma could be caused by infection or vasculitis.

Cardiac or vascular neoplasm
PET/CT uptake with FDG and some other radiopharmaceuticals is nonspecific for infection, inflammation, or malignancy, so abnormal or focal activity must be interpreted in the appropriate clinical setting.

Differential considerations for suspected cardiac neoplasm include normal variation in myocardial activity, uptake in the left atrial appendage, and lipomatous hypertrophy of the intra-atrial septum. Although lipomatous hypertrophy of the intra-atrial septum can show increased FDG activity and enlargement of the intra-atrial septum resembling a neoplastic process, corresponding fat density on CT confirms the diagnosis.

Differential considerations for focal vascular uptake include atherosclerosis, aneurysm, dissection, intramural hematoma, and infection.

Cardiac or vascular infection

As previously described, PET/CT uptake with FDG and some other radiopharmaceuticals is nonspecific for infection, inflammation, or malignancy so must be interpreted in the appropriate clinical setting. Vascular grafts can show uptake related to chronic inflammation and thrombus[29,48] versus infection.

Vasculitis

The differential for vasculitis is atherosclerotic uptake.

Differential diagnoses are summarized in **Table 3**.

Pearls, Pitfalls, Variants

- FDG-PET is nonspecific for infection, inflammation, and malignancy and studies must be interpreted in the appropriate clinical setting
- Motion artifact can mimic lesions; non–attenuation-corrected images may be helpful, particularly in the brain and heart
- Stress must be adequate for myocardial perfusion imaging to avoid false-negatives
- Proper dietary preparation is essential to maximize study yield
- Images should be properly windowed to identify cardiac neoplasms
- Knowledge of normal variants and common benign findings is essential for accurate interpretation; common variants include lipomatous hypertrophy of the intra-atrial septum and vascular graft uptake

What Referring Physicians Need to Know

- PET/CT myocardial perfusion imaging effectively evaluates the coronary vasculature
- Viability PET/CT can evaluate for hibernating myocardium in patients who are potential candidates for revascularization procedures
- PET/CT can evaluate the metabolic and anatomic involvement of a variety of inflammatory, infectious, and malignant cardiovascular disorders
- PET/CT can identify cardiac involvement in sarcoidosis and amyloidosis

Table 3
Differential diagnoses

Diagnosis	Differential Diagnoses
Atherosclerosis	Metastases, vasculitis
Hibernating myocardium	Myocardial infarction
Cardiac sarcoidosis	Tumor
Cardiac amyloidosis	Subtypes of cardiac amyloidosis
Cerebrovascular disease	Prior insult, metastases
Acute aortic syndromes	Infection, vasculitis
Cardiac or vascular neoplasm	Infection, inflammation, atherosclerosis, normal/benign uptake
Cardiac or vascular infection	Inflammation, malignancy

- Novel targeted radiopharmaceutical agents and novel use of established techniques show promise in diagnosing and monitoring cardiovascular diseases

SUMMARY

PET/CT can evaluate the metabolic and anatomic involvement of a variety of inflammatory, infectious, and malignant cardiovascular disorders. PET/CT is useful in evaluating coronary vasculature, hibernating myocardium, cardiac sarcoidosis, cardiac amyloidosis, cerebrovascular disease, acute aortic syndromes, cardiac and vascular neoplasms, cardiac and vascular infections, and vasculitis. Novel targeted radiopharmaceutical agents and novel use of established techniques show promise in diagnosing and monitoring cardiovascular diseases.

REFERENCES

1. Mozaffarian D, Benjamin EJ, Go AS, et al. Heart disease and stroke statistics–2015 update: a report from the American Heart Association. Circulation 2015; 131(4):e29–322.
2. Brunken RC. Promising new 18F-labeled tracers for PET myocardial perfusion imaging. J Nucl Med 2015;56(10):1478–9.
3. Lapa C, Reiter T, Kircher M, et al. Somatostatin receptor based PET/CT in patients with the suspicion of cardiac sarcoidosis: an initial comparison to cardiac MRI. Oncotarget 2016;7(47):77807–14.
4. Minoshima S, Drzezga AE, Barthel H, et al. SNMMI procedure standard/EANM practice guideline for amyloid PET imaging of the brain 1.0. J Nucl Med 2016; 57(8):1316–22.
5. Lhommel R, Sempoux C, Ivanoiu A, et al. Is 18F-flutemetamol PET/CT able to reveal cardiac amyloidosis? Clin Nucl Med 2014;39(8):747–9.
6. Garcia-Gonzalez P, Cozar-Santiago MD, Maceira AM. Cardiac amyloidosis detected using 18F-florbetapir PET/CT. Rev Esp Cardiol (Engl Ed) 2016;69(12): 1215.
7. Law WP, Wang WY, Moore PT, et al. Cardiac amyloid imaging with 18F-florbetaben PET: a pilot study. J Nucl Med 2016;57(11):1733–9.
8. Gagliardi C, Tabacchi E, Bonfiglioli R, et al. Does the etiology of cardiac amyloidosis determine the myocardial uptake of [18F]-NaF PET/CT? J Nucl Cardiol 2017; 24(2):746–9.
9. Van Der Gucht A, Galat A, Rosso J, et al. [18F]-NaF PET/CT imaging in cardiac amyloidosis. J Nucl Cardiol 2016;23(4):846–9.
10. Skali H, Schulman AR, Dorbala S. 18F-FDG PET/CT for the assessment of myocardial sarcoidosis. Curr Cardiol Rep 2013;15(4):352.
11. Iannuzzi MC, Rybicki BA, Teirstein AS. Sarcoidosis. N Engl J Med 2007;357(21): 2153–65.
12. Okumura W, Iwasaki T, Toyama T, et al. Usefulness of fasting 18F-FDG PET in identification of cardiac sarcoidosis. J Nucl Med 2004;45(12):1989–98.
13. Ahmadian A, Pawar S, Govender P, et al. The response of FDG uptake to immunosuppressive treatment on FDG PET/CT imaging for cardiac sarcoidosis. J Nucl Cardiol 2017;24(2):413–24.
14. Miller CT, Sweiss NJ, Lu Y. FDG PET/CT evidence of effective treatment of cardiac sarcoidosis with adalimumab. Clin Nucl Med 2016;41(5):417–8.
15. Maurer AH, Burshteyn M, Adler LP, et al. How to differentiate benign versus malignant cardiac and paracardiac 18F FDG uptake at oncologic PET/CT. Radiographics 2011;31(5):1287–305.

16. Wittstein IS, Thiemann DR, Lima JA, et al. Neurohumoral features of myocardial stunning due to sudden emotional stress. N Engl J Med 2005;352(6):539–48.
17. Merlini G, Bellotti V. Molecular mechanisms of amyloidosis. N Engl J Med 2003; 349(6):583–96.
18. Sperry BW, Vranian MN, Hachamovitch R, et al. Subtype-specific interactions and prognosis in cardiac amyloidosis. J Am Heart Assoc 2016;5(3):e002877.
19. Williams G, Kolodny GM. Suppression of myocardial 18F-FDG uptake by preparing patients with a high-fat, low-carbohydrate diet. AJR Am J Roentgenol 2008; 190(2):W151–6.
20. Rinuncini M, Zuin M, Scaranello F, et al. Differentiation of cardiac thrombus from cardiac tumor combining cardiac MRI and 18F-FDG-PET/CT imaging. Int J Cardiol 2016;212:94–6.
21. Yan J, Zhang C, Niu Y, et al. The role of 18F-FDG PET/CT in infectious endocarditis: a systematic review and meta-analysis. Int J Clin Pharmacol Ther 2016; 54(5):337–42.
22. Pizzi MN, Roque A, Fernandez-Hidalgo N, et al. Improving the diagnosis of infective endocarditis in prosthetic valves and intracardiac devices with 18F-fluordeoxyglucose positron emission tomography/computed tomography angiography: initial results at an infective endocarditis referral center. Circulation 2015;132(12):1113–26.
23. Granados U, Fuster D, Pericas JM, et al. Diagnostic accuracy of 18F-FDG PET/CT in infective endocarditis and implantable cardiac electronic device infection: a cross-sectional study. J Nucl Med 2016;57(11):1726–32.
24. Honnorat E, Seng P, Riberi A, et al. Late infectious endocarditis of surgical patch closure of atrial septal defects diagnosed by 18F-fluorodeoxyglucose gated cardiac computed tomography (18F-FDG-PET/CT): a case report. BMC Res Notes 2016;9(1):416.
25. Asmar A, Ozcan C, Diederichsen AC, et al. Clinical impact of 18F-FDG-PET/CT in the extra cardiac work-up of patients with infective endocarditis. Eur Heart J Cardiovasc Imaging 2014;15(9):1013–9.
26. Ben-Haim S, Kupzov E, Tamir A, et al. Changing patterns of abnormal vascular wall F-18 fluorodeoxyglucose uptake on follow-up PET/CT studies. J Nucl Cardiol 2006;13(6):791–800.
27. Mehta NN, Torigian DA, Gelfand JM, et al. Quantification of atherosclerotic plaque activity and vascular inflammation using [18-F] fluorodeoxyglucose positron emission tomography/computed tomography (FDG-PET/CT). J Vis Exp 2012;(63):e3777.
28. Pasha AK, Moghbel M, Saboury B, et al. Effects of age and cardiovascular risk factors on (18)F-FDG PET/CT quantification of atherosclerosis in the aorta and peripheral arteries. Hell J Nucl Med 2015;18(1):5–10.
29. Hayashida T, Sueyoshi E, Sakamoto I, et al. PET features of aortic diseases. AJR Am J Roentgenol 2010;195(1):229–33.
30. Rudd JH, Warburton EA, Fryer TD, et al. Imaging atherosclerotic plaque inflammation with [18F]-fluorodeoxyglucose positron emission tomography. Circulation 2002;105(23):2708–11.
31. Basu S, Beheshti M, Alavi A. Value of (18)F NaF PET/CT in the detection and global quantification of cardiovascular molecular calcification as part of the atherosclerotic process. PET Clin 2012;7(3):329–39.
32. Basu S, Hoilund-Carlsen PF, Alavi A. Assessing global cardiovascular molecular calcification with 18F-fluoride PET/CT: will this become a clinical reality and a

challenge to CT calcification scoring? Eur J Nucl Med Mol Imaging 2012;39(4): 660–4.

33. Janssen T, Bannas P, Herrmann J, et al. Association of linear (1)(8)F-sodium fluoride accumulation in femoral arteries as a measure of diffuse calcification with cardiovascular risk factors: a PET/CT study. J Nucl Cardiol 2013;20(4):569–77.

34. Derlin T, Toth Z, Papp L, et al. Correlation of inflammation assessed by 18F-FDG PET, active mineral deposition assessed by 18F-fluoride PET, and vascular calcification in atherosclerotic plaque: a dual-tracer PET/CT study. J Nucl Med 2011; 52(7):1020–7.

35. Dunphy MP, Freiman A, Larson SM, et al. Association of vascular 18F-FDG uptake with vascular calcification. J Nucl Med 2005;46(8):1278–84.

36. Wykrzykowska J, Lehman S, Williams G, et al. Imaging of inflamed and vulnerable plaque in coronary arteries with 18F-FDG PET/CT in patients with suppression of myocardial uptake using a low-carbohydrate, high-fat preparation. J Nucl Med 2009;50(4):563–8.

37. Harisankar CN, Mittal BR, Agrawal KL, et al. Utility of high fat and low carbohydrate diet in suppressing myocardial FDG uptake. J Nucl Cardiol 2011;18(5): 926–36.

38. Bala G, Blykers A, Xavier C, et al. Targeting of vascular cell adhesion molecule-1 by 18F-labelled nanobodies for PET/CT imaging of inflamed atherosclerotic plaques. Eur Heart J Cardiovasc Imaging 2016;17(9):1001–8.

39. Tahara N, Kai H, Ishibashi M, et al. Simvastatin attenuates plaque inflammation: evaluation by fluorodeoxyglucose positron emission tomography. J Am Coll Cardiol 2006;48(9):1825–31.

40. Sakalihasan N, Hustinx R, Limet R. Contribution of PET scanning to the evaluation of abdominal aortic aneurysm. Semin Vasc Surg 2004;17(2):144–53.

41. Reeps C, Pelisek J, Bundschuh RA, et al. Imaging of acute and chronic aortic dissection by 18F-FDG PET/CT. J Nucl Med 2010;51(5):686–91.

42. Ryan A, McCook B, Sholosh B, et al. Acute intramural hematoma of the aorta as a cause of positive FDG PET/CT. Clin Nucl Med 2007;32(9):729–31.

43. Tezuka D, Haraguchi G, Ishihara T, et al. Role of FDG PET-CT in Takayasu arteritis: sensitive detection of recurrences. JACC Cardiovasc Imaging 2012;5(4):422–9.

44. Mehta NN, Yu Y, Saboury B, et al. Systemic and vascular inflammation in patients with moderate to severe psoriasis as measured by [18F]-fluorodeoxyglucose positron emission tomography-computed tomography (FDG-PET/CT): a pilot study. Arch Dermatol 2011;147(9):1031–9.

45. Rose S, Sheth NH, Baker JF, et al. A comparison of vascular inflammation in psoriasis, rheumatoid arthritis, and healthy subjects by FDG-PET/CT: a pilot study. Am J Cardiovasc Dis 2013;3(4):273–8.

46. Naik HB, Natarajan B, Stansky E, et al. Severity of psoriasis associates with aortic vascular inflammation detected by FDG PET/CT and neutrophil activation in a prospective observational study. Arterioscler Thromb Vasc Biol 2015;35(12): 2667–76.

47. Powers WJ, Zazulia AR. PET in cerebrovascular disease. PET Clin 2010;5(1): 83106.

48. Sah BR, Husmann L, Mayer D, et al. Diagnostic performance of 18F-FDG-PET/CT in vascular graft infections. Eur J Vasc Endovasc Surg 2015;49(4):455–64.

49. Husmann L, Sah BR, Scherrer A, et al. (1)(8)F-FDG PET/CT for therapy control in vascular graft infections: a first feasibility study. J Nucl Med 2015;56(7):1024–9.

50. Makis W, Stern J. Chronic vascular graft infection with fistula to bone causing vertebral osteomyelitis, imaged with F-18 FDG PET/CT. Clin Nucl Med 2010; 35(10):794–6.
51. Hagenaars JC, Wever PC, Vlake AW, et al. Value of 18F-FDG PET/CT in diagnosing chronic Q fever in patients with central vascular disease. Neth J Med 2016;74(7):301–8.
52. Hsiao E, Laury A, Rybicki FJ, et al. Images in vascular medicine. Metastatic aortic intimal sarcoma: the use of PET/CT in diagnosing and staging. Vasc Med 2011; 16(1):81–2.
53. von Falck C, Meyer B, Fegbeutel C, et al. Imaging features of primary sarcomas of the great vessels in CT, MRI and PET/CT: a single-center experience. BMC Med Imaging 2013;13:25.
54. Naswa N, Kumar R, Bal C, et al. Vascular thrombosis as a cause of abdominal pain in a patient with neuroendocrine carcinoma of pancreas: findings on (68) Ga-DOTANOC PET/CT. Indian J Nucl Med 2012;27(1):35–7.
55. Malik D, Basher R, Vadi S, et al. Cardiac metastasis from lung cancer mimicking as perfusion defect on N-13 ammonia and FDG myocardial viability PET/CT scan. J Nucl Cardiol 2016. https://doi.org/10.1007/s12350-016-0609-x.

Gut Microbiome in Health and Disease
Emerging Diagnostic Opportunities

Aonghus Lavelle, MB, PhD[a], Colin Hill, MSc, PhD, DSc[b],*

KEYWORDS

- Microbiome • Colorectal cancer • Fecal microbiota transplantation
- Inflammatory bowel disease • Cancer immunotherapy • Personalized medicine
- Biomarkers

KEY POINTS

- Microbiome science has developed to the point where translation of pre-clinical observations into the clinical arena is imminent.
- Challenges facing the development of microbiome laboratory diagnostics include biological and environmental sources of variation, methodological standardization and the definition of health.
- Both gastrointestinal and extra-intestinal conditions are demonstrating great promise for microbiome-based diagnostics and therapeutics.
- Microbiome diagnostics may serve as biomarkers for disease risk or therapeutic efficacy, as companion diagnostics for microbiome-based therapies such as Fecal Microbiota Transplant or as a gateway to personalized interventions when integrated with other forms of personalized data.

INTRODUCTION

The gut microbiome encompasses the bacterial, viral, archaeal, fungal, and protozoal communities that live within our gastrointestinal tract. These communities significantly extend our complement of genes, allowing fermentation of otherwise inaccessible dietary food sources, providing a source of vitamins and allowing the metabolism of xenobiotics, in addition to playing a fundamental role in our metabolic homeostasis, immune education, and susceptibility to disease. However, numerous challenges have restricted our efforts to translate microbiome findings into routine diagnostic

This article originally appeared in *Gastroenterology Clinics*, Volume 48, Issue 2, June 2019.
Disclosure Statement: The authors have nothing to disclose.
[a] Department of Medicine, APC Microbiome Ireland, University College Cork, Coláiste na hOllscoile, Corcaigh College Road, Cork T12 K8A, Ireland; [b] School of Microbiology, APC Microbiome Ireland, University College Cork, Coláiste na hOllscoile, Corcaigh College Road, Cork T12 K8A, Ireland
* Corresponding author.
E-mail address: c.hill@ucc.ie

monitoring. Here, the authors describe the unique features of the microbiome that make clinical translation a challenge and identify several key areas where early progress has been or is likely to be made.

ACQUISITION, ASSEMBLY, AND ESTABLISHED COMMUNITIES

At birth, humans rapidly become colonized with microbes in an essentially stochastic manner. Microbial exposure is essential for normal immune development, with a requirement for specific microbial functions at critical time points, the absence of which can lead to long-term effects on immune development.[1] Characteristic microbiomes based on body site are not present at birth,[2] with community structure and function rapidly consolidating to their respective niches by 6 weeks of age.[3] Although most neonatal body sites and fluids resemble maternal skin and vaginal communities, meconium, the first pass of intestinal contents, has a distinct microbial composition, which may suggest that limited first microbial contact may actually occur in utero.[4]

Succession of gut microbial species toward an adult microbiome takes place over the following 1 to 3 years[5] and is almost certainly influenced by preterm delivery and antibiotic use,[6] feeding,[7] maternal health,[8] and delivery mode.[9] Succession of bacterial communities is a nonrandom process, with changes in diet, particularly discontinuation of breast feeding[5] and the commencement of solid foods resulting in defined transitions, an increase in diversity, and convergence toward an adult configuration.[10]

By adulthood, the distal gut microbiome contains an estimated 10^{10} to 10^{11} bacteria per gram of feces,[11] dominated by the phyla Bacteroidetes and Firmicutes, with varying contributions from other phyla, including Proteobacteria, Actinobacteria, and Verrucomicrobia.[12] Combined data from the Flemish Gut Flora Project, the LLDeep cohort in Holland, the human microbiome project (HMP), and the UK twins study described 664 genera, with an estimate of 784 ± 40 genera total richness in western populations.[13] Adding data from New Guinea, Peru, and Tanzania, 14 core genera were present in greater than 95% of individuals across the dataset, suggesting a global core bacterial microbiome.

NONBACTERIAL COMPONENTS

In addition to bacteria, large communities of viruses exist within the gut microbiome. Bacteriophages, viruses with a bacterial host, dominate this population and exist at approximately 10^{10} to 10^{11} particles per gram of feces,[14] with potentially higher quantities on mucosal surfaces.[15] In ecological communities, such as marine environments, phage and their hosts interact in a cycle of bacterial infection, replication, cell lysis, and resistance, leading to an evolutionary "arms race." This lytic cycle contrasts with the predominant behavior of phages within the gut, where a temperate or lysogenic cycle leads to incorporation of phage DNA within the host genome, reverting to lytic behavior under certain stresses.[16] Phages can thus have direct and indirect effects on their host communities.[17] Succession dynamics,[18] temporal stability,[19] and interindividual variation[20] appear broadly similar to bacterial communities, and although the complete role of phages within the gut remains to be determined, they have been associated with certain disease, including inflammatory bowel disease (IBD),[21] and show potential as biomarkers and therapeutic tools.[22]

Microbial eukaryotes, such as diverse fungal species, are also important and are biologically relevant, although accounting for a numerically small portion of the total microbial community. The gut "mycobiome" is dominated by yeast, prominently Saccharomyces, Malassezia, and Candida spp in the HMP cohort, and overall, fungal communities are less diverse.[23] Decreases in certain fungal species with anti-inflammatory properties, such as *Saccharomyces cerevisiae*, as well as increases in potentially pathogenic species, such as *Candida albicans*, have been described in IBD.[24] Interestingly, less temporal stability is observed in terms of fungal communities with a loss of significant interpersonal differentiation over time, contrasting with the case of the gut bacteriome and virome.[23]

SOURCES OF MICROBIOME VARIATION
Biological and Environmental

In terms of the human-associated microbiome, the largest variation in taxonomic composition is consistently between body habitats, whereas within body habitats, there is a large degree of interpersonal variation, as evidenced by the findings of the Human Microbiome Project,[12] with individuals also tending to remain more like themselves than others over time.[25] However, when viewed in terms of the genetic composition of the microbiome, this striking interindividual variation largely disappears, highlighting that the underlying genetic machinery is much more tightly conserved.

Interpersonal variability does not appear to be strongly shaped by host genetic makeup or microbiome heritability but is markedly influenced by environmental exposures, as recently demonstrated in a large Israeli cohort and validated in a Dutch population.[26] In this landmark study, microbiome composition was additive with host genotype in predicting a range of host phenotypes, including blood markers of glycemic control and high-density lipoprotein cholesterol, body mass index (BMI), and several anthropometric measures. Factors that have been demonstrated to have an association with microbiome composition include diet, stool consistency, medication use, antibiotic prescribing, BMI, household sharing, blood parameters, gender, health, physical activity, and age; these are essential covariates for any large microbiome study[13,26,27] (**Fig. 1**A).

Methodological

In addition to biological variation, variation in technical approach is a significant obstacle to comparability between studies (**Fig. 1**B). Various DNA sequencing methodologies have been used, including 454 pyrosequencing and Illumina technologies, whereas third-generation sequencing platforms are emerging, such as PacBio and MinION.[28] At the other end of the spectrum, polymerase chain reaction (PCR) can identify specific members of the community, whereas in between, microarray technology has been used to develop the HITchip, a fixed phylogenetic array.[29] In addition, agreed protocols for acquisition, storage, DNA extraction, amplification, sequencing, and bioinformatic analysis of biological samples are beginning to be published. To tackle variations between approaches, the Microbiome Quality Control Project (www.mbqc.org/) has published their first round of protocols for the handling and bioinformatic analysis of metagenomic and amplicon sequencing of gut samples.[30,31] Notably, DNA extraction, handling laboratory and bioinformatics pipeline all have effects, at times comparable to biological sources of variation. Bioinformatic approaches have also been applied to the important issue of microbial contamination, and a Bayesian method, SourceTracker, has been developed.[32] It should be noted that variation in methodologies is to be expected in a rapidly developing area, and it is important that standardization does not impede innovations in method development.

DEFINING HEALTH

One of the major challenges in microbiome science (and other areas of medicine) involves defining health. Given the sources of variation described above and the

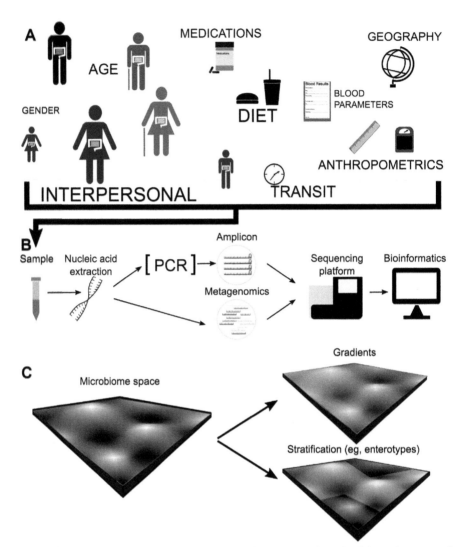

Fig. 1. (*A*) Biological and environmental sources of variation. (*B*) Methodological sources of variation. (*C*) Representation of the microbiome landscape, with alternate interpretations of gradients or stratification (equivalent to enterotypes).

"landscape of possible microbiome configurations,"[33] this has been challenging (**Fig. 1C**). Enterotypes, defined as "densely populated areas in a multidimensional space of community composition," were associated initially with 1 of 3 key indicator taxons, namely *Prevotella*, *Bacteroides*, or *Ruminococcaceae*.[34] Definition of these densely populated areas does depend on the statistical methodology applied and may change with geographic source, reflecting data biased in favor of Western countries.[33,34] However, enterotypes, particularly those associated with *Prevotella* and *Bacteroides*, have been widely reproduced, demonstrate enterotype-specific enrichments of functional gene categories, and have been associated with host disease phenotypes.[33] Such a proposal allows for stratification of individuals and may facilitate numerous clinical applications, including biomarker discovery and personalized interventions. However, further large-scale studies are required to determine if different enterotypes are linked to meaningful clinical differences. In addition, as de novo clustering is dependent on the current sample set, potential clinical applications require a reference "enterotype-space" to assure samples are correctly assigned to their true cluster. In discovery projects, ordination results are highly dependent on the statistical method applied, the number of samples, and the sequence coverage,[35] and underlying all these efforts remains the requirement for strict standardization of sample acquisition and processing in studies that are to be directly compared with one another.

Although enterotypes provide a mechanism of recovering structure across the microbiome landscape, direct comparison between disease and health in case-control studies remains an important tool for identifying disease-associated microbiome alterations. Many disease-associated confounders exist however, as demonstrated in the case of type II diabetes mellitus (T2DM), where the purported disease-associated alterations were subsequently attributed to metformin, a common oral hypoglycemic agent used in the treatment of T2DM.[36] A large Flemish population study (the Flemish Gut Flora Project) has estimated that between 400 and 900 individuals per group would be required to adequately power microbiome studies depending on the circumstance and background covariates.[13] These results suggest that many studies comparing disease and control subjects are underpowered, leading to the conclusions that reference datasets with heavily phenotyped control subjects for matching will be invaluable for future microbiome discovery projects.

CLINICAL OPPORTUNITIES

Although the factors detailed above represent significant challenges to universal diagnostic microbiome tests, certain clinical scenarios show great promise for translational applications. The authors describe several of these, in both gastrointestinal and non-gastrointestinal disorders, to illustrate the scope and application of potential microbiome-based diagnostics (**Box 1**).

Colorectal Cancer

Although clinically isolated strains of gut bacteria, such as *Streptococcus bovis* bacteremia, have been associated with colorectal cancer (CRC),[37] culture-

---

Box 1
Opportunities for microbiome-based diagnostics

Microbiome-based biomarkers may improve population screening for colorectal cancer and precancerous lesions.

Microbiome-based diagnostics may inform therapeutic pathways in CD, particularly suitability for treatment deescalation and risk-stratification for postoperative recurrence.

Coupling microbiome diagnostics and therapeutics will become important, particularly in the era of FMT and may aid rational matching of donors-recipients in clinical trials for IBD.

Identification of patients with cancer at risk of nonresponse to immunotherapy and subsequent expansion of specific bacterial populations may improve response rates to checkpoint inhibitors.

Personalized dietary interventions, incorporating microbiome analysis, represent a prototype for integrated approaches to personalized therapeutics.

independent sequencing technologies have provided many insights into compositional changes associated with CRC, and there is mounting evidence to suggest that the intestinal microbiota may play a key role in its pathogenesis. Specific bacteria that have been associated with CRC tumorigenesis include *Escherichia coli*,[38] enterotoxigenic *Bacteroides fragilis*,[39] and, most commonly, *Fusobacterium nucleatum*.

F nucleatum is an invasive gram-negative bacterium, important in polymicrobial biofilms associated with periodontitis,[40] and is notably also increased in IBD, where it may be more invasive.[41] *F nucleatum* has been found to be increased in CRC,[42,43] precancerous lesions,[44,45] and fecal samples in CRC[46] and has even been detected in CRC metastases.[43] *Fusobacterium* carriage may also have prognostic relevance and has been associated with lymph-node metastases[42,47] and reduced overall survival.[48,49] These findings have strong mechanistic underpinnings, with *F nucleatum* known to activate β-catenin signaling via a surface adhesin, FadA, binding to E-cadherin. Furthermore, *F nucleatum* can enhance progression of tumors by causing an increase in tumor-infiltrating myeloid cells within the tumor microenvironment.[50,51] Despite this, it is likely that *Fusobacterium* spp are only associated with a subset of CRCs.[43]

Other associations with oral pathogens have also been demonstrated. Using a Dirichlet Multinomial Model, investigators in China identified 5 metacommunities associated with different phenotypes (controls, adenomas, and CRC). Interestingly, the metacommunity with the strongest association with CRC was characterized by enrichment of *F nucleatum* and other periodontal pathogens.[52] Associations with periodontal disease and CRC have been described,[53] and increased prevalence of pathogenic oral bacteria groups, including *Peptostreptococcus*, *Prevotella*, *Steptococcus*, *Parvimonas*, and *Porphyromonas*, has been associated with reduced colonic abundance of *Lachnospiraceae*.[54,55]

These findings allowed investigators to demonstrate that microbiome-based screening can supplement current noninvasive biomarkers, such as fecal occult blood (FOB)[56] tests or fecal immunohistochemical tests (FIT),[54] to improve detection of early colorectal neoplasia (**Fig. 2A**). Using quantitative PCR of the butyryl-CoA dehydrogenase gene from *F nucleatum* and the rpoB gene from *Parvimonas micra* determined by cross-ethnic validation, investigators achieved a true-positive detection rate (TPR) of 0.723 with a false-positive rate (FPR) of 0.073 without the use of FOB or FIT.[57] Adding oral microbiota to stool allowed Irish researchers to improve detection of CRC, with a TPR of 0.76 and an FPR of 0.05.[55]

Therapeutic Strategies in Crohn's Disease

Many studies have demonstrated microbiome alterations associated with IBD, most prominently Crohn's disease (CD), and specifically, ileal CD, with a common theme being a reduction in overall bacterial diversity.[58] Reductions in butyrate-producing species, particularly *Faecalibacterium prausnitzii* in CD[58,59] as well as selected members of the *Lachnospiraceae*,[58] have been consistently described, with increases in adherent and invasive *E coli* demonstrated in the ileum of ileal CD patients.[60] Increased prevalence of *Ruminococcus gnavus*, Proteobacteria, *Veillonella*, and *Fusobacterium* spp has also been described.[61,62] Notably, children with new onset CD before treatment demonstrated much more dramatic microbiome alterations when mucosal biopsy samples were sequenced compared with stool samples, with predictive power for 6-month disease activity, suggesting that the diagnostic and prognostic viability of microbiome-based biomarkers in IBD may be enhanced by mucosal biopsy sampling.[62]

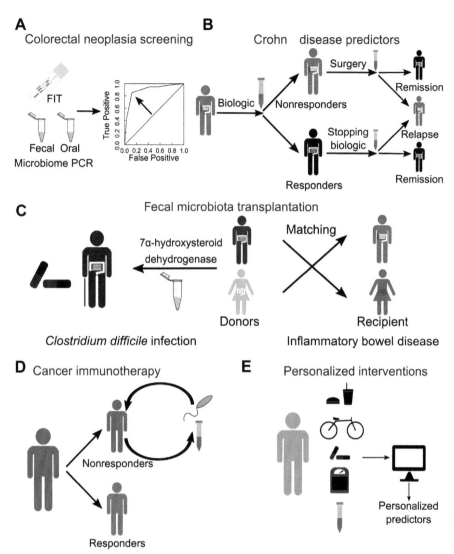

Fig. 2. Promising applications of microbiome-based diagnostics based on seminal research findings discussed in the text. (*A*) Improving sensitivity and specificity of noninvasive colorectal neoplasia detection. (*B*) Potential microbiome predictors in CD. (*C*) Applications of FMT in CDI and IBD. (*D*) Microbiome assessment as a potential source of nonresponse in cancer immunotherapy with potential for targeted modulation. (*E*) Integrating personalized microbiome data with other data types to develop personalized prediction algorithms.

Microbiome analysis has also demonstrated efficacy in predicting anastomotic recurrence of CD following surgical resection,[63] a common problem that can affect more than half of patients who undergo this procedure and occurs following restoration of the fecal stream[64] (**Fig. 2**B). Recovery of mucosal microbiome composition at 6-months postsurgery was associated with remission, while putative fecal biomarkers of disease recurrence presurgery were also noted.[63] In addition, in a parallel evaluation of the pivotal POCER (Post-Operative Crohn's Disease Recurrence) study, evaluating strategies for preventing postoperative recurrence of CD, levels of *Faecalibacterium* and *Proteus*, in combination with smoking status, were moderately predictive of early recurrence.[65]

In a therapeutic setting, PCR-based microbiome analysis predicted relapse independently of the inflammatory marker CRP following withdrawal of therapy with infliximab in CD, a question of huge clinical relevance given the cost and potential side effects of long-term biologic therapy.[66] More recently, in a multiethnic Chinese and Western cohort, microbial species could predict response to infliximab therapy with 86.5% accuracy, improving to 93.8% when combined with the stool marker fecal calprotectin.[67] These findings are extremely promising in identifying microbiome-based diagnostics, which are additive with markers of inflammatory burden that have traditionally been associated with response prediction.

Fecal Microbiota Transplantation

Fecal microbiota transplantation (FMT) has become a standard treatment of recurrent *Clostridium difficile* infection (CDI), a major health care challenge associated with antibiotic use.[68] Recurrent CDI occurs in approximately 20% of CDI cases, associated with a marked loss of microbiome diversity and an inability of the native microbiome to "reboot" following treatment of CDI with specific antibiotics, such as vancomycin, metronidazole, and fidaxomicin. Just a single dose of the antibiotic clindamycin results in a profound loss of diversity in the gut microbiota of mice and a resulting enhanced susceptibility to CDI,[69] presumably because of the commensal microbiota providing a significant barrier via colonization resistance. First-line antibiotic treatments, such as vancomycin, can result in profound and persistent collateral effects on the microbiome, which may be associated with subsequent risk of pathogen expansion and is remediated by FMT.[70] FMT is commonly performed at endoscopy, where healthy donor fecal suspensions that have been prescreened for pathogens are infused into the recipient. Donor feces can be acquired from healthy volunteers or increasingly from donor banks, such as OpenBiome. Extensive screening of donor samples is required to prevent pathogen transmission, and extended host phenotype exclusion criteria and standardized screening protocols will become important.[71] Phase 3 clinical trials on commercially prepared products are also underway, including SER-109, a capsule made by Seres Therapeutics, and RBX2660, an enema bag made by Rebiotix.

Incorporating microbiome parameters into models has also helped improve classification of CDI, and a combination of clinical and microbiome variables may better predict at-risk hospitalized patients.[72] Furthermore, specific molecular mechanisms have been elucidated, identifying that the microbiota also provides resistance to CDI through bile acid metabolism.[73] Investigators have identified loss of a specific bacterial species, *Clostridium scindens*, which provides colonization resistance to CDI due to expression of the secondary bile acid biosynthesis gene, 7α-hydroxysteroid dehydrogenase, detectable by PCR.[74] Recovery of resistance to CDI occurred with administration of this bacterium, pointing toward a potential combination of PCR-based diagnosis and targeted therapeutic expansion (**Fig. 2**C).

FMT is also being investigated in other conditions, notably IBD. Some promise has been demonstrated in ulcerative colitis, where several randomized controlled trials have demonstrated variable efficacy in induction of remission,[75–77] although not all.[78] Interestingly, the potential for certain healthy donors to be better at inducing remission was suggested ("superdonors"). Higher donor richness,[79] the presence of conspecific or shared species,[80] and increased butyrate production, with lower levels of Bacteroidetes and Proteobacteria in donors,[81] were associated with induction of remission, suggesting that refined selection of donors and potential matching strategies may improve remission rates.

Cancer Immunotherapy

The gut microbiome plays a fundamental role in the education of innate and adaptive immune responses as well as in maintenance of immune homeostasis. Cancer immunotherapy seeks to inhibit tumor-derived immunosuppression via immune checkpoint inhibitors against programmed cell death protein-1 (PD-1) and its ligand, PD-L1, as well as CTLA-4, although response rates are variable. In patients treated with checkpoint inhibitors, response phenotype can be transferred to germ-free mice from patients by fecal transplant, suggesting a pivotal role for the microbiome in clinical response to immunotherapy.[82] Germ-free or antibiotic-treated murine cancer models show a significantly reduced response to a range of chemotherapeutic and anticancer treatments, whereas in humans, a reduction in the efficacy of PD-1/PD-L1 inhibitors has been demonstrated following antibiotic administration across a range of cancer types. Specific bacteria associated with response include the presence of *Akkermansia muciniphila*, *Alistipes*, and members of the Firmicutes.[83] Similar findings have been reported for CTLA-4 inhibitors, although this was associated with specific *Bacteroides* species, notably *B fragilis*.[84] Further associations include increased presence of *Enterococcus hirae* in response to both PD-1/PD-L1 inhibition and cyclophosphamide therapy.[85] In another seminal study, melanoma xenograft mice (C57Bl/6) demonstrated differences in tumor growth rate depending on vendor, attributable to differences in intratumoral T-cell response.[86] Cohousing, or appropriately directed transplant of fecal suspensions, could ameliorate the effects on tumor growth and tumor immune response. *Bifidobacterium* was most strongly associated with an increased immune response; therapeutic administration of *Bifidobacterium* species from different sources reduced tumor growth. *Bifidobacterium longum* was also found to be increased in responders to checkpoint inhibitors, in addition to *Collinsella aerofaciens* and *Enterococcus faecium*.[82] Although there is a lack of consistency between studies as to which bacterial species mediate these effects, multiple lines of evidence point toward microbiome-mediated response to immunotherapy in cancer, opening the door to a promising field of coupled diagnostic and therapeutic interventions to improve response to cancer immunotherapy[87] (**Fig. 2D**).

Personalized Dietary Interventions

Host metabolism is intrinsically linked to the gut microbiome, and numerous foundational studies have demonstrated that the microbiome plays a key role in energy harvest, obesity, and metabolic syndrome.[88–90] As described throughout this review, interpersonal variation is consistently the most significant variable in terms of gut microbiome composition. Researchers in Israel have demonstrated that postprandial glycemic response (PPGR) is also highly variable between individuals.[91] Using a cohort of more than 800 individuals with continuous blood glucose tracking, combined with dietary, lifestyle, medical, anthropometric, and microbiome analysis, the researchers were able to predict PPGR using a machine-learning algorithm far more accurately than by meal carbohydrate content. The improved prediction of PPGR was validated in a subsequent cohort and was the basis of a successful trial, where personalized diets were comparable when administered by an expert or by the algorithm. Both the expert and the algorithm had access to continuous glucose monitoring data for the prior week, although only the algorithm could make inferences about previously unobserved meals, while additionally being able to leverage information on other lifestyle covariates. Interestingly, despite the variation in microbiome composition between individuals, some conserved patterns were noted in response to the short-term dietary intervention (which involved 1 week of a "good" diet and 1 week of a "bad" diet), including increases in *Roseburia inulinivorans*, *Eubacterium eligens*, *Alistipes putredinis*, and *Bacteroides vulgatus* and reductions in *Bifidobacterium adolescentis* and Anaerostipes following the "good" diet, largely consistent with previous literature. In a smaller study looking at white bread in comparison to sourdough bread, the same group demonstrated similar findings, although in this case, they were able to accurately predict PPGR based on initial microbiome composition alone.[92]

These pivotal studies have demonstrated that interpersonal variation in the microbiome can be a gateway into personalized dietary interventions, with an enormous potential for extension into personalized diagnostics and therapeutics (**Fig. 2**E). Importantly, they also provide a template for the manner in which data from microbiome studies may be integrated with lifestyle, dietary, and medical data, to provide a personalized model of microbiome and host response to interventions.

SUMMARY

A new horizon of microbiome-based diagnostic tools is in sight, ranging from assays to improve noninvasive population screening in conditions like CRC, to complementary biomarkers of disease progression and therapeutic response in IBD. Focused microbiome analysis may help identify individuals at risk of CDI and allow for targeted rescue of colonization resistance, as well as informing rational matching strategies for emerging FMT indications, such as in IBD. More broadly, extensive microbiome characterization may be integrated into a personalized portfolio of features, allowing for tailored intervention strategies in a range of conditions. Large-scale population cohorts, adequately powered studies, applications of data science, and universal standardization of pipelines will be required to realize these ambitious goals in the coming years.

ACKNOWLEDGEMENTS

APC Microbiome Ireland is funded with financial support by Science Foundation Ireland (SFI) under Grant Number SFI/12/RC/2273.

REFERENCES

1. Gomez de Aguero M, Ganal-Vonarburg SC, Fuhrer T, et al. The maternal microbiota drives early postnatal innate immune development. Science 2016; 351(6279):1296–302.
2. Dominguez-Bello MG, Costello EK, Contreras M, et al. Delivery mode shapes the acquisition and structure of the initial microbiota across multiple body habitats in newborns. Proc Natl Acad Sci U S A 2010;107(26):11971–5.
3. Chu DM, Ma J, Prince AL, et al. Maturation of the infant microbiome community structure and function across multiple body sites and in relation to mode of delivery. Nat Med 2017;23:314.
4. Collado MC, Rautava S, Aakko J, et al. Human gut colonisation may be initiated in utero by distinct microbial communities in the placenta and amniotic fluid. Sci Rep 2016;6:23129.
5. Bäckhed F, Roswall J, Peng Y, et al. Dynamics and stabilization of the human gut microbiome during the first year of life. Cell Host Microbe 2015;17(6):852.
6. Gibson MK, Wang B, Ahmadi S, et al. Developmental dynamics of the preterm infant gut microbiota and antibiotic resistome. Nat Microbiol 2016;1:16024.

7. Bokulich NA, Chung J, Battaglia T, et al. Antibiotics, birth mode, and diet shape microbiome maturation during early life. Sci Transl Med 2016;8(343):343ra82.

8. Hu J, Nomura Y, Bashir A, et al. Diversified microbiota of meconium is affected by maternal diabetes status. PLoS One 2013;8(11):e78257.

9. Azad MB, Konya T, Maughan H, et al. Gut microbiota of healthy Canadian infants: profiles by mode of delivery and infant diet at 4 months. CMAJ 2013;185(5): 385–94.

10. Koenig JE, Spor A, Scalfone N, et al. Succession of microbial consortia in the developing infant gut microbiome. Proc Natl Acad Sci U S A 2011;108(Suppl 1):4578–85.

11. Vandeputte D, Kathagen G, D'Hoe K, et al. Quantitative microbiome profiling links gut community variation to microbial load. Nature 2017;551(7681):507–11.

12. The Human Microbiome Consortium. Structure, function and diversity of the healthy human microbiome. Nature 2012;486(7402):207–14.

13. Falony G, Joossens M, Vieira-Silva S, et al. Population-level analysis of gut micro-biome variation. Science 2016;352(6285):560–4.

14. Shkoporov AN, Ryan FJ, Draper LA, et al. Reproducible protocols for metage-nomic analysis of human faecal phageomes. Microbiome 2018;6(1):68.

15. Barr JJ, Auro R, Furlan M, et al. Bacteriophage adhering to mucus provide a non-host-derived immunity. Proc Natl Acad Sci U S A 2013;110(26):10771–6.

16. Fuhrman JA. Marine viruses and their biogeochemical and ecological effects. Na-ture 1999;399:541.

17. Manrique P, Dills M, Young M. The human gut phage community and its implica-tions for health and disease. Viruses 2017;9(6):141.

18. Breitbart M, Haynes M, Kelley S, et al. Viral diversity and dynamics in an infant gut. Res Microbiol 2008;159(5):367–73.

19. Minot S, Bryson A, Chehoud C, et al. Rapid evolution of the human gut virome. Proc Natl Acad Sci U S A 2013;110(30):12450–5.

20. Minot S, Sinha R, Chen J, et al. The human gut virome: inter-individual variation and dynamic response to diet. Genome Res 2011;21(10):1616–25.

21. Norman JM, Handley SA, Baldridge MT, et al. Disease-specific alterations in the enteric virome in inflammatory bowel disease. Cell 2015;160(3):447–60.

22. Dalmasso M, Hill C, Ross RP. Exploiting gut bacteriophages for human health. Trends Microbiol 2014;22(7):399–405.

23. Nash AK, Auchtung TA, Wong MC, et al. The gut mycobiome of the Human Micro-biome Project healthy cohort. Microbiome 2017;5:153.

24. Sokol H, Leducq V, Aschard H, et al. Fungal microbiota dysbiosis in IBD. Gut 2017;66(6):1039–48.

25. Costello EK, Lauber CL, Hamady M, et al. Bacterial community variation in human body habitats across space and time. Science 2009;326(5960):1694–7.

26. Rothschild D, Weissbrod O, Barkan E, et al. Environment dominates over host ge-netics in shaping human gut microbiota. Nature 2018;555:210.

27. Maier L, Pruteanu M, Kuhn M, et al. Extensive impact of non-antibiotic drugs on human gut bacteria. Nature 2018;555:623.

28. Cao Y, Fanning S, Proos S, et al. A review on the applications of next generation sequencing technologies as applied to food-related microbiome studies. Front Microbiol 2017;8:1829.

29. Rajilić-Stojanović M, Heilig HGHJ, Molenaar D, et al. Development and applica-tion of the human intestinal tract chip, a phylogenetic microarray: analysis of uni-versally conserved phylotypes in the abundant microbiota of young and elderly adults. Environ Microbiol 2009;11(7):1736–51.

30. Sinha R, Abu-Ali G, Vogtmann E, et al. Assessment of variation in microbial community amplicon sequencing by the Microbiome Quality Control (MBQC) project consortium. Nat Biotechnol 2017;35(11):1077–86.
31. Costea PI, Zeller G, Sunagawa S, et al. Towards standards for human fecal sample processing in metagenomic studies. Nat Biotechnol 2017;35(11):1069–76.
32. Knights D, Kuczynski J, Charlson ES, et al. Bayesian community-wide culture-independent microbial source tracking. Nat Methods 2011;8(9):761–3.
33. Costea PI, Hildebrand F, Arumugam M, et al. Enterotypes in the landscape of gut microbial community composition. Nat Microbiol 2018;3(1):8–16.
34. Arumugam M, Raes J, Pelletier E, et al. Enterotypes of the human gut microbiome. Nature 2011;473(7346):174–80.
35. Kuczynski J, Liu Z, Lozupone C, et al. Microbial community resemblance methods differ in their ability to detect biologically relevant patterns. Nat Methods 2010;7(10):813–9.
36. Forslund K, Hildebrand F, Nielsen T, et al. Disentangling type 2 diabetes and metformin treatment signatures in the human gut microbiota. Nature 2015;528:262.
37. Corredoira JC, Alonso MP, Garcia JF, et al. Clinical characteristics and significance of Streptococcus salivarius bacteremia and Streptococcus bovis bacteremia: a prospective 16-year study. Eur J Clin Microbiol Infect Dis 2005;24(4): 250–5.
38. Arthur JC, Perez-Chanona E, Mühlbauer M, et al. Intestinal inflammation targets cancer-inducing activity of the microbiota. Science 2012;338(6103):120–3.
39. Toprak NU, Yagci A, Gulluoglu BM, et al. A possible role of Bacteroides fragilis enterotoxin in the aetiology of colorectal cancer. Clin Microbiol Infect 2006; 12(8):782–6.
40. Signat B, Roques C, Poulet P, et al. Fusobacterium nucleatum in periodontal health and disease. Curr Issues Mol Biol 2011;13(2):25–36.
41. Strauss J, Kaplan GG, Beck PL, et al. Invasive potential of gut mucosa-derived Fusobacterium nucleatum positively correlates with IBD status of the host. Inflamm Bowel Dis 2011;17(9):1971–8.
42. Castellarin M, Warren RL, Freeman JD, et al. Fusobacterium nucleatum infection is prevalent in human colorectal carcinoma. Genome Res 2012;22(2):299–306.
43. Kostic AD, Gevers D, Pedamallu CS, et al. Genomic analysis identifies association of Fusobacterium with colorectal carcinoma. Genome Res 2012;22(2):292–8.
44. McCoy AN, Araújo-Pérez F, Azcárate-Peril A, et al. Fusobacterium is associated with colorectal adenomas. PLoS One 2013;8(1):e53653.
45. Miki I, Shinichi K, Katsuhiko N, et al. Association of Fusobacterium nucleatum with clinical and molecular features in colorectal serrated pathway. Int J Cancer 2015; 137(6):1258–68.
46. Ahn J, Sinha R, Pei Z, et al. Human gut microbiome and risk for colorectal cancer. J Natl Cancer Inst 2013;105(24):1907–11.
47. Li YY, Ge QX, Cao J, et al. Association of Fusobacterium nucleatum infection with colorectal cancer in Chinese patients. World J Gastroenterol 2016;22(11): 3227–33.
48. Flanagan L, Schmid J, Ebert M, et al. Fusobacterium nucleatum associates with stages of colorectal neoplasia development, colorectal cancer and disease outcome. Eur J Clin Microbiol Infect Dis 2014;33(8):1381–90.
49. Mima K, Nishihara R, Qian ZR, et al. Fusobacterium nucleatum in colorectal carcinoma tissue and patient prognosis. Gut 2016;65(12):1973–80.

50. Rubinstein Mara R, Wang X, Liu W, et al. *Fusobacterium nucleatum* promotes colorectal carcinogenesis by modulating E-Cadherin/β-Catenin signaling via its FadA adhesin. Cell Host Microbe 2013;14(2):195–206.
51. Kostic Aleksandar D, Chun E, Robertson L, et al. *Fusobacterium nucleatum* potentiates intestinal tumorigenesis and modulates the tumor-immune microenvironment. Cell Host Microbe 2013;14(2):207–15.
52. Nakatsu G, Li X, Zhou H, et al. Gut mucosal microbiome across stages of colorectal carcinogenesis. Nat Commun 2015;6:8727.
53. Momen-Heravi F, Babic A, Tworoger SS, et al. Periodontal disease, tooth loss and colorectal cancer risk: results from the Nurses' Health Study. Int J Cancer 2017; 140(3):646–52.
54. Baxter NT, Ruffin MT, Rogers MA, et al. Microbiota-based model improves the sensitivity of fecal immunochemical test for detecting colonic lesions. Genome Med 2016;8(1):37.
55. Flemer B, Warren RD, Barrett MP, et al. The oral microbiota in colorectal cancer is distinctive and predictive. Gut 2018;67(8):1454–63.
56. Zeller G, Tap J, Voigt AY, et al. Potential of fecal microbiota for early-stage detection of colorectal cancer. Mol Syst Biol 2014;10(11):766.
57. Yu J, Feng Q, Wong SH, et al. Metagenomic analysis of faecal microbiome as a tool towards targeted non-invasive biomarkers for colorectal cancer. Gut 2017; 66(1):70–8.
58. Willing BP, Dicksved J, Halfvarson J, et al. A pyrosequencing study in twins shows that gastrointestinal microbial profiles vary with inflammatory bowel disease phenotypes. Gastroenterology 2010;139(6):1844–54.e1.
59. Sokol H, Pigneur B, Watterlot L, et al. Faecalibacterium prausnitzii is an anti-inflammatory commensal bacterium identified by gut microbiota analysis of Crohn's disease patients. Proc Natl Acad Sci U S A 2008;105(43):16731–6.
60. Darfeuille-Michaud A, Boudeau J, Bulois P, et al. High prevalence of adherent-invasive Escherichia coli associated with ileal mucosa in Crohn's disease. Gastroenterology 2004;127(2):412–21.
61. Quince C, Ijaz UZ, Loman N, et al. Extensive modulation of the fecal metagenome in children with Crohn's disease during exclusive enteral nutrition. Am J Gastroenterol 2015;110(12):1718–29 [quiz: 1730].
62. Gevers D, Kugathasan S, Denson LA, et al. The treatment-naive microbiome in new-onset Crohn's disease. Cell Host Microbe 2014;15(3):382–92.
63. Mondot S, Lepage P, Seksik P, et al. Structural robustness of the gut mucosal microbiota is associated with Crohn's disease remission after surgery. Gut 2016; 65(6):954–62.
64. D'Haens GR, Geboes K, Peeters M, et al. Early lesions of recurrent Crohn's disease caused by infusion of intestinal contents in excluded ileum. Gastroenterology 1998;114(2):262–7.
65. Wright EK, Kamm MA, Wagner J, et al. Microbial factors associated with postoperative Crohn's disease recurrence. J Crohn's Colitis 2017;11(2):191–203.
66. Rajca S, Grondin V, Louis E, et al. Alterations in the intestinal microbiome (dysbiosis) as a predictor of relapse after infliximab withdrawal in Crohn's disease. Inflamm Bowel Dis 2014;20(6):978–86.
67. Zhou Y, Xu ZZ, He Y, et al. Gut microbiota offers universal biomarkers across ethnicity in inflammatory bowel disease diagnosis and infliximab response prediction. mSystems 2018;3(1) [pii:e00188-17].
68. van Nood E, Vrieze A, Nieuwdorp M, et al. Duodenal infusion of donor feces for recurrent Clostridium difficile. N Engl J Med 2013;368(5):407–15.

69. Buffie CG, Jarchum I, Equinda M, et al. Profound alterations of intestinal microbiota following a single dose of clindamycin results in sustained susceptibility to Clostridium difficile-induced colitis. Infect Immun 2012;80(1):62–73.

70. Isaac S, Scher JU, Djukovic A, et al. Short- and long-term effects of oral vancomycin on the human intestinal microbiota. J Antimicrob Chemother 2017;72(1): 128–36.

71. Ding NS, Mullish BH, McLaughlin J, et al. Meeting update: faecal microbiota transplantation—bench, bedside, courtroom? Frontline Gastroenterol 2018; 9(1):45–8.

72. Schubert AM, Rogers MAM, Ring C, et al. Microbiome data distinguish patients with Clostridium difficile infection and Non-C. difficile-associated diarrhea from healthy controls. MBio 2014;5(3). e01021-14.

73. Weingarden AR, Chen C, Bobr A, et al. Microbiota transplantation restores normal fecal bile acid composition in recurrent Clostridium difficile infection. Am J Physiol Gastrointest Liver Physiol 2014;306(4):G310–9.

74. Buffie CG, Bucci V, Stein RR, et al. Precision microbiome reconstitution restores bile acid mediated resistance to Clostridium difficile. Nature 2015;517(7533): 205–8.

75. Moayyedi P, Surette MG, Kim PT, et al. Fecal microbiota transplantation induces remission in patients with active ulcerative colitis in a randomized controlled trial. Gastroenterology 2015;149(1):102–9.e6.

76. Paramsothy S, Kamm MA, Kaakoush NO, et al. Multidonor intensive faecal microbiota transplantation for active ulcerative colitis: a randomised placebo-controlled trial. Lancet 2017;389(10075):1218–28.

77. Costello SP, Waters O, Bryant RV, et al. Short duration, low intensity, pooled fecal microbiota transplantation induces remission in patients with mild-moderately active ulcerative colitis: a randomised controlled trial. Gastroenterology 2017; 152(5):S198–9.

78. Rossen NG, Fuentes S, van der Spek MJ, et al. Findings from a randomized controlled trial of fecal transplantation for patients with ulcerative colitis. Gastroenterology 2015;149(1):110–8.e4.

79. Vermeire S, Joossens M, Verbeke K, et al. Donor species richness determines faecal microbiota transplantation success in inflammatory bowel disease. J Crohn's Colitis 2016;10(4):387–94.

80. Li SS, Zhu A, Benes V, et al. Durable coexistence of donor and recipient strains after fecal microbiota transplantation. Science 2016;352(6285):586–9.

81. Fuentes S, Rossen NG, van der Spek MJ, et al. Microbial shifts and signatures of long-term remission in ulcerative colitis after faecal microbiota transplantation. ISME J 2017;11(8):1877–89.

82. Matson V, Fessler J, Bao R, et al. The commensal microbiome is associated with anti–PD-1 efficacy in metastatic melanoma patients. Science 2018;359(6371): 104–8.

83. Routy B, Le Chatelier E, Derosa L, et al. Gut microbiome influences efficacy of PD-1–based immunotherapy against epithelial tumors. Science 2018; 359(6371):91–7.

84. Vétizou M, Pitt JM, Daillère R, et al. Anticancer immunotherapy by CTLA-4 blockade relies on the gut microbiota. Science 2015;350(6264):1079–84.

85. Daillere R, Vetizou M, Waldschmitt N, et al. Enterococcus hirae and Barnesiella intestinihominis facilitate Cyclophosphamide-induced therapeutic immunomodulatory effects. Immunity 2016;45(4):931–43.

86. Sivan A, Corrales L, Hubert N, et al. Commensal *Bifidobacterium* promotes anti-tumor immunity and facilitates anti–PD-L1 efficacy. Science 2015;350(6264): 1084–9.
87. Zitvogel L, Ma Y, Raoult D, et al. The microbiome in cancer immunotherapy: diagnostic tools and therapeutic strategies. Science 2018;359(6382):1366–70.
88. Turnbaugh PJ, Ley RE, Mahowald MA, et al. An obesity-associated gut microbiome with increased capacity for energy harvest. Nature 2006;444(7122): 1027–31.
89. Le Chatelier E, Nielsen T, Qin J, et al. Richness of human gut microbiome correlates with metabolic markers. Nature 2013;500:541.
90. Ridaura VK, Faith JJ, Rey FE, et al. Gut microbiota from twins discordant for obesity modulate adiposity and metabolic phenotypes in mice. Science 2013; 341(6150). https://doi.org/10.1126/science.1241214.
91. Zeevi D, Korem T, Zmora N, et al. Personalized nutrition by prediction of glycemic responses. Cell 2015;163(5):1079–94.
92. Korem T, Zeevi D, Zmora N, et al. Bread affects clinical parameters and induces gut microbiome-associated personal glycemic responses. Cell Metab 2017; 25(6):1243–53.e5.

Metabolomics and the Microbiome as Biomarkers in Sepsis

Jisoo Lee, MD[a,b,*], Debasree Banerjee, MD, MS[a,b]

KEYWORDS

- Metabolomics • Pharmaco-metabonomics • Microbiome • Gut microbiota
- Dysbiosis • Personalized medicine

KEY POINTS

- Technologic advancements in mass spectrometry offer opportunities to study metabolite profiles using targeted and untargeted approaches.
- Metabolomics provides new ways of exploring the diagnosis, mechanism, and prognosis of sepsis via novel biomarkers.
- The use of pharmaco-metabonomics in predicting drug response may enable patient stratification and precision medicine.
- Microbiome composition changes dramatically in sepsis, as the diversity of microbiota decreases, and potential pathogens become dominant.
- Understanding the complex interactions of the host's metabolomics and microbiome can provide novel preventive and therapeutic strategies against sepsis.

INTRODUCTION

Sepsis remains a clinical challenge to physicians and researchers alike, given its heterogeneity in presentation, from diagnosis, pharmacologic and nonpharmacological interventions, and prognostication. Sepsis is defined as a "life-threatening organ dysfunction due to a dysregulated host response to infection."[1] Decades of research in sepsis has revealed that the pathways and outcomes of sepsis is largely affected by the interactions of 2 factors: the host genetics and environmental factors. Advances in technology have allowed us to delve further into the cellular and subcellular pathologic changes that occur in a septic host. The study of "Omics" comprises genomics, transcriptomics, proteomics, and metabolomics, and refers to the systemic measurement

This article originally appeared in *Critical Care Clinics*, Volume 36, Issue 1, January 2020.
Disclosure Statement: None.
[a] Division of Pulmonary, Critical Care and Sleep Medicine, The Warren Alpert School of Medicine at Brown University, Providence, RI, USA; [b] Division of Pulmonary, Critical Care & Sleep Medicine, Rhode Island Hospital, POB Suite 224, 595 Eddy Street, Providence, RI 02903, USA
* Corresponding author. Division of Pulmonary, Critical Care, & Sleep Medicine, Rhode Island Hospital, POB Suite 224, 595 Eddy Street, Providence, RI 02903.
E-mail address: jisoo_lee@brown.edu

of an entire class of biochemical species at the DNA, RNA, protein, and metabolite levels.[2] The host's genome, transcriptome, and proteome are all reflected in the metabolome, a snapshot of the metabolites in the host at any specific time point during the disease process.[3] Similarly, emerging technologies have allowed more in-depth understanding of environmental factors that influence sepsis outcome, particularly the microbiome and its role in nosocomial and opportunistic infection, a well-described sequelae of sepsis. Metabolomics and the study of the microbiome together provide new possibilities in the quest for personalized medicine in sepsis through the integration of host and environmental factors.

THE DEFINITION OF METABOLOMICS

Metabolomics is the study of the metabolome, which is a collection of small molecules produced by cells that are responsible for metabolic processes in organisms.[4] Metabolomics is a relatively new concept that has appeared in the past decade. Metabolomics, unlike genomics, transcriptomics, and proteomics, serve as direct biomarkers of biochemical activity, and are thus easier to directly correlate with phenotypes.[5]

There are targeted and untargeted approaches to studying the metabolome. The targeted metabolomics studies focus on measuring a specified number of metabolites in the pathway of interest.[5] This approach allows researchers to ask a specific biochemical question based on a hypothesis. Although it is an effective way to obtain deeper insights of a specific hypothesis, the success of the study depends on the strength of preexisting data and knowledge.[6] The untargeted metabolomics, or "global metabolomics," on the other hand, uses an unbiased screening method to identify thousands of metabolites in a single experiment, and thus enables exploratory studies of unknown metabolites.[7] The metabolic profile is then compared in 2 conditions or across a population in order to discover a novel metabolite.[6] The untargeted approach allows a broad and comprehensive inspection into the metabolome. **Fig. 1** describes the workflow of targeted and untargeted approaches of liquid chromatography–mass spectrometry (LC-MS), one of the tools used to identify metabolites from specimens.[5]

Metabolomics is increasingly used in a wide variety of research, such as to identify biomarkers, identify drug activities, or drug-induced toxicity and metabolism.[8] The application of metabolomics in various scientific fields is depicted in **Fig. 2**.[6]

THE PLATFORMS OF METABOLOMICS

There are several platforms that enable metabolomics experiments. In targeted metabolomics, triple quadrupole mass spectrometry is used to target a list of metabolites to be screened for a disease or biochemical pathway.[5] This is a highly sensitive method that enables absolute quantification of low-concentration metabolites.[5] In untargeted metabolomics, platforms such as nuclear magnetic resonance (NMR), gas chromatography-mass spectrometry (GC-MS), and LC-MS are used. Each of these platforms have strengths and weaknesses, as shown in **Table 1**. These platforms are often used in various combinations in experiments.

NMR spectroscopy measures the signals from the nuclei of isotopes of certain atoms, such as hydrogen-1 (^{1}H), and it can elucidate more detailed molecular structures of compounds in the solution state compared with mass spectrometry.[4,7] NMR enables real-time reaction monitoring at controlled temperatures[6]; however, it has lower sensitivity compared with mass spectrometry. Mass spectrometry measures the mass-to-charge ratio of charged molecules or molecular fragments, and identifies the ionized metabolites by separating technology involving gas or liquid

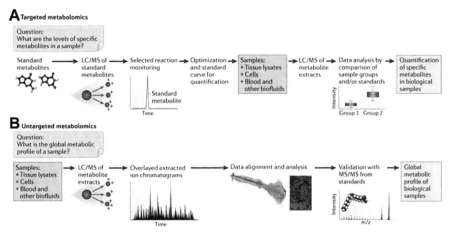

Fig. 1. The targeted and untargeted workflow for LC-MS–based metabolomics. (*A*) Targeted methods are established based on standard metabolites. The metabolites are then extracted from samples such as tissue lysates, cells, or blood and other biofluids. The metabolites are analyzed, and the data output provides quantification of these metabolites by comparing to the previously built standard methods. (*B*) Untargeted method takes the biologic samples, such as tissue lysates, cells, or blood and other biofluids, which are separated using liquid chromatography. These samples are subsequently analyzed by mass spectrometry for data acquisition. The results are processed by bioinformatic software to generate global metabolic profile of biological samples. (*From* Patti GJ, Yanes O, Siuzdak G. Innovation: Metabolomics: the apogee of the omics trilogy. Nat Rev Mol Cell Biol. 2012 Mar 22;13(4):263-9. https://doi.org/10.1038/nrm3314; with permission.)

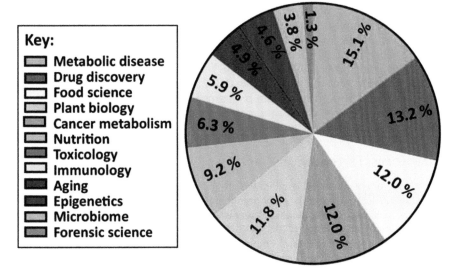

Trends in Biochemical Sciences

Fig. 2. The distribution of recent publications on applications of metabolomics by scientific field. (*From* Liu X, Locasale JW. Metabolomics: A Primer. Trends Biochem Sci. 2017 Apr;42(4):274-284. https://doi.org/10.1016/j.tibs.2017.01.004. Epub 2017 Feb 11; with permission.)

Table 1
Platforms of metabolomics: the mechanism, pros, and cons

	NMR	GC-MS	LC-MS
Mechanism	Measures the signals from the nuclei of isotopes of atoms	Measures the mass-to-charge ratio of charged metabolites; metabolites are separated by gas chromatography	Measures the mass-to-charge ratio of charged molecules; metabolites are separated by liquid chromatography
Pros	• Real-time measurements • Nondestructive • More detailed molecular structures • Quantitative	• Good sensitivity • Broad metabolite detection coverage • Good for analysis of gases or volatile metabolites	• Highest sensitivity • Broad metabolite detection coverage • Easy sample preparation
Cons	• Low sensitivity	• Destructive • Labor-intensive sample preparation • Limited to volatile metabolites • Potential noise from derivatization • Nonquantitative	• Destructive • Limited to organic compounds that form molecular ions • Nonquantitative

Abbreviations: GC-MS, gas chromatography–mass spectrometry; LC-MS, liquid chromatography–mass spectrometry; NMR, nuclear magnetic resonance.

chromatography.[7] GC-MS has good sensitivity, but sample preparation is labor-intensive.[9] Because the use of GC-MS is limited to metabolites that are volatile and stable enough to pass through the heated separation column, some metabolites needs a derivatization process to make them suitable to test.[10] LC-MS has the highest sensitivity with wider metabolite detection coverage, but it is more difficult to identify metabolites compared with NMR or GC-MS[9]; however, LC-MS does not require extraction or derivatization processes like GC-MS.[10] With the advancements of these platforms and metabolomic software programs such as MathDAMP, MetAlign, and MzMine, there has been significant progress in the identification, interpretation, and analysis of massive metabolomic profiles.[5]

METABOLOMICS EXPERIMENTS IN SEPSIS

Early management of sepsis is critical in preventing progression to septic shock and improving mortality. Therefore, early detection is crucial; however, diagnosing sepsis remains a challenge. The diagnosis of sepsis is aided by the presence of microbiologic cultures in the body, but only 30% to 40% of patients with severe sepsis or septic shock yield positive test results.[11] The current understanding of sepsis progression involves various proinflammatory and anti-inflammatory pathways that are activated by a specific pathogen and affect the individual host.[4] Critical illness, such as sepsis, disrupts the metabolomic profile, and identification of these metabolites can lead to useful innovations to detect and treat sepsis.[3]

In humans, serum, plasma and urine samples can be used to study the metabolome. In the article by Su and colleagues,[12] a total of 65 patients (35 patients with sepsis, 15 patients with systemic inflammatory response syndrome [SIRS], and 15 healthy subjects) were studied to identify and differentiate metabolic biomarkers involved in the different stages of sepsis. Patients' serum samples from venipuncture were used to measure metabolites by LC-MS technique. The investigators found that the metabolic profiling of the healthy controls, patients with SIRS, and patients with sepsis were markedly different. Patients with sepsis had significantly lower levels of lactitol dehydrate and S-phenyl-D-cysteine and higher levels of S-(3-methylbuta-noyl)-dihydrolipoamide-E and N-nonanoyl glycine, when compared with patients with SIRS. Although further studies are required for validation, the identification of these metabolites can provide the basis for future study in distinguishing sterile from infected inflammatory responses in patients. This study also showed that 2-phe-nylacetamide, dimethyllysine, glyceryl-phosphoryl-ethanolamine, and D-cysteine were related to the severity of sepsis. Furthermore, 4 metabolites, S-(3-methylbutanoyl)-dihydrolipoamide-E, PG (22:2(13Z,16Z)0:0), glycerophosphocholine, and S-succinyl-glutathione, were elevated within the 48 hours before death, indicating their possible use in predicting mortality.

Another study by Stringer and colleagues[13] used NMR spectroscopy to study the metabolome of patients with sepsis-induced acute lung injury. This study looked at 6 healthy controls and 13 patients with sepsis-induced acute lung injury (ALI), and identified 4 metabolites that were significantly different. Total glutathione associated with oxidant stress, adenosine associated with the loss of ATP homeostasis, phos-phatidylserine associated with apoptosis, were all significantly elevated in the sepsis-induced ALI group compared with the healthy control group. On the other hand, sphingomyelin, which is associated with disruption of endothelial barrier function, was significantly decreased in the sepsis-induced ALI group compared with the healthy control group.

Schmerler and colleagues[14] used targeted metabolomics to identify lipids that could differentiate sepsis from SIRS. The LC-MS platform was used to study a total of 186 metabolites from 6 analyte classes (acylcarnitines, amino acids, biogenic amines, glycerophospholipids, sphingolipids, and carbohydrates) were determined in 74 patients with SIRS and 69 patients with sepsis. This study determined that the activities of acylcarnitine C10:1 and glycerophospholipid PCaaC32:0 were signifi-cantly different in patients with sepsis compared with patients with SIRS. Using the 2 markers, C10:1 and PCaaC32:0, the investigators were able to correctly classify SIRS and sepsis in 80% of patients in the training set and 70% of patients in the test set for validation.

METABOLOMICS IN THERAPEUTIC OUTCOMES OF SEPSIS

Metabolomics has been widely explored in evaluating therapeutic outcomes. Drug ef-fects are widely varied in individuals, which is determined not only by the genetic vari-ation but also by environmental influences such as nutritional status, gut microbiota, age, illness, and drug-drug interactions.[10] Although pharmacogenomics has led to significant improvements in correlating drugs responses with host genetic polymor-phisms,[15] pharmacogenomics does not take environmental factors into account. The "pharmaco-metabonomic" approach is defined as "the prediction of the outcome of a drug or xenobiotic intervention in an individual based on a mathematical model of pre-intervention metabolite signatures."[10] The pharmaco-metabonomics has the po-tential to identify metabolites that could predict responses of clinical drugs based on the individual's baseline metabolic profile. Furthermore, comparing the metabolic pro-files of an individual's pretreatment and posttreatment can reveal novel drug mecha-nisms and their metabolic pathways.[8] The advancements in the metabolomics and pharmaco-metabonomics may lead to tailored therapy, enabling optimization of therapeutic outcome.[7]

The clinical application of pharmaco-metabonomics is exemplified by a study by Clayton and colleagues.[16] In this study, ^{1}H NMR spectroscopy was used to compare the urinary metabolite profiles in 99 healthy male volunteers before and after a standard dose of acetaminophen. The investigators found that elevated levels of predose *para*-cresol sulfate was associated with decreased postdose ratios of acetaminophen sulfate to acetaminophen glucuronide. *Para*-cresol is thought to originate from bacteria in the gut microbiome, and thus the investigators conclude that individual's gut microbiome with different levels of *para*-cresol leads to different systemic effect of acetaminophen. This illustrates how pharmaco-metabonomics enables deeper insight into the interplay of metabolomics and microbiome in the efficacy of drug treatment.

Despite recent advancements of technologies enabling rapid and efficient profiling of the metabolome, there are many limitations of metabolomics at this time, which include lack of validation, limited clinical experience and research data, and dearth of standardized technologies and software used as a gold standard for the study of the metabolome.

MICROBIOME IN SEPSIS

Although metabolomics increases the depth of understanding of the host's response to disease, understanding its relationship with environmental factors (ie, microbiome) is equally crucial in developing targeted therapies. The microbiome of an individual changes according to the severity of the illness.[17] It has been shown that when the diverse and balanced gut microbiota is disturbed, it leads to altered host immunity to pathogens, causing increased susceptibility of sepsis.[18] This is described as "dysbiosis," which is a state that the composition and diversity of microbiome is distorted.[19]

Dysbiosis of the gut microbiome affects sepsis outcomes. The upper gastrointestinal (GI) tract becomes a reservoir of pathogens, such as *Escherichia coli, Pseudomonas aeruginosa, Enterococcus*, as it loses acidity for protective microbiomes.[17] In the lower GI tract, the diversity of the microbiome decreases, and the intestinal mucus layer is thinned and disrupted and allows for pathogens to grow in abundance.[17] The bacterial content of the gut determines the severity of systemic injury in sepsis. The inflammation and injury sustained by organs is lessened when the bacterial burden is lowered. Lowering bacterial burden is done primarily by defecation, however this process is slowed in critical illness due to disturbances of glucose and electrolyte levels, endogenous opioid production, as well as by therapeutic interventions such as sedatives, opioids, and catecholamines.[17]

The respiratory microbiome is also severely altered in patients with sepsis. The oropharyngeal microbes migrate to the lungs in critical illness, and the pathogenic bacteria of the oropharynx such as *Klebsiella pneumoniae, Pseudomonas aeruginosa* and Proteobacteria increase the risk of infection in the lungs.[17,20] Normal lungs are usually not a favorable place for microbes given the lack of nutrition and presence of a lipid-rich surfactant.[17] As the alveoli become filled with oropharyngeal microbes, the lungs become a reservoir and source of nutrition for the pathogens to disrupt the systemic immunity. Furthermore, during lung injury from critical illness such as sepsis or acute respiratory distress syndrome, the surfactant becomes inactivated, mucociliary clearance is impaired, and the influx of edema creates steep oxygen gradients, which all help facilitate bacterial growth.[17,21–23] Thus, in the lungs in critical illness, there is increased migration of microbiota from the gut to the lungs, decreased elimination, and increased growth of potential pathogens. Molecular stress signals from catecholamines and inflammatory cytokines also increase the likelihood of the growth of pathogens. Increased alveolar catecholamine concentrations were shown to correlate with the disruption of microbiome in human bronchoalveolar lavage samples, thus creating dominant species, such as *Pseudomonas aeruginosa*, *Streptococcus pneumoniae*, *Staphylococcus aureus*, and *Klebsiella pneumoniae*.[17]

Microbiota of patients alter significantly with disease severity and pharmacologic and nonpharmacological interventions and procedures done to the patient. Understanding the relationships of microbiota and host resistance can lead to significant innovations to preventive and therapeutic strategies against sepsis.

MICROBIOME MODULATION IN SEPSIS MANAGEMENT

There are attempts to use microbiome modulation for sepsis management in several stages; prevention, treatment, and recovery.[18] In a systemic review and meta-analysis of 30 trials of 2972 patients,[24] it showed that probiotics were associated with reduced infection. The study also noted a reduction in the incidence of ventilator-associated pneumonia, but did not see any effect on mortality, length of stay, or diarrhea.

Synbiotics, which is "a combination of probiotics and prebiotics: dietary components that enhance the growth of these species," is a promising therapy to restore dysbiosis.[19] A randomized, double-blinded placebo-controlled trial in rural India looked at more than 4500 infants at least 35 weeks of gestation without signs of sepsis or other morbidity and administered oral symbiotic preparation of *Lactobacillus plantarum* and a fructooligosaccharide versus placebo.[25] Administration of the symbiotic preparation resulted in a significant reduction in the primary outcome (the combination of sepsis and death). This study also showed that the treatment group had significantly reduced incidence of lower respiratory tract infections, as well as culture-positive and culture-negative sepsis.

Decolonization strategies, such as selective decolonization of the digestive tract (SDD), selective oropharyngeal decontamination (SOD), and topical oropharyngeal chlorhexidine were studied to determine its effect on mortality.[26] SDD uses nonabsorbable antibiotics, such as polymyxin, tobramycin, and amphotericin, that are applied as a paste during routine mouth care, in combination with a short course of intravenous antibiotics.[26] SOD applies the antibiotic paste to the oropharynx only without empirical intravenous antibiotics. The systemic review and meta-analysis of Price and colleagues[26] revealed that SDD and SOD had favorable effects on mortality in adults patients in the intensive care units, however chlorhexidine was associated with increased mortality.

Fecal microbiota transplantation (FMT) is another means of trying to regain homeostasis of the microbiome and is commonly used in recurrent *Clostridium difficile* infection. Its use has been expanded and explored in the treatment of diarrhea and sepsis as well. A case report from China showed that FMT was successful in treating septic shock and diarrhea in a 44-year-old woman who presented with polymicrobial septic shock in the setting of severe watery diarrhea.[27] The analysis of patient's fecal microbiota before FMT showed significant intestinal microbiota dysbiosis with dominant pathogenic Proteobacteria. After the FMT, there was a significant modification in the patient's microbiota, with enrichment of commensal Firmicutes and depletion of opportunistic Proteobacteria and thus restoring the disrupted microbiota. Another ongoing study is aiming to find the efficacy of auto-FMT for prevention of infection in a cohort of patients receiving allo-hematopoietic cell transplantation (clinicaltrials.gov: NCT02269150).

SUMMARY

Although there have been significant improvements in sepsis management and outcomes, understanding the pathophysiology and mechanism of sepsis progression as well as attempts to personalize sepsis treatment remain a big challenge. Metabolomics provides a unique approach to study the impact of sepsis on the host's metabolite profiles at specific time points during illness. Furthermore, the dysbiosis caused in the host's microbiome severely affects the host's vulnerability to pathogens and thus the severity of sepsis. With new technologies to better identify and study novel biomarkers in metabolomics and study interventions for modulating the microbiome, these fields are emerging areas of interest and show promise for ways to diagnose and treat sepsis.

REFERENCES

1. Shankar-Hari M, Phillips GS, Levy ML, et al. Developing a new definition and assessing new clinical criteria for septic shock: for the third international consensus definitions for sepsis and septic shock (Sepsis-3). Jama 2016;315:775–87.
2. Itenov TS, Murray DD, Jensen JUS. Sepsis: personalized medicine utilizing 'omic' technologies-a paradigm shift? Healthcare (Basel) 2018;6:1–9.
3. Beloborodova NV, Olenin AY, Pautova AK. Metabolomic findings in sepsis as a damage of host-microbial metabolism integration. J Crit Care 2018;43:246–55.
4. Ludwig KR, Hummon AB. Mass spectrometry for the discovery of biomarkers of sepsis. Mol Biosyst 2017;13:648–64.
5. Patti GJ, Yanes O, Siuzdak G. Innovation: metabolomics: the apogee of the omics trilogy. Nat Rev Mol Cell Biol 2012;13:263–9.
6. Liu X, Locasale JW. Metabolomics: a primer. Trends Biochem Sci 2017;42: 274–84.
7. Everett JR. Pharmacometabonomics in humans: a new tool for personalized medicine. Pharmacogenomics 2015;16:737–54.
8. Vincent JL, Brealey D, Libert N, et al. Rapid diagnosis of infection in the critically ill, a multicenter study of molecular detection in bloodstream infections, pneumonia, and sterile site infections. Crit Care Med 2015;43:2283–91.
9. Li B, He X, Jia W, et al. Novel applications of metabolomics in personalized medicine: a mini-review. Molecules 2017;22:2–10.
10. Clayton TA, Lindon JC, Cloarec O, et al. Pharmaco-metabonomic phenotyping and personalized drug treatment. Nature 2006;440:1073–7.
11. Levy MM, Fink MP, Marshall JC, et al. 2001 SCCM/ESICM/ACCP/ATS/SIS international sepsis definitions conference. Crit Care Med 2003;31:1250–6.
12. Su L, Huang Y, Zhu Y, et al. Discrimination of sepsis stage metabolic profiles with an LC/MS-MS-based metabolomics approach. BMJ Open Respir Res 2014;1: e000056.
13. Stringer KA, Serkova NJ, Karnovsky A, et al. Metabolic consequences of sepsis-induced acute lung injury revealed by plasma (1)H-nuclear magnetic resonance quantitative metabolomics and computational analysis. Am J Physiol Lung Cell Mol Physiol 2011;300. L4–I11.
14. Schmerler D, Neugebauer S, Ludewig K, et al. Targeted metabolomics for discrimination of systemic inflammatory disorders in critically ill patients. J Lipid Res 2012;53:1369–75.
15. Weinshilboum R, Wang L. Pharmacogenomics: bench to bedside. Nat Rev Drug Discov 2004;3:739–48.

16. Clayton TA, Baker D, Lindon JC, et al. Pharmacometabonomic identification of a significant host-microbiome metabolic interaction affecting human drug metabolism. Proc Natl Acad Sci U S A 2009;106:14728–33.
17. Dickson RP. The microbiome and critical illness. Lancet Respir Med 2016;4: 59–72.
18. Haak BW, Prescott HC, Wiersinga WJ. Therapeutic potential of the gut microbiota in the prevention and treatment of sepsis. Front Immunol 2018;9:2042.
19. Haak BW, Levi M, Wiersinga WJ. Microbiota-targeted therapies on the intensive care unit. Curr Opin Crit Care 2017;23:167–74.
20. Johanson WG, Pierce AK, Sanford JP. Changing pharyngeal bacterial flora of hospitalized patients. Emergence of gram-negative bacilli. N Engl J Med 1969; 281:1137–40.
21. Gunther A, Siebert C, Schmidt R, et al. Surfactant alterations in severe pneumonia, acute respiratory distress syndrome, and cardiogenic lung edema. Am J Respir Crit Care Med 1996;153:176–84.
22. Nakagawa NK, Franchini ML, Driusso P, et al. Mucociliary clearance is impaired in acutely ill patients. Chest 2005;128:2772–7.
23. Albenberg L, Esipova TV, Judge CP, et al. Correlation between intraluminal oxygen gradient and radial partitioning of intestinal microbiota. Gastroenterology 2014;147:1055–63.e8.
24. Manzanares W, Lemieux M, Langlois PL, et al. Probiotic and synbiotic therapy in critical illness: a systematic review and meta-analysis. Crit Care 2016;19:262.
25. Panigrahi P, Parida S, Nanda NC, et al. A randomized synbiotic trial to prevent sepsis among infants in rural India. Nature 2017;548:407–12.
26. Price R, MacLennan G, Glen J. Selective digestive or oropharyngeal decontamination and topical oropharyngeal chlorhexidine for prevention of death in general intensive care: systematic review and network meta-analysis. BMJ 2014;348: g2197.
27. Li Q, Wang C, Tang C, et al. Successful treatment of severe sepsis and diarrhea after vagotomy utilizing fecal microbiota transplantation: a case report. Crit Care 2015;19:37.

Precision Medicine in Pediatric Oncology

Kieuhoa T. Vo, MD, MAS[a], D. Williams Parsons, MD, PhD[b],
Nita L. Seibel, MD[c],*

KEYWORDS

- Genomic profiling • Next-generation sequencing • Pediatric cancer
- Precision medicine • Targeted therapy

KEY POINTS

- The ultimate goal of precision medicine in pediatric oncology is to develop more effective and less toxic therapies in children, adolescents, and young adults with cancer.
- Precision clinical trials designed to assess the impact of molecularly targeted therapies in pediatric oncology are ongoing in the United States and Europe.
- Our understanding of the cancer genomic landscape, advancement in genomic technologies, and drug development in enhanced targeted therapies, may lead to future opportunities for precision medicine in pediatric oncology.

INTRODUCTION

Dramatic improvements in clinical outcomes have been seen for children and adolescents with cancer over the past 5 decades.[1] The improvement in survival is attributed primarily to risk-stratification of therapies and treatment intensification with cytotoxic chemotherapy and multimodal approaches. However, accelerating the progress of pediatric oncology requires both therapeutic advances and attention to diminishing the late effects of standard cytotoxic therapies. The ultimate goal of precision medicine in pediatric oncology is to develop more effective and less toxic therapies in children, adolescents, and young adults with cancer. With

This article originally appeared in *Surgical Oncology Clinics*, Volume 29, Issue 1, January 2020.
Disclosure: D.W. Parsons is the co-inventor on current and pending patents related to cancer genes discovered through sequencing of several adult cancer types and participates in royalty sharing related to those patents. The other authors have nothing to disclose.
[a] Department of Pediatrics, University of California San Francisco School of Medicine, Benioff Children's Hospital, 550 16th Street, 4th Floor, Box 0434, San Francisco, CA 94158, USA;
[b] Section of Hematology/Oncology, Department of Pediatrics, Baylor College of Medicine, Texas Children's Hospital, 1102 Bates Avenue, Suite 1030.15, Houston, TX 77030, USA; [c] Division of Cancer Treatment and Diagnosis, Clinical Investigations Branch, National Cancer Institute, 9609 Medical Center Drive, 5W340, MSC9737, Bethesda, MD 20892, USA
* Corresponding author. National Cancer Institute, 9609 Medical Center Drive, 5W340, MSC9737, Bethesda, MD 20892, USA.
E-mail address: Seibelnl@mail.nih.gov

the advancement in diagnostic and molecular profiling technologies, precision medicine trials using clinical molecular testing are becoming more common for adult malignancies. Similarly, there is an interest in how these technologies can be applied to tumors in children and adolescents to expand our understanding of the biology of pediatric cancers and evaluate the clinical implications of genomic testing for these patients, with the ultimate goal of improving survival for pediatric malignancies. This article reviews the early studies in pediatric oncology showing the feasibility of this approach, describes future plans to evaluate the clinical implications in multicenter clinical trials, and identifies the challenges of applying genomics in the patient population.

Feasibility of Precision Medicine in Pediatric Oncology

Biomarker-driven directed therapies have been used in pediatric oncology; however, combining this treatment approach with individualized genomic analysis is in its nascent phase.[2–4] Over the last 5 years, several pediatric oncology studies have explored the feasibility and use of genomics-driven precision medicine and provided the foundation for pursuing this approach. These pilot studies have explored different features of precision medicine and used various study designs, including patient population, timing of specimen acquisition, and inclusion of routine germline analysis. Of note, none of the published studies included prospective treatment arms as part of the study, although several studies include clinical follow-up to assess therapy response and outcomes to genomics-based recommendations.

The Baylor College of Medicine Advancing Sequencing in Childhood Cancer Care study completed enrollment of a primary cohort of 287 newly diagnosed and previously untreated patients with solid, including central nervous system (CNS), tumors.[5] Whole-exome sequencing (WES) was performed both on tumor samples and peripheral blood. In the report of the first 150 patients (<18 years), in whom 121 tumors were sequenced, 33 patients (27%) were found to have somatic mutations of established or potential clinical use. An additional 24 patients (20%) were found to have mutations in consensus cancer genes that were not classified as targetable. Diagnostic germline findings related to patient phenotype (either cancer or other diseases or both) were discovered in 15 (10%) of 150 cases, including 13 (8.6%) with pathogenic or likely pathogenic mutations in known cancer susceptibility genes. Treatment decisions or recommendations were not part of this study.

The University of Michigan Pediatric Michigan Oncology Sequencing study is modeled after the sequencing experience in adults with cancer.[6] The preliminary results of a cohort of 102 pediatric and young adult participants (25 years and younger) with refractory or relapsed cancer and newly diagnosed patients with high-risk or rare cancer types have been published.[6] Patients with both hematopoietic malignancies and solid tumors were included. A total of 91 patients underwent genomic analyses with WES of tumor and germline DNA, as well as RNA sequencing (RNA-seq) of tumor. A multidisciplinary tumor board provided clinical recommendations. They identified 42 patients (46%) with potentially actionable findings that were not identified by standard diagnostic tests, which did not include sequencing. Nine of the patients had germline findings, 10 had somatic actionable gene fusions found through RNA-seq, and 2 had their diagnosis changed because of the analyses. A total of 23 patients had an individualized care decision made based on either tumor or germline sequencing results. Fourteen of the patients had a change in therapy, 9 underwent genetic counseling, and 1 required both. Of the 14 patients, 9 had a clinical response to the change in therapy lasting more than 6 months. The median turnaround time for return of the results was 54 days.

The individualized cancer therapy (iCAT) study is a multicenter study led by investigators at the Dana-Farber Cancer Institute/Boston Children's Hospital to assess the feasibility of identifying actionable alterations and making individualized cancer therapy recommendations in pediatric and young adult patients (30 years and younger) with relapsed, refractory, or high-risk extracranial solid tumors.[7] A multidisciplinary expert panel reviewed the profiling results, and iCAT treatment recommendations were made if an actionable alteration was present, and an appropriate drug was available. Of the 100 participants, 31 had tumor submitted only from diagnosis, whereas the rest had tumor submitted from recurrence or local control or multiple specimens from recurrence and diagnosis. Tumor profiling was successful in specimens from 89 patients. Overall, 31 (31%) patients received an iCAT treatment recommendation and 3 received matched therapy. There were 0no objective responses. Three patients had a change in their diagnosis based on the tumor profiling. Six patients had an actionable alteration, but an appropriate drug was not available through a clinical trial or as a Food and Drug Administration (FDA)-approved therapy with an age-appropriate dose and formulation, and so an iCAT recommendation could not be made. Finally, 43 (43%) participants had results with potential clinical significance but not resulting in iCAT treatment recommendations were identified, including mutations indicating the possible presence of a cancer predisposition syndrome (if also found in the germline).

The Precision in Pediatric Sequencing Program at Columbia University Medical Center instituted a prospective clinical next-generation sequencing (NGS) for high-risk pediatric cancer and hematologic disorders.[8] WES and RNA-seq were performed on tumor and normal tissue from 101 high-risk pediatric patients. Results were initially reviewed by a molecular pathologist and subsequently by a multidisciplinary molecular tumor board. Potentially actionable alterations were identified in 38% of patients, of which 16% subsequently received matched therapy. In an additional 38% of patients, the genomic data provided clinically relevant information of diagnostic, prognostic, or pharmacogenomic significance. RNA-seq was clinically impactful in 37 of 65 patients (57%), providing diagnostic and/or prognostic information for 17 patients (26%) and identified therapeutic targets in 15 patients (23%). Known or likely pathogenic germline alterations were discovered in 18 of 90 patients (20%), with 14% having germline alternations in cancer predisposition genes. American College of Medical Genetics secondary findings were identified in 6 patients.

The Individualized Therapy for Relapsed Malignancies in Childhood project is a nationwide German program for children and young adults with refractory, relapsed cancers, which aims to identify therapeutic targets on an individualized basis.[9] In the report of the pilot phase, 57 patients aged 1 to 40 years with hematopoietic and solid malignancies were enrolled. Seven patients for whom no standard therapy was available were enrolled at the time of primary diagnosis. Tumor specimens were analyzed by WES, low-coverage whole-genome, and RNA-seq, as well as methylation and expression microarray analyses. A customized 7-step scoring algorithm was used to prioritize molecular targets and reviewed by an interdisciplinary molecular tumor board before returning the results to the treating physician. Germline DNA was screened on each patient for damaging alterations in a predefined list of known cancer predisposition genes. Turnaround time was 28 days. Of 52 patients, 26 (50%) with NGS data on their tumors harbored a potentially actionable alteration with a prioritization score of intermediate or higher. Ten patients received targeted therapy based on these results, with responses seen in some of the previously treated patients, although systematic follow-up was not an objective of this study. Underlying cancer predisposition was detected in 2 patients (4%). Comparative primary tumor–

relapsed tumor analysis revealed substantial tumor evolution in addition to detection in one case of an unsuspected secondary malignancy.

The Institut Curie reported their 1-year experience of genetic analysis and molecular biology tumor board discussions for targeted therapies in pediatric solid tumors.[10] Tumor tissue from 60 pediatric patients (aged up to 21.5 years) with poor prognosis or relapsed or refractory solid, including CNS, tumors were analyzed with panel-based NGS and array comparative genomic hybridization. The most recently available tumor tissue was analyzed but, where there was inadequate material, a new biopsy was not requested and the initial diagnostic biopsy specimen was used. Recommendations from the molecular biology tumor board were given to the treating physicians. The mean turnaround time from patient referral to the molecular biology tumor board and release of results was 42 ± 16 days. Of the 58 patients in whom molecular profiling was feasible, 23 (40%) had a potentially actionable finding with high-grade gliomas having the highest number of targetable alterations. Of the 23 patients, 6 received a matched targeted therapy, with 5 being enrolled in a clinical trial and 1 by compassionate use. Two patients had a partial response. Despite having a targetable lesion, 4 patients could not receive therapy owing to lack of available clinical trials with the agents. The remaining 13 patients did not receive targeted therapy because of pursuit of conventional chemotherapy or change in health status. The investigators concluded that this approach is feasible, but only a small proportion of patients were able to receive the targeted therapy.

A single-institutional feasibility study (MOSCATO-01) at Gustave Roussy in France prospectively characterized genomic alterations in recurrent or refractory solid tumors of pediatric patients for selection of targeted therapy. Seventy-five patients underwent tumor biopsy or surgical resection of primary or metastatic tumor site on study. Tumor samples were analyzed by comparative genomic hybridization array NGS for 75 target genes, WES, and RNA-seq. Biological significance of the alterations and recommendation of targeted therapies available were discussed in a multidisciplinary tumor board. All patients were pretreated, 37% had CNS tumors, and 63% had an extracranial solid tumor. Successful molecular analysis in 69 patients detected an actionable alteration in various oncogenic pathways in 61% of patients, and a change in diagnosis was seen in 3 patients. Fourteen patients received 17 targeted therapies. This study demonstrated the feasibility of research biopsies in advanced pediatric malignancies for NGS and matching potential actionable mutations with targeted therapies.

These initial pilot studies demonstrated the feasibility of clinical sequencing for patients with childhood cancers and set the stage for subsequent precision medicine trials that prospectively assess the impact of molecularly targeted therapies in pediatric oncology. Our evolving understanding of the landscape of the cancer genome of pediatric cancers also necessitates the inclusion of unique genomic technologies, such as RNA analysis for fusion detection, and analyses of germline mutations for cancer susceptibility risk determination in forthcoming studies.

National Cancer Institute-Children's Oncology Group Pediatric Molecular Analysis for Therapeutic Choice: New Era of Precision Medicine in Pediatric Oncology

In collaboration with, and supported by, the National Cancer Institute (NCI), the Children's Oncology Group (COG) is leveraging the information gained from earlier precision medicine studies a step further in their design of a histology agnostic trial in which eligibility to treatment arms is determined based on predefined lists of genomic aberration(s), or actionable mutation(s) of interest (aMOI). Pediatric MATCH (Molecular Analysis for Therapeutic Choice) is a national clinical trial under a single IND (NCT03155620; **Fig. 1**). Relapsed tumor tissue from pediatric and young adult patients

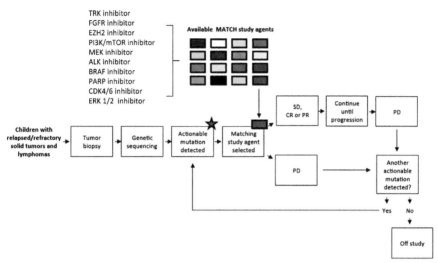

Fig. 1. NCI-COG Pediatric Molecular Analysis for Therapeutic Choice (MATCH) trial schema. ALK, anaplastic lymphoma kinase; CR, complete response; ERK, extracellular signal-regulated kinase; EZH2, enhancer of zeste homolog 2; FGFR, fibroblast growth factor receptor; PARP, poly-ADP ribose polymerase; PD, progressive disease; PI3K/mTOR, phosphoinositide 3-kinase/mammalian target of rapamycin; PR, partial response; SD, stable disease; TRK, tyrosine receptor kinase. (*From* Allen CE, Laetsch TW, Mody R, et al. Target and Agent Prioritization for the Children's Oncology Group-National Cancer Institute Pediatric MATCH Trial. *J Natl Cancer Inst.* 2017;109(5); with permission.)

with recurrent or refractory tumors including CNS tumors, as well as lymphomas and histiocytic disorders, is submitted for molecular profiling. To provide broader access to precision medicine trials for the adolescent and young adult oncology population, patients aged up to of 21 years are eligible to enroll on Pediatric MATCH.

Similar to the NCI MATCH study for adults, if an aberration is identified that has been defined as a driver mutation for a Pediatric MATCH study drug targeting the identified aberration, then the patient will have the opportunity to enroll onto the relevant single-agent treatment arm. Consequently, the trial is providing access to the study agent(s) for each patient in addition to tumor genomic analysis and treatment assignment. This trial will screen over 1000 patients for multiple targets and evaluate investigational targeted therapies for clinical activity in patients carrying specific mutations that can inform future trials. This is the largest pediatric oncology trial for all solid tumors to identify the molecular aberration(s) in the tumor and provide the investigational agent for the treatment of the identified molecular aberrations within the same trial. Similar to the NCI MATCH study for adults, Pediatric MATCH uses an analytically validated NGS-targeted assay of more than 4000 different mutations (single nucleotide variants, indels, copy-number alterations, and gene fusions) across more than 140 genes.[11] This type of basket or umbrella hybrid trial uses a rules-based treatment assignment, based on available preclinical and clinical data, which has not been used in the other pediatric trials.[12] This offers the advantage of predefining treatment based on the presence of a molecular aberration, ensures availability of agents within the context of a trial, and negates assignment bias because all patients with a predefined aMOI are assigned a given treatment.

The primary aims of the study are to determine the objective response rate in pediatric patients with advanced solid tumors and lymphomas harboring a priori specified genomic alterations treated with pathway-targeting agents, and to determine the proportion of pediatric patients whose tumors have pathway alterations that can be targeted by existing anticancer drugs. A total of 20 patients will be enrolled per treatment arm (or stratum within the arm) depending on the aMOIs, and the agent will be considered of interest for further development if 3 or more patients of 20 show a response. The arms may be expanded in the trial to enroll additional patients if activity is seen for a particular agent. The study will have the flexibility to open and close arms. A patient's tumor that progresses while on treatment will be eligible to go on another treatment arm if the tumor has additional genetic aberrations that are being targeted with another Pediatric MATCH agent.

The molecular targets and study drugs selected for the trial were identified and prioritized by the Pediatric MATCH Target and Agent Prioritization (TAP) committee consisting of representatives from COG disease committees from 10 children's hospitals, the NCI, and the FDA. The TAP committee systematically reviewed target and agent pairs for inclusion in the Pediatric MATCH trial. Criteria used to prioritize the target and agent pairs included the frequency of the alterations in the target in pediatric malignancies, the strength of the evidence linking the target to the activity of the agent, whether the target can be detected with the testing platform, clinical and preclinical evidence for the specific agent, and other ongoing or planned biomarker-defined clinical studies. Details of this process have been described previously.[13] Two criteria established for identifying specific agents to be considered for inclusion in Pediatric MATCH were demonstrated activity against tumors with a particular genomic alteration, and the establishment of an adult-recommended phase 2 dose. The same levels of evidence for drug selection used in NCI MATCH were applied for Pediatric MATCH.[11] Neither a completed pediatric phase 1 study nor a pediatric formulation was required to be considered for Pediatric MATCH trial. However, in the case of an oral agent, appropriately sized capsules or tablets were required to dose pediatric patients. Currently, the Pediatric MATCH trial has opened 10 treatment arms with the goal of investigating a total of 15 to 20 single agents based on ongoing review of new data and as agents become available based on the identified targets.

In a report of the first 422 patients enrolled from 93 COG sites on the Pediatric MATCH screening protocol, the median age is 13 years (range 1–21).[14] A tumor sample was submitted for 390 patients, sequencing was attempted for 370 patients (95%), and results were confirmed for 357 patients (92%). The median turnaround time for the tumor genomic results was 15 days. An aMOI for at least one of the 10 current treatment arms was identified in approximately 25% of patients with tumor submitted for the Pediatric MATCH screening protocol. These patients are assigned to a treatment arm and must meet the eligibility criteria to enroll on therapy.

There are some notable differences for Pediatric MATCH compared with NCI MATCH or similar precision medicine protocols. The number of molecular aberrations seen in pediatric tumors (∼10%) is predicted to be much less than identified in adult malignancies.[15,16] These projections are based primarily on actionable mutation frequencies in newly diagnosed tumors. However, the Pediatric MATCH aMOI detection rate is currently higher than predicted.[14] In comparison, this Pediatric MATCH aMOI detection rate is higher than the match rate of for NCI MATCH for the first 10 treatment arms (approximately 9%).[11] One reason for this may be that patients with known targetable mutations from previous molecular testing are enrolling on the screening study at a higher rate on Pediatric MATCH. In addition, the Pediatric MATCH study is optimizing the chances of finding a targetable aberration in a patient's tumor by requiring the submission of tumor specimen from a biopsy done after recurrence or progression and as close to the time of genomic analysis, because tumors are likely to acquire more mutations over time.[17–20] In fact, in some studies in adults, it is recommended that a metastatic (as opposed to primary) lesion is biopsied.[21,22] To provide access for as many children and adolescents as possible, and because the risks associated with biopsies in children differ from adults, there is more flexibility with the timing of the biopsy (need not be obtained just before study enrollment as long as it is from a recurrence) or in the case of brain stem gliomas from the time of diagnosis in the Pediatric MATCH study. Finally, although tumors occurring in adults may have a larger number of mutations (on average), many of those mutations are passenger mutations that have been acquired over time and that may have little relevance to the biology (or treatment) of the tumor. Thus, the number of targetable mutations might be more similar in children and adults than initially projected based on total number of mutations.

Pediatric cancers harbor a different spectrum and frequency of mutations compared with adult cancers. For example, frequent targetable kinase alterations seen in lung cancer and breast cancer, such as EGFR and HER2, respectively, rarely occur in pediatric tumors. Therefore, such agents would not meet the selection criteria as treatment arms in Pediatric MATCH. Drug availability is another challenge, because agents are not yet available to target many of the recurrent aberrations identified in pediatric tumors. Based on the small number of pediatric cancers, and even smaller subgroups of molecular aberrations identified in the tumors, agents have not been developed to target some of the detectable molecular aberrations, such as epigenetic alterations.

Similar to several of the pediatric studies described earlier, germline DNA is collected and analyzed from all patients enrolled on Pediatric MATCH. In contrast, NCI MATCH does not evaluate germline molecular aberrations. By including germline analysis using the same panel as for tumor sequencing, it is possible to determine which mutations are of interest and which actionable mutations of interest represent germline variants in cancer susceptibility genes. Clinical genomics laboratories interpret the germline findings and provide a report back to the treating oncologist identifying whether any of the genomic aberrations included in the tumor sequencing report represent pathogenic or likely pathogenic germline variants in cancer susceptibility genes. The results of the germline analysis are not used for treatment assignment and are not meant to provide a comprehensive cancer susceptibility evaluation. However, based on the results, the treating pediatric oncologist may recommend formal genetic testing and counseling for the patient/family.

Other Precision Medicine Trials in Pediatric Oncology

There is a similar precision medicine initiative for the conduct of a genomically driven basket study for children and adolescents with relapsed or refractory cancers in Europe. The European Proof-of-Concept Therapeutic Stratification Trial of Molecular Anomalies in Relapsed or Refractory Tumors in Children uses genomic data derived from multiple panels from several ongoing sequencing studies in Europe.[23] In contrast to Pediatric MATCH, which uses predefined levels of evidence linking variants to targeted therapies, sequencing data are reviewed at a multidisciplinary molecular tumor board to determine whether an actionable variant is present and whether the variant is a match for one of the ESMART treatment arms or other targeted agent trials. At present, ESMART has 7 treatment arms for 5 genomic targets/pathways. Each of the treatment arms are conducted as individual clinical trials, with a phase 1 dose escalation phase and a phase 2 expansion phase. In contrast to Pediatric MATCH, which thus far includes only single agents, many of the treatment arms in ESMART combines targeted agents with chemotherapy.

The initial results for the European pediatric precision medicine initiative have been reported.[24] From 2016 to 2017, 174 patients with a median age of 13 years (range, 1–32) were included in the European molecular profiling trial (MAPPYACTS). Currently, the analysis for 104 patients has been completed. Seventy-six percent of patients had at least one "actionable" variant. Based on the detected alteration, 21 patients were included in the ESMART trial since it opened in August 2016, with 2 patients enrolling on 2 different treatment arms: CDK4/6 inhibitor ribociclib plus chemotherapy (1) or everolimus (5); DNA repair interfering combinations WEE1 inhibitor AZD1775 plus chemotherapy (4) and PARP inhibitor olaparib plus chemotherapy (1); dual mammalian target of rapamycin inhibitor vistusertib alone (1) or with chemotherapy (5); or nivolumab and cyclophosphamide (6).[24]

Umbrella trials focusing on specific diseases or histologies in pediatric oncology are currently underway in patients with relapsed and refractory or newly diagnosed cancers. These studies require a good understanding of the gene variants to be encountered in a specific diagnosis and its activity to targeted agents. Moreover, the feasibility of conducting these studies requires that the frequency of variants is sufficient to justify a clinical trial within a disease group. Examples of these studies are shown in **Table 1**.

A major challenge with these precision medicine clinical trials is that the treatment regimens are tailored to an increasingly smaller subset of genomically defined

Table 1
Examples of the range of precision medicine trials in pediatric oncology

Study Design	Clinical Trial	Sponsor	NCT
Relapsed or refractory cancers			
Basket studies across multiple histologies	Pediatric MATCH	NCI-COG	
	AcSé-ESMART	Gustave Roussey	NCT02813135
Histology-specific umbrella studies	NEPENTHE (neuroblastoma)	CHOP	NCT02780128
	Ruxolitinib or Dasatinib + chemotherapy in Ph-like ALL	MD Anderson	NCT02420717
	RELPALL (ALL)	St. Jude	NCT03515200
Newly diagnosed cancers			
Histology-specific umbrella studies	Dasatinib + chemotherapy for Ph-like ALL	COG	NCT02883049
	Ruxolitinib + chemotherapy for CRLF2/JAK/STAT mutations in ALL	COG	NCT02723994
	Crizotinib + chemotherapy in ALK aberrant neuroblastoma	COG	NCT03126916
	Total therapy XVII JAK/STAT mutations in ALL/lymphoma	St. Jude	NCT03117751
	Clinical/Molecular Risk-Directed Therapy in Medulloblastoma	St. Jude	NCT01878617
	BIOMEDE (DIPG)	Gustave Roussy	NCT02233049

Abbreviations: AcSé-ESMART, European Proof-of-Concept Therapeutic Stratification Trial of Molecular Anomalies in Relapsed or Refractory Tumors; ALK, anaplastic lymphoma kinase; ALL, acute lymphoblastic leukemia; CHOP, Children's Hospital of Philadelphia; COG, Children's Oncology Group; DIPG, diffuse intrinsic pontine glioma; NCT, ClinicalTrials.gov Identifier/Number.

patients. Clinical trials such as these are intended to be screening trials to detect a signal in a histology agnostic cohort based on the genetic marker. Additional studies will need to be designed to assess the true activity of an agent in a prespecified cohort. Likewise, future study designs and statistical methods will need to address these issues as we analyze clinical trial results and consider incorporating this information into standard of care therapies.

SUMMARY

Molecular characterization has the potential to advance the management of pediatric cancer malignancies. The clinical integration of genome sequencing into standard clinical practice has been limited. Although there are still many obstacles remaining as precision medicine is applied to pediatric oncology, these studies represent the first step in exploring this application of genomic-directed treatment of patients with childhood cancer.

ACKNOWLEDGEMENT

Pediatric MATCH (APEC1621) is supported by NCTN Operations Center Grant U10CA180886 to the Children's Oncology Group from the National Cancer Institute of the National Institutes of Health.

REFERENCES

1. Siegel RL, Miller KD, Jemal A. Cancer statistics, 2016. CA Cancer J Clin 2016; 66(1):7–30.
2. Schultz KR, Bowman WP, Aledo A, et al. Improved early event-free survival with imatinib in Philadelphia chromosome-positive acute lymphoblastic leukemia: a children's oncology group study. J Clin Oncol 2009;27(31):5175–81.
3. Mosse YP, Lim MS, Voss SD, et al. Safety and activity of crizotinib for paediatric patients with refractory solid tumours or anaplastic large-cell lymphoma: a Children's Oncology Group phase 1 consortium study. Lancet Oncol 2013;14(6): 472–80.
4. Schultz KR, Carroll A, Heerema NA, et al. Long-term follow-up of imatinib in pediatric Philadelphia chromosome-positive acute lymphoblastic leukemia: Children's Oncology Group study AALL0031. Leukemia 2014;28(7):1467–71.
5. Parsons DW, Roy A, Yang Y, et al. Diagnostic yield of clinical tumor and germline whole-exome sequencing for children with solid tumors. JAMA Oncol 2016;2(5): 616–24.
6. Mody RJ, Wu YM, Lonigro RJ, et al. Integrative clinical sequencing in the management of refractory or relapsed cancer in youth. JAMA 2015;314(9):913–25.
7. Harris MH, DuBois SG, Glade Bender JL, et al. Multicenter feasibility study of tumor molecular profiling to inform therapeutic decisions in advanced pediatric solid tumors: the individualized cancer therapy (iCat) study. JAMA Oncol 2016; 2(5):608–15.
8. Oberg JA, Glade Bender JL, Sulis ML, et al. Implementation of next generation sequencing into pediatric hematology-oncology practice: moving beyond actionable alterations. Genome Med 2016;8(1):133.
9. Worst BC, van Tilburg CM, Balasubramanian GP, et al. Next-generation personalised medicine for high-risk paediatric cancer patients - The INFORM pilot study. Eur J Cancer 2016;65:91–101.

10. Pincez T, Clement N, Lapouble E, et al. Feasibility and clinical integration of molecular profiling for target identification in pediatric solid tumors. Pediatr Blood Cancer 2017;64(6). https://doi.org/10.1002/pbc.26365.

11. Conley BA, Gray R, Chen A, et al. Abstract CT101: NCI-molecular analysis for therapy choice (NCI-MATCH) clinical trial: interim analysis. Cancer Res 2016; 76(14 Supplement):CT101.

12. Takebe N, Yap TA. Precision medicine in oncology. Curr Probl Cancer 2017;41(3): 163–5.

13. Allen CE, Laetsch TW, Mody R, et al. Target and agent prioritization for the Children's Oncology Group-National Cancer Institute Pediatric MATCH trial. J Natl Cancer Inst 2017;109(5). https://doi.org/10.1093/jnci/djw274.

14. Parsons DW, Janeway KA, Patton D, et al. Identification of targetable molecular alterations in the NCI-COG Pediatric MATCH trial. J Clin Oncol 2019;37(suppl) [abstract: 10011].

15. Lawrence MS, Stojanov P, Polak P, et al. Mutational heterogeneity in cancer and the search for new cancer-associated genes. Nature 2013;499(7457):214–8.

16. Vogelstein B, Papadopoulos N, Velculescu VE, et al. Cancer genome landscapes. Science 2013;339(6127):1546–58.

17. Schleiermacher G, Javanmardi N, Bernard V, et al. Emergence of new ALK mutations at relapse of neuroblastoma. J Clin Oncol 2014;32(25):2727–34.

18. Eleveld TF, Oldridge DA, Bernard V, et al. Relapsed neuroblastomas show frequent RAS-MAPK pathway mutations. Nat Genet 2015;47(8):864–71.

19. Schramm A, Koster J, Assenov Y, et al. Mutational dynamics between primary and relapse neuroblastomas. Nat Genet 2015;47(8):872–7.

20. Padovan-Merhar OM, Raman P, Ostrovnaya I, et al. Enrichment of targetable mutations in the relapsed neuroblastoma genome. PLoS Genet 2016;12(12): e1006501.

21. Gerlinger M, Rowan AJ, Horswell S, et al. Intratumor heterogeneity and branched evolution revealed by multiregion sequencing. N Engl J Med 2012;366(10): 883–92.

22. Le Tourneau C, Kamal M, Tsimberidou AM, et al. Treatment algorithms based on tumor molecular profiling: the essence of precision medicine trials. J Natl Cancer Inst 2016;108(4). https://doi.org/10.1093/jnci/djv362.

23. Moreno L, Pearson ADJ, Paoletti X, et al. Early phase clinical trials of anticancer agents in children and adolescents - an ITCC perspective. Nat Rev Clin Oncol 2017;14(8):497–507.

24. Geoerger B, Schleiermacher G, Pierron G, et al. Abstract CT004: European pediatric precision medicine program in recurrent tumors: first results from MAPPYACTS molecular profiling trial towards AcSe-ESMART proof-of-concept study. Cancer Res 2017;77(13 Supplement):CT004.

Precision Medicine and Targeted Therapies in Breast Cancer

Ian Greenwalt, MD[a], Norah Zaza, BA[b], Shibandri Das, MD[a],
Benjamin D. Li, MD, MBA[c],*

KEYWORDS

- Breast cancer • Precision medicine • Targeted therapy • Endocrine therapy • HER2
- Multigene array • Genomics • Radiomics

KEY POINTS

- Discuss the current state of breast cancer care including endocrine therapy, anti-HER2 therapy and chemotherapy.
- Discuss the current state of precision medicine including molecular subtyping and gene expression profiles.
- Discuss the role of genomics and radiomics in precision medicine and breast cancer care.

INTRODUCTION

Progress made in our understanding of genomics, proteomics, and cancer biology has led to a deeper appreciation for the complexity and variability in a tumor's genotypic and phenotypic expression, and the complex malignant transformation known as cancer. Consequently, cancer treatment has also begun to evolve toward a more individualized, precise and targeted approach for each patient and the specific cancer that has been diagnosed, based on the complexity of the molecular profile of the tumor and the patient. This has marked the beginning of the era toward precision medicine and targeted therapeutics.

The evolution in breast cancer therapy serves as a prime example for this nascent journey. In the following article, a review of the history of targeted therapy in breast cancer, an update on its current state, and the role precision medicine has played in breast cancer care are highlighted. The overarching goal is to provide an overview

This article originally appeared in *Surgical Oncology Clinics*, Volume 29, Issue 1, January 2020.
Disclosure Statement: The authors have nothing to disclose.
[a] University Hospitals Cleveland Medical Center, MetroHealth Hospitals, Louis Stokes Veterans Administration Hospital, Case Western Reserve University, Cleveland, OH, USA; [b] Case Western Reserve University, Cleveland, OH, USA; [c] MetroHealth System, Case Western Reserve University, Cancer Care Pavilion, Suite C2100, 2500 MetroHealth Drive, Cleveland, OH 44109-1998, USA
* Corresponding author.
E-mail address: bli@metrohealth.org

of how precision medicine has impacted breast cancer management as an example of the early progress made in precision medicine and targeted therapy in cancer care.

TARGETED THERAPIES IN BREAST CANCER
Endocrine Therapy

Tamoxifen is the earliest and best studied example of targeted therapy in our anticancer armamentarium. As a selective estrogen receptor modulator that can competitively bind to the estrogen receptor (ER) on cell surfaces of breast cancer cells, tamoxifen has been shown to improve disease-free survival in premenopausal and postmenopausal women with breast cancer since the 1970s.[1,2] In postmenopausal women, response rates of the cancer were on the order of 50% to 70% for those with ER-positive ± progesterone receptor (PR)-positive tumors. In contrast, there is a less than 10% response rate for those patients with ER-negative/PR-negative tumors. In the adjuvant setting, pooling the results of multiple clinical trials, the Early Breast Cancer Trialists' Collaborative Group (EBCTCG) reported the impact of tamoxifen on patients with ER-positive breast cancer. These findings showed an improvement in 10-year survival by 10.9% for node-positive (61.4% vs 50.5% survival, $P<.00001$) and 5.6% for node-negative (78.9% vs 73.3% survival, $P<.00001$) breast cancer.[3] In male breast cancer, in which the disease is rare but has been found to be more likely positive for ERs, tamoxifen has an overall response rate of 50% in unselected male patients but increases to 71% in patients with ER-positive tumors. Finally, the EBCTCG also reported that adjuvant tamoxifen therapy reduced the risk of development of contralateral breast cancer by 39% compared with no adjuvant therapy.[2]

Aromatase inhibitors (AI) offered the next development in targeting hormone receptor–positive breast cancers. Aromatase catalyzes the conversion of androgens to estrogens and can be used to decrease levels of circulating estrogen, specifically in postmenopausal women.[1,4] The 2 categories of AI are Type 1 steroidals and Type II nonsteroidals. Type I steroidals include formestane and exemestane. These bind competitively to aromatase enzyme. Type II nonsteroidals, such as anastrozole and letrozole, bind reversibly to aromatase and require continued drug presence in the body for sustained inhibition.

Today, the 3 most commonly used and orally available agents are emestane, anastrozole, and letrozole. There have been 2 large randomized phase 3 trials: (1) the North American trial and (2) TARGET trial. These 2 trials compared tamoxifen versus AI efficacy in reducing cancer recurrence. In TARGET, anastrozole 1 mg/d orally showed equivalence with comparison to tamoxifen 20 mg/d orally in terms of median time to disease progression and clinical benefit rate. In the North American trial, the results showed a significant improvement in median time to disease progression of 11.1 months with anastrozole, compared with 5.6 months with tamoxifen. In addition, in a phase 3 head-to-head trial, Mouridsen and colleagues[5] demonstrated that letrozole achieved better results when compared with tamoxifen alone. Women treated with letrozole had a 3-month improvement in time to progression, as well as longer time to chemotherapy when compared with tamoxifen.[4]

Human Epidermal Growth Factor Receptor 2 Therapy

The discovery of trastuzumab, a monoclonal antibody (MAB) that inhibits the extracellular domain of the human epidermal growth factor receptor 2 (HER2) receptor, is seen as the beginning of a new era in targeted therapy for breast cancer.[1] HER2 can homodimerize or heterodimerize, both of which lead to activation of PI3K/AKT pathways.

The addition of trastuzumab, either concurrently or sequentially, to chemotherapy regimens improves both overall survival (OS) and disease-free progression (DFS) (hazard ratio [HR] 0.66; 95% confidence interval [CI] 0.57–0.77, $P<.00001$; and HR 0.60; 95% CI 0.50–0.71, $P<.00001$, respectively).[6] Pertuzumab is another MAB that acts on HER2. It inhibits the heterodimerization domain and in tumor models, trastuzumab and pertuzumab have been found to have synergistic antitumor activity. This was subsequently confirmed in the CLEOPATRA trial. In this study, patients with HER2-positive, metastatic disease with no prior treatment were randomly assigned to trastuzumab and docetaxel, plus either pertuzumab or placebo. There was an increase in progression-free survival (PFS) of 6 months and OS of 16 months when pertuzumab was added to trastuzumab.[7]

MAB targeting of HER2 also has made inroads in the adjuvant management of breast cancer. Pertuzumab was evaluated as an addition to adjuvant trastuzumab and chemotherapy in patients with HER2-positive, nonmetastatic, breast cancer after surgical resection. The adjuvant therapy regimen was initiated within 8 weeks of surgery. Patients were assigned to standard chemotherapy and trastuzumab plus pertuzumab or standard chemotherapy and trastuzumab plus placebo for 1 year. Pertuzumab and trastuzumab with chemotherapy led to a 94.1% rate of DFS. It was 93.2% in the placebo group. In the cohort of patients with node-positive disease, the 3-year rate of invasive DFS was 92.0% in the pertuzumab group compared with 90.2% in the placebo group (HR for invasive-disease event, 0.77; 95% CI 0.62–0.96; $P = .02$).[8]

Another role for anti-HER2 therapies in the adjuvant setting is the novel combination of trastuzumab with a cytotoxic chemotherapeutic agent, emtansine (TDM1). This conjugate works by inhibiting HER2 signaling (via trastuzumab) and also prevents microtubule function (via DM1). A study investigated the risk of recurrence of invasive breast cancer in those with residual invasive disease treated with TDM1 and trastuzumab compared with trastuzumab alone in the adjuvant setting. The study group was made up of patients with HER2-positive, nonmetastatic breast cancer treated with neoadjuvant therapy with residual disease found on surgical pathology. The group then received the 2 adjuvant regimens. Comparative results demonstrated that those treated with adjuvant TDM1 had a 50% lower risk of recurrence or death than those with trastuzumab alone.[9]

RECENT DEVELOPMENTS IN TARGETED THERAPY INVOLVING OTHER MOLECULAR PATHWAYS
Mammalian Target of Rapamycin Pathway Inhibitors

In studying patients with hormone receptor–positive, advanced stage breast cancer who developed resistance to endocrine therapies, it was discovered that their tumors had upregulation of the mammalian target of rapamycin (mTOR) kinase pathway.[1] Based on this discovery, it was later found that a combination of mTOR inhibition along with anti-endocrine therapies, had resulted in improved survival in patients with breast cancer. As Baselga and colleagues[10] demonstrated, the use of mTOR inhibitors with AIs created a synergistic effect that can cease proliferation and induce apoptosis of hormone receptor–positive tumors in patients with advanced disease. Through this combination of everolimus with AI, there was improved PFS from 2.8 to 6.9 months when compared with AI alone (HR 0.43; 95% CI 0.35–0.54; $P<.001$).

This therapeutic strategy was then applied to the management of disease initially refractory to endocrine therapies. In patients with unfavorable response to first-line AI agents, such as letrozole or anastrozole, combining exemestane with everolimus provided improved PFS. This was supported by the results of the phase 2, randomized controlled trial BOLERO-6 study of everolimus plus exemestane versus everolimus alone (PFS HR of 0.74, 90% CI 0.57–0.97).[11]

Inhibition of the mTOR pathway has further applications in delaying or preventing resistance to endocrine therapies. Royce and colleagues[12] postulated that dual inhibition targeting mTOR and hormone receptor–positive tumors could delay or prevent endocrine resistance by weeding out hormone independent cell lines with early dual therapy. This multicenter, phase 2 clinical trial demonstrated PFS of 22 months (95% CI 18.1–25.1 months) with the use of everolimus and letrozole compared with letrozole alone. Before this study, PFS was typically 9.0 to 9.4 months.

Cyclin Dependent Kinase 4 and 6 Pathway Inhibitors

Another targeted therapy strategy involves the Cyclin Dependent Kinase 4 and 6 (CDK 4/6) pathway. CDK 4/6 plays a central role in the phosphorylation of the Rb protein, which allows the progression of G1 to S phase in the cell cycle.[1] Upregulating the phosphorylation of the Rb protein has been demonstrated in hormone-resistant breast cancer cells. Medications such as ribociclib, abemaciclib, and palbociclib are small molecules that can inhibit the CDK 4/6 pathway, shutting down the cell cycle, and leading to apoptosis of cancer cells. Similar to the combination of mTOR inhibitors and AI, the dual use of CDK 4/6 inhibitors with AI has a synergistic effect on hormone receptor–positive breast cancers. There has been a demonstrable improvement in PFS with the use of palbociclib and letrozole compared with letrozole alone in patients with hormone receptor–positive, HER2-negative, advanced stage breast cancer. Finn and colleagues[13] showed this in PALOMA-1/TRIO-18 with a PFS of 20.2 months in the palbociclib and letrozole arm compared with PFS of 10.2 months in the letrozole group.

There also appears to be an application for CDK 4/6 inhibition in breast cancers that have displayed endocrine resistance. In patients with hormone receptor–positive, HER2-negative breast cancer with advanced disease that had demonstrated previous resistance to endocrine therapies, Sledge and colleagues[14] reported that the combined use of abemaciclib with fulvestrant resulted in a PFS of 16.4 months versus 9.3 months with fulvestrant alone (HR 0.553; 95% CI 0.449–0.681). There was also tumor size reduction with a mean decrease in tumor size of 62.5% for the abemaciclib and fulvestrant arm compared with 32.8% for the control arm.

Poly ADP-Ribose Polymerase Inhibitors

Poly ADP-Ribose Polymerase (PARP) is one of the means by which cells attempt to maintain genomic integrity. In the presence of single-strand DNA breaks, PARP is activated and acts as both a signal and a platform for DNA repair proteins.[15] Otherwise, the damage may result in cell death. BRCA1 and BRCA2 gene products are proteins important in the repair of double-strand DNA breaks. BRCA gene mutations can lead to errors in DNA repair that can eventually result in breast cancer formation in normal breast cells. When subjected to enough damage in DNA and where the mechanisms of repair are severely compromised, cell death, even among cancer cells, can occur.

PARP inhibitors block the repair of single-strand DNA breaks. If these unrepaired nicks persist during DNA replication, double-strand breaks can form. In breast cancer with BRCA mutations, these double breaks cannot be efficiently repaired. As a result, the breast cancer cells die. Normal breast cells without BRCA mutation still have their repair mechanism intact. Thus, they can survive the inhibition of PARP.

PARP inhibitors, such as olaparib and talazoparib, have been shown to improve the outcomes for patients with BRCA-positive breast cancer.[15] Robson and colleagues[16] and Litton and colleagues[17] illustrated the efficacy of PARP inhibitors in patients with metastatic BRCA-positive breast cancer by achieving improved PFS as well as decreased risk of disease progression, decreased risk of death, and delay in time to clinical deterioration. Specifically, the median PFS for the olaparib group was 2.8 months longer than the standard chemotherapy group (HR for disease progression or death of 0.58; 95% CI 0.43–0.80; $P<.001$).

THE ROLE OF PRECISION MEDICINE IN DETERMINING TREATMENT

In 2011, the National Research Council released a consensus study report with the proposal to redefine disease based on molecular and environmental determinants, rather than using traditional signs, symptoms, and traditional histology.[18] The potential for harnessing big data networks and expanding molecular signatures to redefine disease, tailoring a personalized treatment regimen based on an individual's unique molecular profile along with other determinants, can result in far more efficacious treatments, and with far fewer treatment-related complications. This very concept is being tested out in a nascent manner in cancer therapy, more specifically, in our approach to breast cancer treatment.

Molecular Subtyping and Treatment Decision

In the previous section, examples of targeted agents in response to actionable mutations in critical molecular pathways were exploited to inhibit or kill tumor cells. Molecular subtyping of cancer also can aid in the decision of whether standard systemic therapy, such as standard cytotoxic chemotherapy, should be part of adjuvant therapy in breast cancer. Although cytotoxic chemotherapy has demonstrated benefits in DFS and OS, these benefits are not universal in the population treated; nor are the degree and susceptibility for adverse events experienced equally. The tumor's biology, the patient's constitution, and the clinical setting all play a role in maximizing the benefits of treatment, and in minimizing the potential for morbid or toxic outcomes. We are just beginning to appreciate and to stratify some of these determinants.

In breast cancer, examples of some such early developments and applications are in the multigene arrays now quite routinely applied to tumor specimens. These include the 3 most commonly used multigene arrays in clinical use today: Oncotype DX, MammaPrint, and PAM50 (Predication Analysis of Microarrays) (**Table 1**). They each represent the next step in individualizing the decision making for chemotherapy for patients with breast cancer.

In Oncotype DX, this multigene array is derived from 21 genes originally studied in patients with ER-positive, lymph node–negative cancers who were treated with tamoxifen. These findings have been extrapolated to patients with early-stage breast cancer and used as a tool to classify patients as low, intermediate, or high risk for recurrence. Based on the risk stratification for recurrence, Oncotype DX results help guide chemotherapy decisions for these patients.[19] This 21-gene array also has been shown to be predictive for locoregional recurrence. As such, Oncotype DX also has a role to play in the selection for adjuvant radiation therapy.

MammaPrint is another multigene array, based on the analysis of 70 genes known to influence tumor growth, signaling, replication, and cell death. MammaPrint is often applied to patients with intermediate risk for recurrent disease. The assay stratifies patients into those with a good versus poor prognostic signature for distant metastasis. Its applicability includes those patients with HER2-positive and node-positive breast cancer. This subset of patients is not usually amenable to Oncotype DX testing alone.

Table 1
Common breast cancer multigene arrays

Test	Composition	Type of Cancer	Application
Oncotype DX	21-gene assay	ER/PR+, node−	Classify early-stage breast cancers into low, intermediate, and high risk of recurrence within 10 y. Help guide use of chemotherapy and radiation.
MammaPrint	70-gene assay	ER/PR+ or ER/PR−	Applied to patient with intermediate risk of recurrence. Stratifies patients into good or poor prognostic risk of metastatic disease.
PAM50	50-gene assay	ER/PR+, node+	Predicts likelihood of recurrence within 10 y.

Abbreviations: ER/PR, estrogen receptor/progesterone receptor, PAM50, Predication Analysis of Microarrays.

MammaPrint is used to aid in the selection of chemotherapies and in providing patients and their treating physicians with additional prognostic information.[19]

Last, PAM50 is an analytical tool designed to classify intrinsic molecular subtyping. The assay estimates a risk for recurrence score to better characterize, classify, and treat patients with early ER-positive, HER2-negative breast cancer. The risk profiling was based on an initial cohort of postmenopausal patients with early ER-positive, HER2-negative tumors, treated with neoadjuvant endocrine therapy, and their related response to neoadjuvant or adjuvant chemotherapy. PAM50 is a microarray of 50 genes.[19]

Gene Expression Profile and Breast Cancer

It can be argued that the era of molecular characterization to determine treatment for breast cancer began when the gene expression profiles of several hundred complementary DNA clones extracted from 78 breast carcinomas were studied in attempt to create a new classification of breast cancer based on the molecular signature obtained.[20] The intent is that a better understanding of a tumor's molecular profile can lead to improved abilities to determine prognosis and enhanced precision in treatment decisions. Since the introduction of breast cancer intrinsic subtype classification, the ability to better predict risk for recurrence, the option to select targeted therapy based on molecular profiling, and a greater degree of precision in therapeutic decision making has resulted in improved clinical outcomes.[21]

Tumor response to treatment is not determined by traditional anatomic prognostic factors, such as tumor size and nodal status. Rather, intrinsic molecular characteristics of each individual tumor, as captured by its array of gene expression, are more informative in predicting treatment response and clinical outcomes. Further developments in the classification of breast cancer based on expression profile will gain in utility and function, as expression profile through microarray and high-throughput analysis become more feasible and prevalent.

Currently, breast tumors can be grouped into 4 molecular subtypes, based on 4 well-established molecular markers. These include hormone receptor ER and PR positivity, HER2 receptor status, and the proliferation index of Ki67. The 4 subtypes identified make up most breast cancers. They are luminal A, luminal B, HER2 overexpression, and basal-like tumors (**Table 2**). Luminal A is described as ER positive with/without PR positivity, HER2-negative, and with less than 14% presence of Ki67.

Table 2
Breast cancer subtypes

Subtype	Molecular Characteristics	Treatment	Response
Luminal A (most common)	ER+, +/− PR, HER2-negative, <14% Ki67	Endocrine therapy	Excellent prognosis. Responds well to Endocrine therapy, not well to chemotherapy.
Luminal B	ER+, +/− PR HER2-positive/negative >14% Ki67	Endocrine and chemotherapy	Worse prognosis. More aggressive than luminal A.
HER2 overexpression	ER and PR-negative HER2-positive, any amount Ki67	Chemotherapy and anti-HER2 therapy	Poor prognosis vs luminal subtypes.
Basal-like	Triple negative, any amount Ki67	Chemotherapy	Very poor prognosis.

Abbreviations: ER, estrogen receptor; HER2, human epidermal growth factor receptor 2; PR, progesterone receptor.

Luminal B is divided into HER2-positive and negative groups, with ER-positive and/or PR-positive hormone status, and a greater than 14% presence of Ki67. The HER2 overexpression tumors are ER and PR negative, HER2 positive, and with any amount of Ki67. Finally, the basal-like subtype has triple negative receptors, with a varying amount of Ki67 presence.[19,20]

Understanding the subtypes and the mutations associated with each provides insight on the prognosis of each subtype, as well as helps in therapeutic decision making. Luminal A is the most common subtype. As an ER-positive and/or PR-positive tumor, it has an excellent prognosis, likely because of the associated low proliferative index score, and a well-differentiated cancer by histologic examination. It responds well to hormone therapy, but poorly to chemotherapy. As such, patients with luminal A breast cancer do well with endocrine therapy and may forego adjuvant chemotherapy.[21]

Luminal B subtype has a higher index of proliferation. It is also associated with a worse prognosis, with a disease course that is significantly more aggressive than luminal A breast cancer. It is more often associated with poorly differentiated histology and a higher frequency for bone metastases. A combined therapeutic strategy of endocrine therapy with chemotherapy is often used to optimize outcomes.[21]

HER2 overexpression subtype has a very high proliferative index and is most often poorly differentiated by histology. Also, in 40% to 80% of the patients, it is associated with the p53 mutation. It has a poor prognosis and a lower survival rate than both luminal subtypes. They are sensitive to anthracycline and taxane-based neoadjuvant chemotherapy though, with a significantly higher pathologic complete response than luminal tumors. However, incomplete tumor eradication by therapy results in early relapse. As these tumors are HER2 positive, patients are candidates for and are responsive to anti-HER2 targeted therapy.[21]

The basal-like subtype is composed of triple negative breast cancer (TNBC). Receptor status of these tumors are ER, PR, and HER2 negative. However, not all TNBCs belong to the basal-like subtype. This subtype of tumors resembles the expression profile of basal epithelial cells in other organs. The cancer tends toward being poorly differentiated, a high proliferative index, mitotic index, and associated with p53 mutations.[22] The patients with this subtype of breast cancer tend to have experienced menarche at a younger age, and being multiparous is not protective like in the luminal subtype. The tumor at presentation tends to be larger, grows more rapidly, and when metastatic, is less likely to be associated with initial node-positive disease. Disseminated disease also tends toward visceral organs.

Overall, the prognosis for this subtype of breast cancer is very poor. Although this subtype is associated with low ER, PR, and HER2 expression, it has high expression for basal markers, such as cytokeratin markers. As basal-like subtype of breast cancer lacks these receptors, it lacks response to the currently available targeted therapy designed for these receptors. Therefore, chemotherapy is the only option in the current treatment armamentarium. Both paclitaxel and doxorubicin-containing neoadjuvant chemotherapies have been shown to produce the best pathologic response among basal-like subtypes.[23]

In general, the luminal subtypes do not appear to be as sensitive to neoadjuvant chemotherapy as the more aggressive subtypes.[23] Caudle and colleagues[24] demonstrated that luminal A and B tumors had significantly lower rates of pathologic complete response (9% and 18%, respectively) compared with patients with HER2 overexpression and basal-like tumors (36% and 38%, respectively).[23] In light of this, preoperative chemotherapy should be strongly considered before surgical intervention for the nonluminal subtypes.

The progression to the use of intrinsic subtype classification in breast cancer in the treatment decision is fundamentally different from the use of tumor markers as prognosticators for cancer outcomes. Using individual prognostic markers as predictors for cancer outcomes do not capture the molecular complexity intrinsic to breast cancer tumors. Gene expression profile using microarray analysis will eventually be able to capture a more precise and comprehensive characterization of the molecular signature of a complex tumor specimen at diagnosis, and as it progresses in its disease course. This allows for adjustment of the therapeutic strategy to a more precise approach to targeted therapy, acting at a specific defective pathway. One such ongoing proof-of-concept trial of matching a defect in a molecular pathway with a specific potential targeted therapy is the recently completed MATCH trial, sponsored by the ECOG-ACRIN group.[25]

Radiomics

Precision medicine to better individualize treatment based on a patient and the tumor's characteristics has applications in radiation therapy. Adjuvant and therapeutic application of radiotherapy is a standard model in breast cancer treatment. At present, individualization of radiotherapy for a patient's tumor involve primarily anatomic precision and imaging features.[26]

Radiomics is a developing science in the extraction of many features from radiographic images using data-characterization algorithms to potentially uncover disease characteristics. With regard to breast cancer, the study of radiomics attempts to correlate a tumor's radiographic features with its intrinsic subtype and molecular profile with the end goal of using this information to help identify clinical outcomes.[26] Specific examples can be seen in the work of Fan and colleagues[27] who reported that with MRI, there is less tumor heterogeneity in less aggressive cancers, like the luminal A subtype. In addition, HER2 overexpression subtype was found to have the highest enhancement value on MRI.

Advancement in breast ultrasound and digital mammography technology also may be used to determine certain biologic characteristics of breast cancer, as well as their Ki67 status. With ultrasound, low-grade tumors tend to have more irregular shapes and are hyperechoic. In contrast, high-grade tumors tend to have a regular shape and are more hypoechoic.[26] Ma and colleagues[28] used 39 features of digital mammography to differentiate subtypes of breast cancer, finding that each tumor subtype was significantly associated with 4 of these features: roundness, concavity, gray mean, and correlation.[26]

Radiomics also plays a role in determining recurrence risk. Drukker and colleagues[29] reported that certain MRI features correlate with recurrent breast cancer. The MRI feature most closely associated with earlier cancer recurrence was the Most Enhancing Tumor Volume (METV). The METV obtained before and after the first cycle of neoadjuvant chemotherapy was reliable in predicting earlier cancer recurrence.

Further application of precision medicine is found at the junction of genomics and radiomics. Investigators have established a genome-adjusted radiation dose (GARD) using gene-expression–based radiation-sensitivity index and a linear quadratic model that describes biological response to radiation.[30] This model is an attempt to facilitate adjustment of radiotherapy dose and predict the effect of radiation therapy. Although this model was tested in several cancers, the breast cancer cohort was further studied to establish a GARD threshold that was associated with better clinical outcomes.[30] Similarly, the MATCH trial mentioned earlier should provide further insight into radiomics, as part of the study design was to examine the potential utility of high-throughput radiologic data in the characterization of tumors and its response to treatment.[25]

Precision Medicine in Breast Surgery

Surgical options in the treatment of breast cancer can be generally simplified into (1) total mastectomy versus partial mastectomy (PM), and (2) nodal staging by sentinel node biopsy (SLN) versus a complete axillary node dissection. The choice of surgery depends on the stage of the breast cancer at presentation, the overall health of the patient, and each patient's preference. That being said, the most commonly performed surgical treatment is PM plus SLN, known commonly as breast conservation surgery (BCS). This is because with the prevalence of the breast cancer screening program, the disease is most commonly diagnosed at a clinically node-negative stage, with a tumor smaller than 5 cm.

Recent studies have begun to investigate clinical outcomes of the different breast cancer subtypes to the various surgical options. Each of the 4 subtypes (luminal A, luminal B, HER2 overexpression, and basal-like) appear to hold different nuances in their response to BCS and radiation therapy. Although all 4 subtypes had a less than 10% recurrence rate at 5 years following BCS, luminal A subtype had a particularly low recurrence rate of 0.8% (luminal B 1.5%, HER2 overexpression 8.4%, basal-like 7.1%).[31] The rate of positive nodes after SLN also varies based on subtype. The highest frequencies of positive SLN were 44.9% and 50.0% among luminal B and HER2 overexpression subtypes, respectively ($P = .0003$).[32] Further improvements in subtyping and more precision in correlation of outcome can potentially lead to the elimination of adjuvant radiation therapy for a specific subtype, or to eliminate the need to perform surgical axillary staging in another subtype.

Radiomics also can potentially impact surgical treatment. As supported by the work of Liu and colleagues,[33] the radiomic signature seen on Dynamic Contrast Enhancement-MRI (DCE-MRI) can suggest the invasiveness of a tumor. Specifically, it was found that the DCE-MRI radiomic signature was an independent risk factor for lymphovascular invasion (odds ratio 2.895; $P = .031$). The presence of nodal disease and lymphovascular invasion identifies patients at higher risk for systemic disease and thus are candidates for neoadjuvant therapy. Based on preoperative evaluation, surgery may be rescheduled, with preference for early initiation of neoadjuvant therapy.

SUMMARY

Advances in breast cancer care over the past several decades have been marked by the development of a large array of therapeutic approaches, leading to multimodal therapy as part of an ever-expanding armamentarium of treatment options. However, much of what we offer in cancer therapy has significant treatment-associated sequelae. Furthermore, the treatment response by each tumor to any given treatment regimen can be highly variable. The good news is that recent developments in therapeutics are getting more and more targeted toward specific tumor-associated molecular defects. Such targeted therapies are generally more precise in their mechanism for tumor inhibition or destruction than traditional cytotoxic chemotherapy. In addition, our understanding of cancer biology continues to evolve. Through the use of multigene assays, molecular and expression profiling, and intrinsic subtyping, each tumor's growth as well as its likelihood to respond to a specific therapy is getting more precise. Together with "big data," such as biometrics gathered through the Internet of things, radiomics, and the rapid advances in high-throughput analysis, there is hope that the future of cancer therapy will continue to evolve toward a more precise approach. Through this improved precision can come greater predictability and efficacy of treatment individualized for each patient, while minimizing the risk of untoward side effects.

REFERENCES

1. Meisel JL, Venur VA, Gnant M, et al. Evolution of targeted therapy in breast cancer: where. Am Soc Clin Oncol Educ Book 2018;38:78–86.
2. Robert NJ. Clinical efficacy of tamoxifen. Oncology (Williston Park) 1997;11(2 Suppl 1):15–20.
3. Early Breast Cancer Trialists' Collaborative Group. Tamoxifen for early breast cancer: an overview of the randomised trials. Lancet 1998;351(9114):1451–67.
4. Schneider RE, Barakat A, Pippen J, et al. Aromatase inhibitors in the treatment of breast cancer in post-menopausal female patients: an update. Breast Cancer (Dove Med Press) 2011;3:113–25.
5. Mouridsen H, Gershanovich M, Sun Y, et al. Phase III study of letrozole versus tamoxifen as first-line therapy of advanced breast cancer in postmenopausal women: analysis of survival and update of efficacy from the international letrozole breast cancer group. J Clin Oncol 2003;21(11):2101–9.
6. Moja L, Compagnoni A, Brambilla C, et al. Trastuzumab containing regimens for metastatic breast cancer. In: Moja L, editor. Cochrane database of systematic reviews. Chichester (United Kingdom): John Wiley & Sons, Ltd; 2006. https://doi.org/10.1002/14651858.CD006242.
7. Nixon N, Verma S. A value-based approach to treatment of HER2-positive breast cancer: examining the evidence. Am Soc Clin Oncol Educ Book 2016;36:e56–63.
8. von Minckwitz G, Procter M, de Azambuja E, et al. Adjuvant pertuzumab and trastuzumab in early HER2-positive breast cancer. N Engl J Med 2017;377(2):122–31.
9. von Minckwitz G, Huang C-S, Mano MS, et al. Trastuzumab emtansine for residual invasive HER2-positive breast cancer. N Engl J Med 2018;380(7):617–28.

10. Baselga J, Campone M, Piccart M, et al. Everolimus in postmenopausal hormone-receptor–positive advanced breast cancer. N Engl J Med 2012;366(6): 520–9.

11. Jerusalem G, De Boer RH, Hurvitz S, et al. Everolimus plus exemestane vs everolimus or capecitabine monotherapy for estrogen receptor-positive, HER2-negative advanced breast cancer: the BOLERO-6 randomized clinical trial. JAMA Oncol 2018;4(10):1367–74.

12. Royce M, Bachelot T, Villanueva C, et al. Everolimus plus endocrine therapy for postmenopausal women with estrogen receptor-positive, human epidermal growth factor receptor 2-negative advanced breast cancer: a clinical trial. JAMA Oncol 2018;4(7):977–84.

13. Finn RS, Crown JP, Lang I, et al. The cyclin-dependent kinase 4/6 inhibitor palbociclib in combination with letrozole versus letrozole alone as first-line treatment of oestrogen receptor-positive, HER2-negative, advanced breast cancer (PALOMA-1/TRIO-18): a randomised phase 2 study. Lancet Oncol 2015;16(1):25–35.

14. Sledge GW, Toi M, Neven P, et al. MONARCH 2: abemaciclib in combination with fulvestrant in women with HR+/HER2-advanced breast cancer who had progressed while receiving endocrine therapy. J Clin Oncol 2017;35(25):2875–84.

15. Faraoni I, Graziani G. Role of BRCA mutations in cancer treatment with Poly(ADP-ribose) polymerase (PARP) inhibitors. Cancers (Basel) 2018;10(12):487.

16. Robson M, Im S-A, Senkus E, et al. Olaparib for metastatic breast cancer in patients with a germline BRCA mutation. N Engl J Med 2017;377(6):523–33.

17. Litton JK, Rugo HS, Ettl J, et al. Talazoparib in Patients with Adavanced Breast Cancer and a Germline BRCA Mutation. N Eng J Med 2018;379(8):753–63.

18. National Research Council. Toward precision medicine: building a knowledge network for biomedical research and a new taxonomy of disease. Washington, DC: National Academic Press; 2011.

19. Harris EER. Precision medicine for breast cancer: the paths to truly individualized diagnosis and treatment. Int J Breast Cancer 2018;2018:1–8.

20. Sørlie T, Perou CM, Tibshirani R, et al. Gene expression profiling can distinguish tumor subclasses of breast carcinomas. In: Hofmann W-K, editor. Gene expression profiling by microarrays, vol. 98. Cambridge (United Kingdom): Cambridge University Press; 2006. p. 132–61. https://doi.org/10.1017/CBO9780511545849.008.

21. Dai XF, Li T, Bai Z, et al. Breast cancer intrinsic subtype classification, clinical use, and future trends. Am J Cancer Res 2015;5(10):2929–43.

22. Koboldt DC, Fulton RS, McLellan MD, et al. The cancer genome atlas network. Nature 2012;490(7418):61–70.

23. Rouzier R, Perou CM, Symmans WF, et al. Breast cancer molecular subtypes respond differently to preoperative chemotherapy. Clin Cancer Res 2005; 11(16):5678–85.

24. Caudle AS, Yu T-K, Tucker SL, et al. Local-regional control according to surrogate markers of breast cancer subtypes and response to neoadjuvant chemotherapy in breast cancer patients undergoing breast conserving therapy. Breast Cancer Res 2012;14(3):R83.

25. Available at: https://www.cancer.gov/about-cancer/treatment/clinical-trials/nci-supported/nci-match. Accessed May 17, 2019.

26. Crivelli P, Ledda RE, Parascandolo N, et al. A new challenge for radiologists: radiomics in breast cancer. Biomed Res Int 2018;2018:1–10.

27. Fan M, Li H, Wang S, et al. Radiomic analysis reveals DCE-MRI features for prediction of molecular subtypes of breast cancer. PLoS One 2017;12(2):1–15.

28. Ma W, Zhao Y, Ji Y, et al. Breast cancer molecular subtype prediction by mammographic radiomic features. Acad Radiol 2019;26(2):196–201.
29. Drukker K, Li H, Antropova N, et al. Most-enhancing tumor volume by MRI radiomics predicts recurrence-free survival "early on" in neoadjuvant treatment of breast cancer. Cancer Imaging 2018;18(1):1–9.
30. Scoot JG, Berglund A, Schell MJ, et al. A Genome-based Model for Adjusting Radiotherapy Dose (GARD): a retrospective, cohort-based study. Lancet Oncology 2017;18(2):202–11.
31. Nguyen PL, Taghian AG, Katz MS, et al. Breast cancer subtype approximated by ER, PR, and Her2 receptors is associated with local-regional and distant failure after breast-conserving therapy. Int J Radiat Oncol 2007;69(3):S26.
32. Mazouni C, Rimareix F, Mathieu MC, et al. Outcome in breast molecular subtypes according to nodal status and surgical procedures. Am J Surg 2013;205(6): 662–7.
33. Liu Z, Feng B, Li C, et al. Preoperative prediction of lymphovascular invasion in invasive breast cancer with dynamic contrast-enhanced-MRI-based radiomics. J Magn Reson Imaging 2019;1–11. https://doi.org/10.1002/jmri.26688.

Precision Medicine in Lung Cancer Treatment

Dhaval R. Shah, MBBS, MD[a], Gregory A. Masters, MD[a,b],*

KEYWORDS

- Lung cancer • Immunotherapy • Targeted therapy • Molecular testing
- Clinical trials

KEY POINTS

- Lung cancer remains leading cause of cancer death in men and women in the United States and more than 80% of these patients have non-small cell lung cancer.
- Platinum-based doublet chemotherapy has been the standard treatment for patients with stage IV non-small cell lung cancer.
- Over the past 5 years, immunotherapy has rapidly changed management of stage IV lung cancer and is now being used as frontline treatment option with or without chemotherapy.
- It is being used as consolidation treatment in management of patients with stage III non-small cell lung cancer after completion of chemotherapy and radiation.
- Immunotherapy is approved for use in patients with extensive stage small cell lung cancer.

INTRODUCTION

Lung cancer is the second most common cancer in men and women, and according to American Cancer Society, approximately 228,150 new cases of lung cancer will be diagnosed in 2019 in the United States. An estimated 142,670 deaths will be attributed to lung cancer in 2019. There are 3 main types of lung cancer, non-small cell lung cancer (NSCLC), small cell lung cancer (SCLC), and lung carcinoid tumor. NSCLC accounts for approximately 85% of new cases, SCLC accounts for approximately 10% to 15% of cases, and carcinoid tumors are less than 5% of new cases.[1] Unfortunately, more than 50% of cases are diagnosed in the advanced stage or stage IV.

Traditionally, the treatment for advanced NSCLC has been chemotherapy. Updated guidelines from the American Society of Clinical Oncology support these recommendations.[2] However, in the past decade, tremendous advances have been made in

This article originally appeared in *Surgical Oncology Clinics*, Volume 29, Issue 1, January 2020.
Disclosure Statement: None.
[a] Helen F. Graham Cancer Center and Research Institute, 4701 Ogletown-Stanton Road, Newark, DE 19713, USA; [b] Thomas Jefferson University Medical School, Philadelphia, PA, USA
* Corresponding author. Helen F. Graham Cancer Center and Research Institute, 4701 Ogletown-Stanton Road, Newark, DE 19713.
E-mail address: Gregory.Masters@usoncology.com

understanding the biology and genetic drivers in NSCLC. As a result, many targeted and immunotherapy drugs are now being used in the management of advanced NSCLC. These drugs are also being incorporated in early stage lung cancer, with the hope of improving outcomes and cure rates in patients with stages I to III lung cancer.

ADVANCED OR STAGE IV NON-SMALL CELL LUNG CANCER

NSCLC is divided into different histologic subtypes, which include adenocarcinoma, large cell carcinoma, and squamous cell carcinoma. Traditionally, platinum-based doublet chemotherapy has been the standard of care in advanced NSCLC. However, Scagliotti and colleagues[3] established the importance of histology in the treatment of advanced NSCLC, showing the advantage of pemetrexed in combination with a platinum agent as first-line treatment in nonsquamous NSCLC histologic subtype. Taxane with a platinum agent is the preferred chemotherapy combination for squamous histology.

Similarly, molecular characterization of NSCLC has become increasingly important as a predictive and prognostic marker to guide therapy. In 2004, an epidermal growth factor receptor (EGFR) mutation was the first molecular target identified in a subgroup of patients with NSCLC, and was associated with significant responses to oral tyrosine kinase inhibitor (TKI) geftinib.[4] Two other TKIs, erlotinib and afatinib, were also shown to be very effective in this subgroup of patients. EGFR TKIs are superior and improve survival as compared with chemotherapy in patients with stage IV NSCLC with certain EGFR mutations. Almost all of these patients will eventually progress and about one-half of them will have a secondary T790M mutation. Osimertinib has been shown to be very effective in T790M mutation, and is the second-line treatment of choice in these patients.[5] In 2018, Soria and colleagues[6] reported superior outcomes with osimertinib compared with first-generation TKIs (erlotinib and geftinib) as first-line treatment for untreated patients with EGFR mutation. Based on this, the US Food and Drug Administration has approved osimertinib for frontline use in EGFR mutant advanced NSCLC.

Similar to the EGFR mutation, EML4-ALK fusion was found to be another targetable gene alteration in small subgroup of patients with advanced nonsquamous NSCLC. EML4-ALK fusion oncogene leads to aberrant activation of EML4-ALK protein and it was first reported in 2007. Crizotinib was the first TKI shown to be effective in this subgroup of patients in 2010.[7] It was then found to be superior to standard chemotherapy in previously untreated ALK-positive NSCLC.[8] Other active TKI drugs include alectinib, certinib, and brigatinib. The ALEX study compared alectinib with crizotinib in untreated patients with EML4-ALK fusion, and showed significant improvement in survival with alectinib.[9] Thus, alectinib is now considered as the preferred first-line treatment option in treatment-naïve patients with this fusion. In patients, who are initially treated with crizotinib, treatment can be changed to second-generation TKIs, such as certinib or brigatinib.

ROS-1 rearrangement and BRAF mutation are other targetable mutations in advanced NSCLC. Crizotinib and certinib are effective in treatment of ROS-1 mutated NSCLC. The combination of dabrafenib and trametinib is considered a first-line or second-line treatment option in patients with advanced NSCLC with BRAF V600E mutation. More recently, larotrectinib has been shown to be a treatment option in patients with NTRK gene fusion,[10] and can be used in patients with lung cancer with this gene fusion.

Given these rapid advancements in the treatment of advanced NSCLC, molecular testing has become very important to choose the correct treatment approach. This molecular testing can be done by different methods, such as hotspot testing for specific genes, or more comprehensive gene sequencing of the tumors. The College of American Pathologists and the International Association for the Study of Lung Cancer recommend upfront testing for EGFR, ALK, and ROS-1 mutations in all patients with advanced nonsquamous NSCLC.[11] Routine testing for BRAF, RET, HER2, KRAS, and MET genes is not considered as a standard, but can be done as part of a gene sequencing panel. The College of American Pathologists/International Association for the Study of Lung Cancer and the American Society of Clinical Oncology guidelines both recommend use of multiplex gene panels (where available) for identifying mutations beyond EGFR, ALK, ROS-1, and BRAF.

Many patients with advanced NSCLC do not have enough biopsy tissue to run all the hotspot or gene sequencing studies listed. Therefore, more recently liquid biopsy or peripheral blood-based genetic testing has been shown to be effective in detection of these gene alterations.[12] The principle behind liquid biopsy is detection of cell free circulating DNA, which is often present in the blood of patients with cancer. This method has most commonly been studied for EGFR mutation, and the US Food and Drug Administration has approved 2 tests for this use. Data are rapidly emerging regarding use of liquid biopsy in testing for other molecular targets.

Despite the advancements in the identification of these molecular targets, the majority of patients with advanced NSCLC do not harbor these mutations. Frontline platinum-based doublet chemotherapy used to be the standard of care for these patients. Immunotherapeutic agents have rapidly changed this standard over the past 5 years. These immune checkpoint inhibitors alter the tumor microenvironment and remove the blockade of the immune system evasion by cancer cells.

One of the mechanisms of the human immune system to eliminate malignant cells is through formation of cancer-specific T cells. Antigen-presenting cells such as natural killer cells and macrophages penetrate the tumor microenvironment, and activate the T cells, which in turn destroy cancer cells. However, in cancer, 2 normal inhibitory pathways (CTLA-4 and programmed death 1 [PD-1] pathways) have been found to suppress this T-cell response. Ipilimumab, an anti–CTLA-4 monoclonal antibody, was the first immune checkpoint inhibitor developed in the treatment of cancer. However, CTLA-4 is an immunoglobulin, which is expressed on activated T cells in many normal and cancer cells, and therefore ipilimumab can be associated with significant inflammatory and autoimmune toxicities. PD-1 receptor pathway is the second mechanism that controls the T-cell immune response. PD-1 gets expressed on the surface of the T cells after persistent antigen exposure, and then interacts with its ligand PD-L1, which is expressed on both immune and cancer cells. This interaction causes inhibition of T-cell activation and response. PD-1 activation normally affects the effector T cells and cytotoxic lymphocytes, which are seen in the lymph node and tumor microenvironment. Inhibition of PD-1 and PD ligand 1 (PD-L1) pathway can therefore lead to prolonged antitumor response and many PD-1 and PD-L1 antibodies have been approved for clinical use.

PD-L1 expression has been found to correlate with response to immunotherapy drugs. In general, higher PD-L1 expression is associated with higher and long-term response.[13] Testing for PD-L1 expression is now standard in all newly diagnosed patients with advanced NSCLC. Tumor mutation burden is the number of mutations seen in the cancer cells' DNA. A higher tumor mutation burden is also associated with better response to immunotherapy. Similarly, microsatellite instability has been shown to be associated with good response to immunotherapy. Most commercial laboratories now report PD-L1 expression, tumor mutation burden, and microsatellite instability status as part of comprehensive gene sequencing report.

Initial studies evaluating immunotherapy drugs in lung cancer were done in the second line setting after progression on platinum doublet chemotherapy. The CheckMate 017 and CheckMate 057 trials showed statistically significant improvement in overall survival with nivolumab compared with docetaxel in squamous and nonsquamous NSCLC, respectively.[14,15] Overall survival was improved by approximately 3 months in both the trials. The KEYNOTE-010 trial showed significant improvement in overall survival with pembrolizumab compared with docetaxel in second line treatment for advanced NSCLC with at least 1% PD-L1 expression in the tumor cells.[16] Based on these trials, initial approval for both nivolumab and pembrolizumab was in the second line setting after progression on first line chemotherapy. Pembrolizumab was approved for patients with PD-L1 overexpression only.

Given the improvement in survival in the second-line setting, pembrolizumab was studied in combination with carboplatin and pemetrexed in first line setting in patients with nonsquamous NSCLC, with no driver mutations. This Keynote 189 trial also included maintenance treatment with pemetrexed and pembrolizumab.[17] Significant improvement in overall survival was noted with addition of pembrolizumab to chemotherapy, and is now considered as the standard of care for first-line treatment in non-squamous advanced NSCLC, irrespective of the PD-L1 status. Pembrolizumab in combination with chemotherapy has also shown to improve survival in patients with metastatic squamous cell NSCLC regardless of PD-L1 expression and is standard of care as a first-line treatment option.[18] The Keynote-042 trial evaluated pembrolizumab alone as first-line therapy versus chemotherapy in stage IV NSCLC, and pembrolizumab was associated with a significant improvement in overall survival. Based on this trial, pembrolizumab alone is also a treatment option for patients with advanced NSCLC and PD-L1 expression or more than 1%. It seems to be most active in tumors with PD-L1 of 50% or greater.

Similarly, the IMpower 150 clinical trial evaluated atezolizumab, which is an anti–PD-L1 antibody, in combination with carboplatin, paclitaxel, and bevacizumab in metastatic nonsquamous NSCLC.[19] This combination also showed improved survival and is another front-line treatment option for patients with nonsquamous NSCLC. Thus, immunotherapy has rapidly changed the management of metastatic NSCLC over the past 5 years.

Despite this rapid progress in the management of NSCLC, most patients eventually have progression of disease; the median survival in these trials is generally 2 years or less. Several trials are ongoing looking at other molecular targets in lung cancer and other solid tumors. Two such large trials are the NCI-MATCH (Molecular Analysis for Therapy Choice) study and American Society of Clinical Oncology's Targeted Agent and Profiling Utilization Registry (TAPUR) study. Similarly the LUNG-MAP (SWOG S1400) study is a multidrug, targeted screening approach for patients with advanced NSCLC. The study matches patients to one of the multiple trial substudies, each testing a different drug based on molecular testing results. This study is a unique collaboration between the National Cancer Institute, academic institutions, and private industry.

MANAGEMENT OF STAGES I TO III NON-SMALL CELL LUNG CANCER

Surgery remains the standard of care of most patients with stage I and stage II NSCLC. However, many patients are not candidates for surgery because of their functional status, medical comorbidities or underlying lung disease. Stereotactic body radiation has rapidly evolved as a treatment option for them and has been shown to have durable disease and long-term control.[20]

In patients who undergo surgery, adjuvant chemotherapy is generally recommended in patients with tumors greater than 4 cm or those with positive lymph nodes. The standard adjuvant chemotherapy is a cisplatin-based combination regimen. Given the success with targeted and immunotherapy in advanced disease, these treatments are now being studied in early stage lung cancer. The ALCHEMIST (Adjuvant Lung Cancer Enrichment Marker Identification and Sequencing Trials) trial is looking at use of EGFR or ALK inhibitors or nivolumab in the adjuvant setting for patients with resected early stage NSCLC. In this trial, patients with EGFR or ALK mutations are randomly assigned to targeted therapy or observation after resection and any adjuvant chemotherapy. Patients without these mutations are randomly assigned to receive nivolumab or observation after resection and adjuvant chemotherapy.

The Keynote-671 trial is evaluating the safety and efficacy of pembrolizumab in combination with platinum doublet chemotherapy in the neoadjuvant and adjuvant settings. In this trial, patients with resectable stage IIB or IIIA NSCLC will be randomized to neoadjuvant chemotherapy with or without pembrolizumab, followed by surgery and then adjuvant pembrolizumab or placebo. This study started in 2018, with anticipated completion in 2024.

The management of patients with stage III NSCLC generally involves a multidisciplinary approach, involving surgical, medical, and radiation oncology. Some patients with early stage IIIA NSCLC undergo surgery, followed by adjuvant chemotherapy with or without radiation. However, patients with unresectable stage IIIA and more advanced stage IIIB and IIIC lung cancers are generally treated with a combination of chemotherapy and radiation. Most of these patients ultimately have progression of disease. To improve outcomes in these patients, the PACIFIC trial looked at using an anti–PDL-1 antibody durvalumab as consolidation therapy in patients with unresectable stage III NSCLC who did not have progression of disease after 2 or more cycles of platinum-based chemoradiotherapy. The trial showed a progression-free survival of 16.8 months for patients who received durvalumab versus a progression-free survival of 5.6 months with placebo. The updated analysis of the trial published in 2018 also showed a significant improvement in overall survival, and consolidation durvalumab is now considered a standard of care after chemotherapy and radiation.[21] New clinical trials will investigate the integration of immunotherapy earlier in a combined modality approach.

MANAGEMENT OF SMALL CELL LUNG CANCER

SCLC is typically divided into limited stage and extensive stage. Limited stage SCLC is treated with a combination of chemotherapy and radiation. Generally, the chemotherapy regimen of choice in this situation is cisplatin and etoposide. However, in older patients, and in patients with renal dysfunction, often carboplatin is used instead of cisplatin.

The management of extensive stage SCLC generally involves combination chemotherapy. Carboplatin and etoposide have been the standard of care for many years. The IMpower133 trial showed improvement in survival with the addition of atezolizumab immunotherapy drug to carboplatin and etoposide. Atezolizumab was given in combination with chemotherapy for the first 4 cycles, and then given as maintenance treatment.[22] This is now a standard of care in the management of extensive stage SCLC.

A similar concept of maintenance treatment is being studied with use of rovalpituzumab tesirine (Rova-T). Rovalpituzumab tesirine is an antibody drug conjugate, which targets the delta-like protein 3 inhibitory notch receptor expressed in SCLC.

Similar other concepts will be studied in the future to improve outcomes in patients with SCLC.

FUTURE

As we move on to the next generation of clinical trials, increasing flexibility will be required to keep up with the rapid advancements in testing and new knowledge. Despite the success seen with immunotherapy, only a small percentage of patients are seeing durable and long-term responses. We therefore need better biomarkers to predict and improve response to immunotherapy. Similarly, combination of antibody–drug conjugates with chemotherapy or immunotherapy will be important to study in the future. In addition, education of community and practicing oncologists will be critical to maximize the benefits to our patients.

SUMMARY

Over the past decade, tremendous progress has been made in understanding the molecular and biologic drivers of lung cancer. Testing for various biomarkers in lung cancer is improving our ability to understand the behavior of different cancers, so we can identify the optimal treatment strategy for each clinical subset of patients. This progress has helped us to deliver individualized precision therapy options for our patients with lung cancer. Ongoing clinical trials will help to improve our ability to offer our patients the most effective treatments to improve their survival and quality of life.

REFERENCES

1. American Cancer Society. Facts & figures 2019. Atlanta (GA): American Cancer Society; 2019.
2. Hanna N, Johnson D, Temin S, et al. Systemic therapy for stage IV non-small-cell lung cancer: American Society of Clinical Oncology clinical practice guideline update. J Clin Oncol 2017;35(30):3484–515.
3. Scagliotti GV, Parikh P, von Pawel J, et al. Phase III study comparing cisplatin plus gemcitabine with cisplatin plus pemetrexed in chemotherapy-naive patients with advanced-stage non-small-cell lung cancer. J Clin Oncol 2008;26:3543–51.
4. Lynch TJ, Bell DW, Sordella R, et al. Activating mutations in the epidermal growth factor receptor underlying responsiveness of non-small-cell lung cancer to gefitinib. N Engl J Med 2004;350(21):2129–39.
5. Goss G, Tsai CM, Shepherd FA, et al. Osimertinib for pretreated EGFR Thr790Met-positive advanced non-small-cell lung cancer (AURA2): a multicentre, open-label, single-arm, phase 2 study. Lancet Oncol 2016;17(12):1643–52.
6. Soria JC, Ohe Y, Vansteenkiste J, et al. Osimertinib in untreated EGFR-mutated advanced non-small-cell lung cancer. N Engl J Med 2018;378(2):113–25.
7. Kwak EL, Bang YJ, Cambridge DR, et al. Anaplastic lymphoma kinase inhibition in non-small-cell lung cancer. N Engl J Med 2010;363(18):1693–703.
8. Solomon BJ, Mok T, Kim DW, et al. First-line crizotinib versus chemotherapy in ALK-positive lung cancer. N Engl J Med 2014;371(23):2167–77.
9. Peters S, Camidge DR, Shaw AT, et al. Alectinib versus Crizotinib in untreated ALK-positive non-small-cell lung cancer. N Engl J Med 2017;377(9):829.
10. Hong DS, Bauer TM, Lee JJ, et al. Larotrectinib in adult patients with solid tumours: a multi-centre, open-label, phase I dose-escalation study. Ann Oncol 2019;30(2):325–31.

11. Lindeman NI, Cagle PT, Aisner DL, et al. Updated molecular testing guideline for the selection of lung cancer patients for treatment with targeted tyrosine kinase inhibitors: guideline from the College of American Pathologists, the International Association for the Study of Lung Cancer, and the Association for Molecular Pathology. J Mol Diagn 2018;20(2):129–59.
12. Aggarwal C, Thompson JC, Black TA, et al. Clinical implications of plasma-based genotyping with the delivery of personalized therapy in metastatic non-small cell lung cancer. JAMA Oncol 2018. https://doi.org/10.1001/jamaoncol.2018.4305.
13. Herbst RS, Soria JC, Kowanetz M, et al. Predictive correlates of response to the anti-PD-L1 antibody MPDL3280A in cancer patients. Nature 2014;515(7528): 563–7.
14. Brahmer J, Reckamp KL, Baas P, et al. Nivolumab versus Docetaxel in advanced squamous-cell non-small-cell lung cancer. N Engl J Med 2015;373:123–35.
15. Borghaei H, Paz-Ares L, Horn L, et al. Nivolumab versus Docetaxel in advanced nonsquamous non-small-cell lung cancer. N Engl J Med 2015;373:1627–39.
16. Herbst RS, Baas P, Kim DW, et al. Pembrolizumab versus docetaxel for previously treated, PD-L1-positive, advanced non-small-cell lung cancer (KEYNOTE-010): a randomised controlled trial. Lancet 2016;387(10027):1540–50.
17. Gandhi L, Rodríguez-Abreu D, Gadgeel S, et al. Pembrolizumab plus chemotherapy in metastatic non-small-cell lung cancer. N Engl J Med 2018;378: 2078–92.
18. Paz-Ares L, Luft A, Vicente D, et al. Pembrolizumab plus chemotherapy for squamous non-small-cell lung cancer. N Engl J Med 2018;379:2040–51.
19. Socinski M, Jotte RM, Cappuzzo F, et al. Atezolizumab for first-line treatment of metastatic nonsquamous NSCLC. N Engl J Med 2018;378:2288–301.
20. Timmerman RD, Paulus R, Pass HI, et al. Stereotactic body radiation therapy for operable early-stage lung cancer: findings from the NRG oncology RTOG 0618 trial. JAMA Oncol 2018;4(9):1263–6.
21. Antonio SJ, Villegas A, Daniel D, et al. Overall survival with durvalumab after chemoradiotherapy in stage III NSCLC. N Engl J Med 2018;379:2342–50.
22. Horn L, Mansfield AS, Szczęsna A, et al. First-line atezolizumab plus chemotherapy in extensive-stage small-cell lung cancer. N Engl J Med 2018;379: 2220–9.

Precision Medicine in the Treatment of Melanoma

Kimberly Aderhold, DO[a], Melissa Wilson, MD, PhD[a],
Adam C. Berger, MD[c],*, Shoshana Levi, MD[b], Joseph Bennett, MD[b]

KEYWORDS

- Melanoma • Precision medicine • Immunotherapy • Driver mutations • Oncogene
- Gene-expression • DecisionDx-melanoma

KEY POINTS

- There are a multitude of possible mutations across tumor genes with varying frequencies. Next-generation sequencing analyzes the tumor cells for all present mutations instead of sequential testing as was standard practice in years past.
- Precision medicine strategies targeting *BRAF*-V600 E/K mutations, with consequent suppression of the mitogen-activated protein kinase signaling pathway, have shown survival benefit in both the adjuvant and metastatic settings.
- MEK inhibitors have shown a small but significant progression-free survival advantage after failure of immunotherapy in *NRAS*-mutant melanoma.
- Immunotherapy with programmed death 1 and/or CTLA-4 inhibition has demonstrated substantial survival advantages in advanced resectable and unresectable melanomas.
- Gene expression profiling may influence postsurgical management by allowing more accurate risk stratification and, hence, more fitting follow-up and diagnostic testing.

Precision treatment of melanoma is rapidly evolving. Before the concept of precision medicine, the treatment of melanoma was limited to dacarbazine and interleukin-2 (IL-2), which achieved only a disappointingly small benefit in few patients with either therapy.[1] Now, however, profoundly more effective treatment options have been discovered that target actionable tumor-specific genetic mutations, including *BRAF*-V600 E/K driver mutations, *NRAS*, and *KIT* oncogenes, as well as immunotherapy with

This article originally appeared in *Surgical Oncology Clinics*, Volume 29, Issue 1, January 2020.
Disclosure Statement: Dr A.C. Berger has received honoraria from Castle Biosciences and Cardinal Health for consulting and speaker's bureau. Dr M. Wilson has received honoraria from BMS and Array Biopharma for advisory boards. The rest of the authors have nothing to disclose.
[a] Sidney Kimmel Medical College, Department of Medical Oncology, 1025 Walnut Street, Suite 700, Philadelphia, PA 19107, USA; [b] Department of Surgery, Christiana Care Health System, 4701 Ogletown Stanton Road, Newark, DE 19713, USA; [c] Rutgers Cancer Institute of New Jersey, 195 Little Albany Street, Room 3005, New Brunswick, NJ 08903, USA
* Corresponding author.
E-mail address: adam.berger@rutgers.edu

programmed death 1 (PD-1) and CTLA-4 inhibition. Often, these mutations are mutually exclusive, usually only 1 mutation is found in a given tumor sample. Next-generation sequencing (NGS) testing has been instrumental in helping to identify large spans of tumor-specific genetic profiles that allow the opportunity to individualize each patient's treatment regimen based on the molecular biology of the tumor cells.

TARGETING BRAF AND MEK

The most common mutation found in melanoma is the *BRAF* driver mutation, with more than 90% of these mutations located at codon 600, termed *BRAF* V600 mutations. Those 10% of mutations not located at codon 600 are referred to as non-V600 *BRAF* mutations and are seen less frequently in melanoma. Additional non-V600 mutations are found in other tumor types, including lung and thyroid cancers.

Within *BRAF* V600 mutations, oncogenic driver mutations *BRAF*-V600 E and *BRAF*-V600 K are by far the most common subtypes in melanoma, having been identified in 40% to 60% of cutaneous melanomas.[2] These mutations within the mitogen-activated protein kinase (MAPK) signaling pathway, along with other pathway aberrations, including the MEK escape mechanisms and *NRAS* mutations, induce constitutive activation of the cell cycle, driving uncontrolled tumor proliferation. Suppression of these signaling pathways has been shown to be an effective strategy in the treatment of melanomas harboring these mutations. Furthermore, the upregulation of MEK 1/2 has been shown to be a prominent escape mechanism, leading to the use of combination therapy with BRAF and MEK inhibition.

BRAF inhibitors, such as dabrafenib and vemurafenib, have demonstrated a survival advantage as both monotherapy and in combination with the MEK inhibitor trametinib in both resectable and unresectable or metastatic melanomas.[3–5] The landmark BRIM-3, and BRIM-8, and coBRIM trials were the first to show the safety and efficacy of using vemurafenib to treat melanomas with *BRAF* V600 E and V600 E mutations.[3,6,7] Extended overall survival (OS) analysis published in 2017 on the 675 subjects studied in the phase III BRIM-3 clinical trial showed that vemurafenib continued to be associated with an improved median OS of 13.6 months versus 9.7 months with dacarbazine in subjects with untreated unresectable stage III or IV melanoma.[7,8]

Data from the breakthrough phase II and phase III clinical trials, BREAK-2 and BREAK-3, conducted in 2012 were the first to demonstrate a safe and effective progression-free survival (PFS) and an OS advantage with dabrafenib monotherapy.[9,10] The 5-year landmark analysis performed in 2017 of the phase III BREAK-3 trial described by Chapman and colleagues[11] showed sustainable and significant 5-year PFS (12% vs 3%) and OS (24% vs 22%) rates with single-agent dabrafenib compared with dacarbazine. A subset of subjects received CTLA-4 (24% vs 24%) and/or PD-1 (8% vs 2%) inhibitors after progression. Thirty-one percent versus 17% did not receive any therapy after long-term follow-up.

Furthermore, a phase III clinical trial conducted in 2015 by Robert and colleagues[5] showed that combination dabrafenib and trametinib had a superior OS rate (72% vs 65%) and PFS (11.4 months vs 7.3 months) when compared with vemurafenib alone in the metastatic setting. Similar results were seen in the metastatic setting in 2018 by Dummer and colleagues,[12] showing that the BRAF inhibitor encorafenib in combination with the MEK inhibitor binimetinib had a longer PFS of 14.9 months compared with 7.3 months with vemurafenib alone.

In adjuvant stage III and resected stage IV disease, the phase III clinical trial performed by Long and colleagues[4] in 2017 showed that combination BRAF and MEK inhibition had a superior 3-year relapse-free survival rate (58% vs 39%) and OS rate

(86% vs 77%) compared with placebo. In 2018, a phase III clinical trial by Maio and colleagues[3] investigated the disease-free survival (DFS) of single-agent vemurafenib compared with placebo in 2 different cohorts. Cohort 1 included stage IIC, IIIA, and IIIB subjects with resectable disease, but the endpoint of median DFS was not reached. Cohort 2 studied stage IIIC resected disease and found a superior DFS of 23.1 months versus 15.4 months with placebo.

TARGETING NRAS

NRAS oncogenic mutations are seen in 15% to 20% of melanomas, and this distinct cohort of melanomas portend a poor prognosis.[13] Melanomas harboring this mutation tend to have more aggressive clinical and pathologic features, including increased mitotic activity, deeper depth of the lesion, and increased rates of nodal metastasis. The mutant allele varies within *NRAS* driver mutations. It is often found on codon Q61 (*NRAS* Q61) or less commonly on codons G12 and G13 (*NRAS* G12 and *NRAS* G13). Although all are considered activating point mutations, they affect the NRAS protein in different ways, leading to different clinical courses.[14]

Owing to the aggressive nature of *NRAS* mutant melanomas, investigation into potential therapeutic agents to target this oncogene has been of interest in the academic community. Preclinical models showed promising tumor response with first-generation MEK inhibitors to treat *NRAS* mutant melanomas. However, several of these trials did not show meaningful efficacy on further investigation.[13] These trials showed significant adverse events, namely ocular and neurologic symptoms that precluded further development of first-generation MEK inhibitors.

Newer second-generation MEK inhibitors subsequently were developed showing more tumor inhibition in preclinical models along with a tolerable safety profile. The first of these was selumetinib. A phase I study of 11 subjects with *NRAS*-mutant melanoma showed only partial response in 1 subject, and stable disease in 7 others. A subsequent phase II trial comparing selumetinib with temozolomide in *NRAS*-unselected subjects and *BRAF*-WT melanomas showed either equivalent or inferior response rates for selumetinib (5.8% vs 9.7%), as well as no benefit in PFS.[15] A second phase II study investigated selumetinib with or without dacarbazine in *BRAF*-WT melanomas but found similarly disappointing responses despite PFS being minimally prolonged (5.6 vs 3.0 months).[16]

Owing to the less than ideal results of selumetinib, development of third-generation MEK inhibitors led to even more promising results because focus shifted to NRAS-mutant melanomas. Dummer and colleagues[17] compared the third-generation MEK inhibitor binimetinib with standard-of-care dacarbazine in advanced or unresectable stage IIIC or IV NRAS-mutant melanomas. The study showed that binimetinib had a small but statistically significant superior median PFS of 2.8 months with binimetinib versus 1.5 months with dacarbazine. The small suboptimal response rates of third-generation MEK inhibitors led to consideration of combination strategies. Combinations of MEK inhibitors with CDK 4/6 inhibitors, RAF, and drugs targeting the EGFR/PI3K pathway have been considered in clinical trials.[14]

TARGETING KIT

Identification of the *KIT* oncogene led to multiple clinical trials studying transmembrane receptor tyrosine kinase as a target in the treatment of melanoma.[1] Binding of the KIT ligand results in activation of multiple downstream signaling pathways, including MAPK, JAK/STAT, and PI3K. Thus, the hypothesis evolved that targeting this mutation may provide an additional target for treatment of melanoma with the tyrosine kinase inhibitor imatinib.

Although several trials have shown efficacy of imatinib in treating melanomas harboring the *KIT* mutation, not all *KIT* mutations are sensitive to imatinib. As with *NRAS* and *BRAF* mutations, *KIT* mutations can vary widely over the genetic coding region, suggesting that not all mutations are equivalent functionally. There is some suggestion that certain mutations may represent passenger mutations instead of driver mutations. Demonstrating this concept, in the trial held by Guo and colleagues,[18] 9 of the 10 subjects who exhibited a response to imatinib had either exon 11 or 13 mutations, whereas there was only 1 of 3 subjects with *KIT* amplification who showed a response. This suggests that more specific molecular selection is necessary for effective targeted treatment with KIT inhibition.

Further defining the concept of more specific allelic selection when using imatinib to treat *KIT* mutant melanomas, 3 phase II studies between 2005 to 2008 revealed negative results, suggesting no benefit from KIT inhibition in metastatic melanoma. However, these studies were performed in molecularly unselected subject populations, and only 1 subject with acral melanoma from the 3 studies had a durable near-complete response. Interestingly, this subject had a splice site *KIT* mutation on exon 15.

Subsequent phase II clinical trials studying imatinib in molecularly selected advanced melanoma showed a small but significant efficacy in a subset of subjects who received imatinib. Carvajal and colleagues[19] showed significant clinical responses in 25 subjects with advanced melanoma, demonstrating an overall durable response rate for imatinib at 16% with a median time to progression of 12 weeks and a median OS of 46.3 weeks in a subset of subjects harboring primary *KIT* mutations. Similar findings were seen by Guo and colleagues,[18] who studied 43 subjects with advanced melanoma harboring *KIT* mutations and found an overall response rate of 23.3%, with a median PFS of 9 months and an OS of 15 months in those subjects who achieved a partial response or stable disease. Nine of the 10 subjects who achieved a partial response harbored *KIT* mutations on exon 11 or 13.

IMMUNOTHERAPY

Immunotherapy has revolutionized the treatment of melanoma and has provided remarkable outcomes for what was previously among most treatment refractory cancers. Immune checkpoint inhibitors play a key role, particularly when no targetable mutations are available. Harnessing the immune system against cancers, which is mediated by cytotoxic lymphocytes and the adaptive immune system, changed the landscape of melanoma therapy. The standard of care in the current era includes immune-modulating modalities such as PD-1 inhibitors (nivolumab and pembrolizumab) and CTLA-4 antibody inhibitors (ipilimumab). Clinical trials investigating these drugs have resulted in unprecedented outcomes in both metastatic and stage III melanomas with improvements in overall and PFS.

The landmark trial in 2010 by Hodi and colleagues[20] changed the way the scientific community approaches melanoma. This phase III study explored the CTLA-4 inhibitor ipilimumab in subjects with metastatic melanoma and found a 10-month improvement in OS, which was monumental compared with the disappointing outcomes seen in prior IL-2 therapies and chemotherapy. The 1-year and 2-year survival rates were 46% and 24%, respectively, compared with 25% and 14%, respectively, in the control group. Immediately after publication of this trial, ipilimumab was approved for the treatment of advanced melanoma.

PD-1 inhibitors have proven to be the most effective immunotherapies in melanoma, especially when combined with the CTLA-4 inhibitor ipilimumab. One of the earliest clinical trials exploring these PD-1 targeted antibodies was with nivolumab in the CheckMate 066 trial. In this trial, 210 subjects with metastatic or unresectable melanoma had a 1-year survival rate of 72.9%, and median PFS was 5.1 months (median OS was not reached).[21] The Keynote-006 trial investigated pembrolizumab at a dosing of every 2 or 3 weeks versus ipilimumab every 3 weeks, and demonstrated a 1-year survival rate of 74.1%, 68.4%, and 58.2%, respectively.[22] Updated long-term analysis of this trial showed durable response to treatment with 91% of subjects who did not progress after 2 years. These trials demonstrated that both nivolumab and pembrolizumab have more favorable safety profiles compared with ipilimumab. Such extraordinary outcomes from PD-1 inhibitors have made these drugs the standard of care for subjects with metastatic or unresectable melanomas.

Furthermore, combination therapy with ipilimumab and PD-1 inhibitors have demonstrated a higher antitumor effect and increased inflammatory cell infiltration compared with ipilimumab alone. Dual blockade with nivolumab plus ipilimumab was first studied in the phase I dose-escalation study, CA209-004, by Wolchok and colleagues.[23] This study was later evaluated in a phase II (CheckMate 069) and phase III (CheckMate 067) clinical trials.[24,25] The objective response rate with combination therapy in the CA209-004 was 40%, which was higher than demonstrated with ipilimumab monotherapy (11%) or nivolumab monotherapy (28%). Updated 3-year analysis of the CA209-004 by Callahan and colleagues[26] in 2018, showed that combination therapy with nivolumab and ipilimumab in subjects with advanced unresectable melanoma had a 3-year OS rate of 63% with median OS not yet reached. The objective response rate was 42% in 3 years with median duration of response 22.3 months. Incidence of grade 3 and 4 toxicities occurred in 59% of subjects over the 3 years.

The phase III clinical trial (CheckMate 067) in 2015 by Larkin and colleagues[27] explored combination treatment with nivolumab and ipilimumab versus nivolumab alone versus ipilimumab alone in untreated unresectable stage III or stage IV subjects. The investigators found that PFS was 11.5 months in the nivolumab-ipilimumab group, but 14 months in subjects with PD-L1 (+) subjects and 11.2 months in PD-L1 (−) subjects. The nivolumab monotherapy cohort had a PFS of 6.9 months overall, with 14 months in the PD-L1 (+) group and 5.3 months in the PD-L1 (−) group. Ipilimumab monotherapy demonstrated a PFS of 2.9 months in the PD-L1 (+) group. In summary, in PD-L1 (+) subjects, combination nivolumab-ipilimumab was essentially equivalent to nivolumab alone but at the price of higher toxicity with the combination. In PD-L1 (−) tumors, nivolumab was superior. Between the 2 monotherapies, nivolumab was superior to ipilimumab. This confirmed the clinical benefit of combination therapy in the treatment of advanced melanomas.

A phase III study in 2015 evaluated immunotherapy in the adjuvant setting and showed that ipilimumab alone improved recurrence-free survival (RFS) by 10 months versus placebo in resected stage III melanomas.[28] Then, in 2017, Weber and colleagues[29] compared nivolumab to ipilimumab in this population and found that nivolumab had a significantly higher 12-month RFS of 70.5%, whereas ipilimumab had a 12-month RFS of 60.8%. In 2018, the PD-1 inhibitor, pembrolizumab, was studied against placebo in subjects with stage III resected melanoma and was found to have a significantly improved 12-month RFS rate of 75.4% with pembrolizumab compared with 61% with placebo.[30–44] The impressive responses seen in these trials led to the approval of PD-1 inhibitors as adjuvant treatment of melanoma.

GENETIC TESTING

A wide array of genetic and genomic aberrations has been identified in melanoma, most commonly *BRAF*, *NRAS*, and *KIT* mutations. Although many are point mutations, various types of genomic abnormalities exist, contributing to the vast heterogenicity of tumor cells. Identifying specific mutations is key to appropriate and effective targeted treatment, and is the backbone behind the concept and value of precision medicine. Traditionally, genetic testing techniques for identifying these aberrations included direct sequencing of DNA, which recognizes point mutations within a given portion of DNA. The single nucleotide extension assay is another molecular study that identifies known point mutations within a specific genetic region of interest; however, this technique will only detect mutations within the genetic region studied. Fluorescence in situ hybridization (FISH) detects greater areas of genomic aberrations, identifying larger gene amplifications, rearrangements, and deletions. There are a multitude of other genomic testing techniques that drive understanding of the genetic signature; however, none stand up to the merit of information made possible by massive parallel sequencing.

Massive parallel sequencing (ie, NGS) transcends the value over traditional molecular testing techniques. It provides simultaneous sequencing of entire exomes and genomes of tumor specimens, thus identifying essentially any subset of genetic and genomic aberration within the cancer cell. As expected, simultaneous sequencing of entire genetic material generates large amounts of data that are, in turn, analyzed and interpreted into the appropriate clinical application. This sophisticated process continues to evolve as research ensues within multiple research laboratories.

The most widely used and researched genomic profiling laboratories include Foundation One Medicine testing and Caris Life Sciences. They use several platforms of molecular and genetic testing for NGS. Analysis is usually performed on frozen tissue sections or blood-based samples. Dynamic light scattering, flow cytometry, fragment analysis, immunohistochemistry, and FISH are available in addition to NGS. In addition to these well-established syndicates, many academic institutions perform their own NGS testing with generalized panels with actionable mutations across all cancer types, whereas some use individualized panels. Exploratory data are often collected based on the institution's modified testing panel, which can be further used in research and institutional clinical trials.

NGS has revolutionized precision medicine and has led to the application of more effective therapies against several different types of cancer. It has helped to construct a comprehensive understanding of the genetic signatures of tumor cells, allowing for targeted treatment and better outcomes. In the study of melanoma, NGS identifies known genomic changes and somatic mutations, such as *BRAF*, *NRAS*, and *KIT* mutations. NGS also prompts the discovery of new genomic aberrations, which continue to be studied and refined as the vast library of data evolves.

Gene Expression Profiling

Another area in which genetic testing is starting to play a bigger role in the care of patients with melanoma is in gene expression profile (GEP) testing, which can provide essential prognostic information for patients with melanoma. The commonly used gene expression profile tests provided by Castle Biosciences stratify samples of both cutaneous and uveal melanomas into high and low risk of recurrence, metastasis, and survival based on the specific gene profile of that individual's melanoma. Although the American Joint Committee on Cancer (AJCC) staging allows for categorization of melanoma into distinct groups based on clinical and pathologic data that predict prognosis, the addition of personalized testing can enhance the accuracy of prognostication. Such results may lead to more informed and effective treatment plans.

The heterogeneity that characterizes the disease progression of melanoma has driven research aimed at identifying those patients with the highest risk of recurrence, metastasis, and mortality. The genetic mutations responsible for conferring malignant potential in melanoma have been investigated for nearly 2 decades as part of this search. Early studies determined that there are reproducible subsets of cutaneous melanoma based on certain genetic profiles.[1] Similarly, distinct classes of uveal melanoma based on gene expression profiles were also identified.[2] Subsets of cutaneous melanomas that included samples with high metastatic potential were further examined, highlighting genes and expressed sequence tags thought to play a role in disease progression and metastasis.[3–9] A comparative, retrospective analysis with samples of primary cutaneous melanoma and their respective metastasis added to the growing knowledge of metastatic pathways for cutaneous melanoma. Additionally, immunohistochemical markers associated with distant metastasis-free survival and OS were identified.[10]

The results from this research led to the development of GEP assays for both uveal and cutaneous melanoma used in clinical practice today. Difficulties in classification and prognostication of uveal melanoma led to rapid adoption of gene profiling. Early testing of a 3-gene signature showed superior prediction of metastatic death when compared with clinical and pathologic prognostic factors such as tumor thickness and presence of invasion, as well as chromosomal aberrations.[2] Additional studies supported these findings[11] and led to the development of a 15-gene GEP assay validated through a prospective multicenter study.[12,13] The studies illustrated a high technical success rate with 97% of cases classified and accurate prognostication of metastasis that outperformed any other prognostic factor (**Fig. 1**). Furthermore, the GEP assay demonstrated net reclassification improvements of 0.43 ($P = .001$) and 0.38 ($P = .004$) over the tumor-node-metastasis (TNM) classification and chromosome 3 status, respectively.

Although TNM staging for cutaneous melanoma provides critical prognostic information to patients and providers, there remains significant variability in the development of disease progression within the different stages.[14] In an effort to address this variability and identify patients at risk of metastases despite reassuring AJCC staging, a 31-gene signature was developed using published genomic anlyses.[15] Archived melanoma samples were classified into 2 groups, with class 1 and class 2 tumors indicating a low and high risk of metastasis, respectively. In a validation set of 104 cases of cutaneous melanoma, the negative predictive value (NPV) and positive predictive value (PPV) were found to be 93% and 72%, respectively. When including only stage I and stage II melanomas, as defined by the AJCC staging system, the NPV and PPV were 94% and 67%, respectively. The GEP assay was found to be an independent predictor of metastatic risk with a hazard ratio of 9.55 ($P = .002$). This compared favorably with the hazard ratio of 5.4 ($P = .002$) for AJCC staging. These findings were supported in follow-up prospective[16,17] and retrospecitve[18,19] trials in which the prognostic accuracy of the 31-gene GEP assay was evaluated. The trials have shown the ability of the assay to accurately risk-stratify patients independent of lymph node status. In a study by Gerami and colleagues[16] with subjects with a class 2 GEP signature, there was no statistical difference in DFS or OS for subjects with positive sentinel lymph nodes and those with negative sentinel lymph nodes (**Fig. 2**). Gene profiling may in fact replace sentinel lymph node status in some cases. A recent study by Vetto and colleagues[20] evaluated the ability of the 31-gene GEP assay to predict lymph node positivity. In subjects with T1-T2 tumors and low-risk gene profiles; that

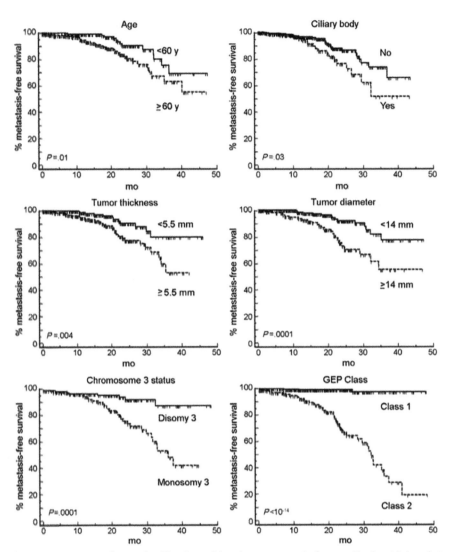

Fig. 1. Comparison of GEP classification with other prognostic factors. Kaplan-Meier plots for the indicated prognostic factors. *P* values were determined by the log-rank method. Age indicates patient's age at the time of the primary tumor diagnosis. Threshold values for dichotomizing continuous variables (tumor thickness and diameter) were determined by receiver operating characteristic analysis. (*From* B. R. Gastman, P. Gerami, S. J. Kurley, et al., Identification of patients at risk of metastasis using a prognostic 31-gene expression profile in subpopulations of melanoma patients with favorable outcomes by standard cirteria. Journal of the American Academy of Dermatology. 2019;1:80:149–157; with permission.)

is, class 1, the rates of sentinel lymph node positivity in those aged greater than or equal to 65 years, 55 to 64 years, and less than 55 years were found to be 1.6%, 4.9%, and 7.6%, respectively. These findings raise the question of whether sentinel lymph node biopsy can be avoided in certain patient populations with low-risk melanomas by GEP assay. The numbers of subjects involved in these studies are still low and require further validation.

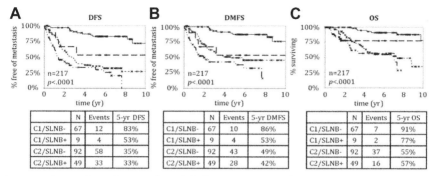

Fig. 2. Kaplan-Meier estimates of DFS (*A*), distant metastasis-free survival (DMFS) (*B*), and OS (*C*) in a cohort of 217 cutaneous melanoma cases with outcomes predicted by sentinel lymph node biopsy (SLNB) procedure in combination with GEP testing. Four subgroups of patients are described and shown after assignment of SLNB and GEP prognostic prediction. (*From* P. Gerami, R. W. Cook, M. C. Russell, et al. Gene expression profiling for molecular staging of cutaneous melanoma in patients undergoing sentinel lymph node biopsy. Journal of the American Academy of Dermatology. 2015; 5:72; 780–785; with permission.)

In terms of prognostic information, GEP for cutaneous melanoma theoretically yields the most benefit for those with low AJCC stages but high metastatic potential. The hope is that by providing personalized evaluation of each melanoma case, clinicians can offer more appropriate treatment plans and follow-up to their patients. In the case of a patient with a stage I or IIA melanoma, a class 2 assignment may provide more realistic prognostic information. National Comprehensive Cancer Network (NCCN) guidelines do not recommend routine imaging as part of follow-up to screen for recurrence or metastasis in stage I or IIA patients, with no evidence of disease after wide local excision and do not recommend the use of GEP testing to inform follow-up screening.[45] It is hypothesized that the addition of class 2 prognostication may influence clinicians to obtain surveillance imaging and evaluate such a patient more regularly, outside of current NCCN algorithms. Additionally, such information may lead to recommendations for inclusion in clinical trials or administration of newer therapies that would not have been previously offered and which have shown improved survival for patients with more advanced disease.

The potential impact of GEP testing can be perceived when assessing outcomes in stage I or IIA patients specifically. In a study evaluating the development of a cutaneous melanoma GEP test, retrospective analysis of the test's predictive value in stage I and II patients was carried out.[46–51] Follow-up was at least 5 years or until a metastatic event. Out of 119 cases of stage I melanoma, 9 cases were found to have documented metastases. Of these 9 cases, 5 (56%) were accurately predicted to have a poor outcome based on being class 2 on GEP testing. Conversely, 5% of stage I patients without a metastatic event were inaccurately over-staged by the GEP assay and assigned to class 2. As the AJCC stage increased, the sensitivity of the GEP test increased but the specificity decreased. For patients with stage IIA ($n = 45$), IIB ($n = 42$), and IIC ($n = 14$) melanomas, 90% (19/21), 96% (27/28), and 100% (11/11), respectively, with metastatic events were appropriately assigned to the class 2 group. At the same time, the number of cases assigned class 2 in which there was no metastatic event by 5 years of follow-up steadily increased across stage II categories; 33% (8/24) of stage IIA, 57% (8/14) of stage IIB, and 67% (2/3) of stage IIC melanomas without metastases were class 2 on GEP testing. Importantly, the staging was not based on the most recent eighth edition of the AJCC system, but the differences between the seventh and eighth editions would not have affected stage II subjects.

Currently, the downstream clinical effects of using GEP testing have not been evaluated and there are no guidelines on how to translate results into decision-making. Thus, looking at the small sample previously described, providers must ask how GEP testing would have affected clinical decision-making for the 164 stage I and IIA patients. Out of those 164 patients, 38 were classified as class 2. Of the 24 stage I and IIA class 2 patients who went on to develop metastasis, would any have been offered additional therapies that would have prevented metastatic events? Or, would the metastatic events be detected earlier, allowing for expedient initiation of systemic therapy? Most importantly, do these changes lead to survival benefit? It is critical to also ask what the effect would have been for the 14 stage I and IIA class 2 patients who did not go on to have metastatic events. Would they have been inappropriately enrolled in clinical trials or received unnecessary therapies? Or would they have only received more regular follow-up and imaging? These are all questions that have yet to be answered.

SUMMARY

Precision medicine has transformed the treatment of melanoma and has provided more meaningful outcomes in a previously treatment-resistant cancer. It has driven changes in molecular testing strategies and clinical trial design, making targeted genetic aberrations the director of therapy for several cancers, notably in melanoma. GEP is helping to identify lower stage patients who may have a higher risk for metastases that may benefit from enhanced surveillance or even treatment. Targeted treatments specific for *BRAF*, *NRAS*, and *KIT* mutations, as well as the use of immunotherapies, have resulted in superior outcomes and survival in both advanced and adjuvant settings. Both monotherapies and combination therapies targeting these mutations have become the standard of care in melanoma, leaving chemotherapy and IL-2 therapy as third-line or greater treatment options when resistance to targeted therapies develops. Further investigations into a multitude of targeted combination therapies may represent opportunities to expand treatment options for patients with melanoma. In conclusion, precision medicine has brought about a new era in the treatment melanoma that continues to improve and evolve each year.

REFERENCES

1. Carvajal RD. Targeting KIT for treatment of advanced melanoma. The Melanoma Letter Winter 2011;29(3).
2. Johnson DB, Flaherty KT, Weber JS, et al. Combined BRAF (Dabrafenib) and MEK Inhibition (Trametinib) in patients with *BRAF* V600 -mutant melanoma experiencing progression with single-agent BRAF inhibitor. J Clin Oncol 2014;32(33): 3697–704.
3. Maio M, Lewis K, Demidov L, et al. Adjuvant vemurafenib in resected, BRAF V600 mutation-positive melanoma (BRIM8): a randomised, double-blind, placebo-controlled, multicentre, phase 3 trial. Lancet Oncol 2018;19(4):510–20.
4. Long GV, Hauschild A, Santinami M, et al. Adjuvant dabrafenib plus trametinib in Stage III *BRAF* -mutated melanoma. N Engl J Med 2017;377(19):1813–23.
5. Robert C, Karaszewska B, Schachter J, et al. Improved overall survival in melanoma with combined dabrafenib and trametinib. N Engl J Med 2015;372(1):30–9.

6. Larkin J, Ascierto PA, Dréno B, et al. Combined vemurafenib and cobimetinib in *BRAF*-mutated melanoma. N Engl J Med 2014;371(20):1867–76.
7. Chapman PB, Hauschild A, Robert C, et al. Improved survival with vemurafenib in melanoma with BRAF V600E mutation. N Engl J Med 2011;364(26):2507–16.
8. Chapman PB, Robert C, Larkin J, et al. Vemurafenib in patients with BRAFV600 mutation-positive metastatic melanoma: final overall survival results of the randomized BRIM-3 study. Ann Oncol 2017;28(10):2581–7.
9. Ascierto PA, Minor D, Ribas A, et al. Phase II trial (BREAK-2) of the BRAF inhibitor dabrafenib (GSK2118436) in patients with metastatic melanoma. J Clin Oncol 2013;31(26):3205–11.
10. Hauschild A, Grob JJ, Demidov LV, et al. Phase III, randomized, open-label, multicenter trial (BREAK-3) comparing the BRAF kinase inhibitor dabrafenib (GSK2118436) with dacarbazine (DTIC) in patients with BRAF ^{V600E}-mutated melanoma. J Clin Oncol 2012;30(18):LBA8500.
11. Chapman PB, Ascierto PA, Schadendorf D, et al. "Updated 5-y landmark analyses of phase 2 (BREAK-2) and phase 3 (BREAK-3) studies evaluating dabrafenib monotherapy in patients with *BRAF* V600–mutant melanoma. J Clin Oncol 2017;35(15_suppl):9526.
12. Dummer R, Ascierto PA, Gogas HJ, et al. Encorafenib plus binimetinib versus vemurafenib or encorafenib in patients with BRAF -mutant melanoma (COLUMBUS): a multicentre, open-label, randomised phase 3 trial. Lancet Oncol 2018; 19(5):603–15.
13. Johnson DB, Lovly CM, Flavin M, et al. Impact of NRAS mutations for patients with advanced melanoma treated with immune therapies. Cancer Immunol Res 2015; 3(3):288–95.
14. Muñoz-Couselo E, Zamora Adelantado E, Ortiz Vélez C, et al. NRAS-mutant melanoma: current challenges and future prospect. Onco Targets Ther 2017;10: 3941–7.
15. Kirkwood JM, Bastholt L, Robert C, et al. Phase II, open-label, randomized trial of the MEK1/2 inhibitor selumetinib as monotherapy versus temozolomide in patients with advanced melanoma. Clin Cancer Res 2012;18(2):555–67.
16. Robert C, Dummer R, Gutzmer R, et al. Selumetinib plus dacarbazine versus placebo plus dacarbazine as first-line treatment for BRAF-mutant metastatic melanoma: a phase 2 double-blind randomised study. Lancet Oncol 2013;14(8): 733–40.
17. Dummer R, Schadendorf D, Ascierto PA, et al. Binimetinib versus dacarbazine in patients with advanced NRAS -mutant melanoma (NEMO): a multicentre, open-label, randomised, phase 3 trial. Lancet Oncol 2017;18(4):435–45.
18. Guo J, Si L, Kong Y, et al. Phase II, open-label, single-arm trial of imatinib mesylate in patients with metastatic melanoma harboring *c-Kit* mutation or amplification. J Clin Oncol 2011;29(21):2904–9.
19. Carvajal RD. KIT as a therapeutic target in metastatic melanoma. JAMA 2011; 305(22):2327.
20. Hodi FS, O'Day SJ, McDermott DF, et al. Improved survival with ipilimumab in patients with metastatic melanoma. N Engl J Med 2010;363(8):711–23.
21. Robert C, Long GV, Brady B, et al. Nivolumab in previously untreated melanoma without *BRAF* mutation. N Engl J Med 2015;372(4):320–30.
22. Robert C, Schachter J, Long GV, et al. Pembrolizumab versus ipilimumab in advanced melanoma. N Engl J Med 2015;372(26):2521–32.
23. Wolchok JD, Kluger H, Callahan MK, et al. Nivolumab plus ipilimumab in advanced melanoma. N Engl J Med 2013;369(2):122–33.

24. Postow MA, Chesney J, Pavlick AC, et al. Nivolumab and Ipilimumab versus Ipilimumab in Untreated Melanoma. N Engl J Med 2015;372(21):2006–17.
25. Hodi FS, Chesney J, Pavlick AC, et al. Combined nivolumab and ipilimumab versus ipilimumab alone in patients with advanced melanoma: 2-year overall survival outcomes in a multicentre, randomised, controlled, phase 2 trial. Lancet Oncol 2016;17(11):1558–68.
26. Callahan MK, Kluger H, Postow MA, et al. Nivolumab plus ipilimumab in patients with advanced melanoma: updated survival, response, and safety data in a phase I dose-escalation study. J Clin Oncol 2018;36(4):391–8.
27. Larkin J, Chiarion-Sileni V, Gonzalez R, et al. Combined nivolumab and ipilimumab or monotherapy in untreated melanoma. N Engl J Med 2015;373(1):23–34.
28. Eggermont AMM, Chiarion-Sileni V, Grob J-J, et al. Adjuvant ipilimumab versus placebo after complete resection of high-risk stage III melanoma (EORTC 18071): a randomised, double-blind, phase 3 trial. Lancet Oncol 2015;16(5):522–30.
29. Weber J, Mandala M, Del Vecchio M, et al. Adjuvant nivolumab versus ipilimumab in resected stage III or IV melanoma. N Engl J Med 2017;377(19):1824–35.
30. Eggermont AMM, Blank CU, Mandala M, et al. Adjuvant pembrolizumab versus placebo in resected stage III melanoma. N Engl J Med 2018;378(19):1789–801.
31. Bittner M, Meltzer P, Chen Y, et al. Molecular classification of cutaneous malignant melanoma by gene expression profiling. Nature 2000;406:536–40.
32. Onken MD, Worley LA, Ehlers JP, et al. Gene expression profiling in uveal melanoma reveals two molecular classes and predicts metastatic death. Cancer Res 2004;64:7205–9.
33. Clark EA, Golub TR, Lander ES, et al. Genomic analysis of metastasis reveals an essential role for RhoC. Nature 2000;406:532–5.
34. Weeraratna AT, Jiang Y, Hostetter G, et al. Wnt5a signaling directly affects cell motility and invasion of metastatic melanoma. Cancer Cell 2002;1:279–88.
35. Haqq C, Nosrati M, Sudilovsky D, et al. The gene expression signatures of melanoma progression. Proc Natl Acad Sci U S A 2005;102:6092–7.
36. Smith AP, Hoek K, Becker D. Whole-genome expression profiling of the melanoma progression pathway reveals marked molecular differences between nevi/melanoma in situ and advanced-stage melanomas. Cancer Biol Ther 2005;4:1018–29.
37. Jaeger J, Koczan D, Thiesen H-J, et al. Gene expression signatures for tumor progression, tumor subtype, and tumor thickness in laser-microdissected melanoma tissues. Clin Cancer Res 2007;13:806–15.
38. Scatolini M, Grand MM, Grosso E, et al. Altered molecular pathways in melanocytic lesions. Int J Cancer 2010;126:1869–81.
39. Mauerer A, Roesch A, Hafner C, et al. Identification of new genes associated with melanoma. Exp Dermatol 2011;20:502–7.
40. Winnepenninckx V, Lazar V, Michiels S, et al. Gene expression profiling of primary cutaneous melanoma and clinical outcome. J Natl Cancer Inst 2006. https://doi.org/10.1093/jnci/djj103.
41. Petrausch U, Martus P, Tö Nnies H, et al. Significance of gene expression analysis in uveal melanoma in comparison to standard risk factors for risk assessment of subsequent metastases. Eye 2008;22:997–1007.
42. Onken MD, Worley LA, Tuscan MD, et al. An accurate, clinically feasible multigene expression assay for predicting metastasis in uveal melanoma. J Mol Diagn 2010;12:461–8.

43. Onken MD, Worley LA, Char DH, et al. Collaborative ocular oncology group report number 1: prospective validation of a multi-gene prognostic assay in uveal melanoma. Ophthalmology 2012. https://doi.org/10.1016/j.ophtha.2012.02.017.

44. Svedman FC, Pillas D, Taylor A, et al. Stage-specific survival and recurrence in patients with cutaneous malignant melanoma in Europe - a systematic review of the literature. Clin Epidemiol 2016;8:109–22.

45. NCCN clinical practice guidelines in oncology (NCCN Guidelines®) for cutaneous melanoma V.2.2019. National Comprehensive Cancer Network, Inc.; 2019. Accessed March 12, 2019.

46. Gerami P, Cook RW, Wilkinson J, et al. Development of a prognostic genetic signature to predict the metastatic risk associated with cutaneous melanoma. Clin Cancer Res 2015. https://doi.org/10.1158/1078-0432.CCR-13-3316.

47. Gerami P, Cook RW, Russell MC, et al. Gene expression profiling for molecular staging of cutaneous melanoma in patients undergoing sentinel lymph node biopsy. J Am Acad Dermatol 2015. https://doi.org/10.1016/j.jaad.2015.01.009.

48. Hsueh EC, DeBloom JR, Lee J, et al. Interim analysis of survival in a prospective, multi-center registry cohort of cutaneous melanoma tested with a prognostic 31-gene expression profile test. J Hematol Oncol 2017;10:152.

49. Zager JS, Gastman BR, Leachman S, et al. Performance of a prognostic 31-gene expression profile in an independent cohort of 523 cutaneous melanoma patients. BMC Cancer 2018;18:130.

50. Gastman BR, Zager JS, Messina JL, et al. Performance of a 31-gene expression profile test in cutaneous melanomas of the head and neck. Head Neck 2019;41: 871–9.

51. Vetto JT, Hsueh EC, Gastman BR, et al. Guidance of sentinel lymph node biopsy decisions in patients with T1–T2 melanoma using gene expression profiling. Future Oncol 2019;15:1207–17.

Personalized Medicine in Gynecologic Cancer
Fact or Fiction?

Logan Corey, MD[a],*, Ana Valente, MD[a,1], Katrina Wade, MD[b]

KEYWORDS

- Personalized medicine • Precision medicine • Targeted therapies
- Gynecologic malignancies

KEY POINTS

- Personalized medicine is an evolving concept that centers around treating cancers based on tumor molecular profiling rather than location of origin.
- Tumor molecular profiling has allowed for several driver mutations to be identified in gynecologic malignancies and subsequent targeted therapies to be created.
- With direct to consumer marketing, patient demand for personalized medicine is increasing.

INTRODUCTION TO PERSONALIZED MEDICINE

Personalized medicine, also known as "precision medicine," is the science of individualizing cancer care by treating tumors based on their genetic makeup rather than their location of origin.[1] Both gene expressional profiling and genome-wide sequencing have played significant roles in making this possible.[2] Knowing a tumor's molecular sequence has allowed for creation of targeted therapies. Examples of current successful oncologic therapies include BRAF inhibitors (vemurafenib) used in melanoma treatment, RET inhibitors (sorafenib) used in advanced renal and hepatocellular carcinomas, and epidermal growth factor receptor or anaplastic lymphoma kinase inhibitors used in non–small-cell lung cancer.[3]

This article originally appeared in *Obstetrics and Gynecology Clinics*, Volume 46, Issue 1, March 2019.

Disclosure Statement: The authors have nothing to disclose.

[a] Department of Obstetrics and Gynecology, Ochsner Clinic Foundation, 2700 Napoleon Avenue, New Orleans, LA 70115, USA; [b] Department of Gynecologic Oncology, Ochsner Clinic Foundation, 2700 Napoleon Avenue, New Orleans, LA 70115, USA

[1] Present address: 1520 Saint Mary Street, Unit D, New Orleans, LA 70130.

* Corresponding author. 209 North Dupre Street, New Orleans, LA 70118.

E-mail address: logan.corey@ochsner.org

In gynecologic oncology, the application of personalized medicine is still a work in progress. Genetic offenders or "driver mutations" have been identified in ovarian cancer (BRCA mutations, NOTCH, P13 K, BRAS/MEK, FOX 1, p53), endometrial cancer (TP53, PTEN, P1K3CA, and KRAS) and cervical cancers (P1K3CA, TP53, RB1).[1] Therapies that target these molecules are being developed and are effective by various mechanisms, including interruption of tumor cell stroma, vasculature, and aberrant signaling mechanisms.[4] Several of these mutations and therapies and their use and challenges are discussed in this article, as we explore the intricacies of personalized medicine in gynecologic malignancy: is it fact or fiction?

DRIVER MUTATIONS

Oncogenic mutations belong to 1 of 2 groups of proteins: oncogenes or tumor suppressor genes. Mutations to oncogenes cause cancer growth, whereas mutations to tumor suppressor genes cause failure of inhibition of cell growth, and therefore indirectly lead to cancer. These oncogenic mutations are known as "driver mutations." Individual oncogenes also contain genetic alterations such as substitutions, insertions, deletions, rearrangements, and loss of heterozygosity. These "passenger mutations" are mutations that are commonly associated with driver mutations that do not themselves cause cancer. Interestingly, there is recent evidence proposed that passenger mutations in cumulative may not be benign bystanders within or around cancer genes and can be harmful to cancer cells.[5]

Identification of driver mutations is of interest because it stands to reason that if either type of driver mutations could be identified and countered, the cancer would be cured or slowed. Successes in such endeavors in other oncology subspecialties, for example, use of the Philadelphia mutation as a target and the use of imatinib in the treatment of chronic myelogenous leukemia, have encouraged expansion of this body of work into other fields including gynecology oncology.[6] Furthermore, the relatively recent capability of researchers to sequence entire cancer genomes in a cost-effective way has allowed for a rapid broadening of the search for driver mutations and the exploration of their utility as possible targets in cancer treatment. Strategies include prediction of function models, machine learning models, and models that are based on the difference in mutation frequencies between driver and passenger mutations.[7] Tumor suppressor genes are generally more difficult to identify as driver mutations than oncogenes. It is much simpler to insert an oncogene into a cell line and evaluate for cancer growth than it is to remove a tumor suppressor gene from a cell line and monitor for cancer growth (ie, knockout models). Occasionally, a single cancer will have multiple driver mutations. This is consistent with the suggestion that some common cancers are thought to require 5 to 7 rate-limiting events on the way to becoming cancerous.[8]

Other ways of identifying driver mutations involve looking for similar mutations in cancers that are present at increased frequency relative to the background genome. This was demonstrated in a large study by the Cancer Genome Atlas that examined more than 400 high-grade serous ovarian adenocarcinomas that used the previous method and found more than 96% of these tumors were characterized by p53 mutations. Additional mutations were identified by cross-referencing other databases. Multiple other mutations were found in most of the tumors along with the p53 mutations, including mutations in *BRAF* (N581S), *PIK3CA* (E545 K and H1047 R), *KRAS* (G12D), and *NRAS* (Q61 R).[8]

Isolating driver mutations in gynecologic cancer has proven difficult. This is most likely due to the complexity and ubiquitous nature of the pathways involved. Multiple pathways are of intense interest at the moment and seem to play a role in development of other cancer types including breast, gastrointestinal, and lung cancers.

TUMOR HETEROGENEITY

Tumor heterogeneity is one of the greatest challenges in the era of personalized medicine. Although studies such as The Cancer Genome Atlas Project (TCGA) and the NCI-Match have helped in our understanding of the molecular basis of gynecologic cancers, they have also highlighted both intertumor and intratumor heterogeneity.[9,10] Intratumor heterogeneity is the concept that multiple biopsies of a single tumor may contain genetic variation and multiple subclonal populations. Studies have highlighted that such extreme molecular diversity can exist in solid tumor biopsies, even when they are collected from the same patient.[11] Whole genome and whole exosome studies have also highlighted genomic heterogeneity during transition from primary tumor to recurrence to metastasis.[12] This presents a unique challenge, especially in attempts to identify curative treatment for advanced disease.[13]

CURRENT TARGETED THERAPIES
Antiangiogenic Therapies

Angiogenesis, or the creation of new vascular supply, plays a key role in successful tumorigenesis. It is a process driven by vascular endothelial growth factor (VEGF). Overexpression of VEGF leads to increased blood supply and subsequent increase in delivery of nutrients and oxygen to tumor beds.[14] Antiangiogenesis therapies target and inhibit VEGF. Bevacizumab is the most studied antiangiogenic agent used in gynecologic cancer treatment.[1] It is a recombinant monoclonal antibody and is the only antiangiogenic therapy approved by the Food and Drug Administration (FDA).[15] Several clinical trials have investigated bevacizumab and demonstrated its efficacy in the treatment of ovarian cancer,[16,17] although overall survival benefit is seen only when bevacizumab is used in combination with standard cytotoxic chemo and then followed by bevacizumab maintenance.[18] In addition, the GOG240 has shown improved progression-free and overall survival when bevacizumab is added to standard chemotherapy in advanced or recurrent cervical cancer.[19]

Poly-ADP-Ribose Polymerase Inhibitors

Poly-ADP-ribose polymerase (PARP) inhibitors are agents that interfere with DNA damage repair. Typically, PARP repairs single-strand DNA breaks.[20] If single-strand DNA breaks are unable to be repaired due to PARP inhibition and accumulate, the DNA replication fork is stalled. In this situation, the cell must rely on double-strand break repair (via the homologous recombination [HR] pathway) to be able to survive, a mechanism that is notoriously absent in BRCA-mutated cells.[1,20] This leads to BRCA-deficient cells being incredibly vulnerable to PARP inhibitors and likewise confers their sensitivity to platinum as HR is required to repair platinum-induced intrastrand and interstrand DNA cross links. Several clinical studies have confirmed PARP inhibitors are effective,[21,22] and have shown significant increase in progression-free survival with their use.[23] Currently, 3 PARP inhibitors are FDA approved: olaparib, rucaparib, and niraparib. The study of PARP inhibitors is still currently under way and the future holds promise that they will not only be reserved for patients with BRCA mutations but may also be used in patients whose tumors have functional defects in other DNA repair proteins.[14]

PHOSPHATIDYL INOSITOL 3-Kinase/AKT/Mammalian TARGET OF RAPAMYCIN/ PHOSPHATASE AND TENSIN HOMOLOG

The phosphatidyl inositol 3-kinase (PI3K)/AKT/mammalian target of rapamycin (mTOR) pathway plays a critical role in the malignant transformation of human tumors and their subsequent growth, proliferation, and metastasis, including ovarian cancers.[24] Characteristic of cell cycle control pathways, there is a normal balance to the activators and inhibitors within these complex pathways and the PI3K/AKT/ mTOR pathway is no different. These interactions are currently being studied for their theoretic druggable and targetable proteins. At the most basic level, the checks and balances are summarized as the following.

Activated PI3K leads to downstream effects to activate AKT. Then AKT can directly activate mTORC1 or indirectly through phosphorylating Tuberin, which inhibits TSC1/ TSC2 complex, which itself is an inhibitor of mTORC1. Activated mTORC1 leads to downstream effects encoding ribosomal proteins, elongation factors, and other proteins required for transition from G1 phase to S phase of cell cycle. Phosphatase and tensin homolog (PTEN) has a role to play in this pathway as a tumor suppressor. PTEN is a negative regulator of the PI3K-dependent AKT signaling and acts as an antagonist of phosphorylation of PIP2 to PIP3.[25]

The understanding of this pathway lends to understanding the separation of targets into 4 main categories: mTOR inhibitors, PI3K inhibitors, dual mTOR/PI3K inhibitors, and AKT inhibitors. Many phase 1 and phase 2 trials are being undertaken with the modest success. A phase III trial by GOG 170-I showed higher response rate to temsirolimus in patients with tumors that exhibited mTOR activity than patients with tumors without mTOR activity. Unfortunately, there seems to be possibility for resistance to inhibitors of the PI3K/AKT/mTOR pathway. The mechanism is unknown but speculated to involve loss of negative feedback loops normally induced when the pathway is active. Proposed mechanisms for combating this is combining these inhibitors with other agents that inhibit at different points of the pathway (**Fig. 1**).[24]

Last, loss of function of PTEN has been detected in ovarian cancer as well as other cancers (eg, Cowden syndrome). This is of interest in PI3K/AKT/mTOR pathway

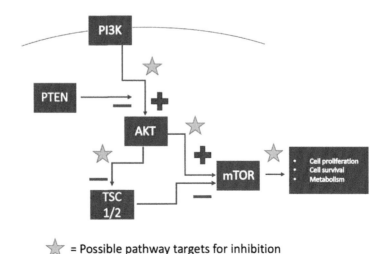

☆ = Possible pathway targets for inhibition

Fig. 1. Simplified PI3K/AKT/mTOR pathway and possible points for inhibition.

because it is believed the ovarian cancer in PTEN knockout mouse models is caused through loss of inhibition of this pathway. Thus, inhibitors of PI3K/AKT/mTOR pathway may be beneficial as chemoprevention in selected patients with known PTEN mutations. It is especially hard to characterize the exact role of PTEN mutations in oncogenesis, as the protein acts in the cytoplasm as well as nucleus, and is also suspected to have antitumor effects by maintaining chromosomal stability, DNA double-strand break repair, and maintaining genome integrity.[26]

Consumer Marketing

The idea of personalized medicine began branching into the consumer market in the mid-2000s (DTC or Direct to Consumer). With the availability of high-throughput genomic sequencing, the price of testing an individual's genomic makeup reached a level affordable to the single consumer. Most of these tests are as simple as buccal or salivary swabs that are sent through the mail to the commercial laboratory. These private genetic laboratories offer testing for simple single-gene disorders (eg, cystic fibrosis) as well as pharmacogenomic tests to individualize drug treatment, including guidance for specific mutation-targeted treatment decisions for patients with cancers. They also include predictive genomic testing for complex disorders and traits such as hypertension and osteoporosis.[27] DTC marketing has become a popular among patients of all fields of medicine and the number of consumers of 23andMe and other similar DTC tests was more than 12 million in 2017. Most pertinent to our field, in March of 2018, the FDA authorized agencies to tell consumers whether they possess 1 of 3 germline mutations in the BRCA1 and BRCA2 genes.[28] **Table 1** lists just a few of the commercially available tumor sequencing assays.

Understanding and knowing BRCA1 and BRCA2 mutations, along with DNA mismatch repair genes of other hereditary cancer syndromes (eg, MLH1, MSH2, MSH6, and PMS2) presents significant opportunities in the treatment and prevention of some gynecologic cancers, including Lynch and Cowden, for example. This information can lead to alterations in screening and treatment plans. However, the

Table 1
Examples of commercially available tumor gene sequencing tests

Tumor Test/Manufacturer	Targets Tested	Tissue	FDA Approval
FD1CDx	BRCA 1/2	Ovary	Yes
MSK-IMPACT	Varied, entire gene sequencing	Multiple	Yes[a]
SOLiD	Varied, entire gene sequencing	Multiple	Yes
Oncomine Dx Target Test	EGFR, BRAF, and ROS1	Lung	Yes
PathVysion	Her2/neu	Breast	Yes
PharmDx	Her2/neu	Breast	Yes
INFORM	Her2/neu	Breast	Yes
Dako	PD-L1	Lung	Yes
MI Profile	Many	Colon, lung	Yes
Solid Tumor Mutation Panel	Many	Multiple	Yes
SmartGenomics	Many	Multiple	Yes
Pervenio Lung NGS Assay	Many	Lung	Yes

Abbreviations: EGFR, epidermal growth factor receptor; FDA, Food and Drug Administration.
[a] Only at Sloan Kettering Memorial.

availability of large population testing of these syndromes due to the DTC genetic testing leads to the idea that in general, the more genes tested, the more nonspecific the results, and the more variants of unknown significance will be found. Genetic counselors are a strained and poorly used source by the users of these genetic testing services. In one study, only 4% reported getting genetic counseling after receiving their genetic sequencing results, and 38% would have seen genetic counseling if one had been available. The risks of testing include increased anxiety or depression from positive results, uncertainty over inconclusive results, financial costs of testing, and difficulty navigating landscape of available testing modalities. Benefits of DTC genomic testing are narrow at this point, but by all accounts have a bright future. Current known benefits include more personalized prognosis, enhanced risk assessment, and improved triage to targeted therapies, such as using PARP inhibitors for BRCA carriers.

Treatment of gynecologic cancer with proprietary drugs, specific cancer therapies, and even specific hospital systems, is also affected by consumer directed advertisers. This is known as cancer related-direct to consumer advertisement (CR-DTCA).[29] CR-DTCA is particularly at risk for not clearly explaining costs, toxicity, and alternatives to patients as demonstrated in a retrospective review of warning letters sent by the FDA for not being fair and balanced, with the most (22%) being sent to CR-DTCA companies. Cancer therapy advertisement has the potential for wide-ranging affects including influencing treatment decisions and affecting the physician-patient relationship. In addition, gynecologic cancer presents challenges for clear information from advertisers to patients and oncologists, as within one general type of cancer (eg, ovarian cancer) there may be multiple potential targets, none of which seem to be singularly better than the other. This is in contrast to other cancers (eg, imatinib in patients with chronic myeloid leukemia with Philadelphia mutation) that have clear and successful treatment targets.

Overall, DTC affects oncologists as much or even more compared with other fields of medicine. Acceptance of the technology allowing for patient-obtained genetic information is necessary to help guide the conversation and inform patients and it would be "futile to try to reverse the course and reduce patients' access."[27] Personalized genetic sequencing tools currently have a role in BRCA and other DNA repair gene identification and can help with risk prediction as well as guide potential roles of chemoprevention. Expansion to more known genetic causes of gynecologic cancers, such as PTEN gene mutations and other homologous recombination-deficient genes, should be future goals of these sequencing tools.

The limiting factor in the usefulness of genetic sequencing tools seems to be with interpretation of the information for the consumers as well as the physicians. This is largely driven by lack of access to genetic counselors. Telemedicine, video chats, or requiring genetic counseling to be offered with the DTC genomic sequencing products may help increase access. Last, CR-DTCA seems to be more susceptible to bias information from marketers than other medical fields. The FDA is already monitoring advertisers but more scrutiny may be required in the future to ensure fair and balanced understanding of cancer therapies advertised to the general public.

PERSONALIZED TUMOR VACCINES

Personalized tumor vaccination is an aspect of treatment in gynecologic malignancies that has come in to play in recent years as we have gained knowledge that tumors may be largely immunogenic. Several studies have highlighted that host antitumor immune response plays a significant role in patient outcomes.[30,31] In ovarian cancer, the presence of tumor infiltrating lymphocytes (TILs) has been associated with increased progression-free survival and overall survival in patients with advanced disease.[30] Specifically, presence of CD-8 TILs has been found to correlate with survival in all stages and histologic types of ovary cancer.

Ovarian cancers are known to express tumor antigens that can serve as targets for peptide vaccination.[32] Peptide vaccinations are designed to target a variety of these antigens including NY-ESO-1, p53, WT-1, HER-2, and VEGF. They are often coadministered with GM-CSF to enhance immune response.[33,34] Whole tumor antigen vaccination is another option in personalized tumor vaccine development that provides for a wider range of tumor antigens.[35]

Dendritic cells (DCs) play a key role in development of cancer vaccination, as they serve as very potent antigen-presenting cells. We have seen in vitro that exposure of T cells to DCs pulsed with ovarian cancer antigens has resulted in the capability to kill autologous tumor cells.[36] Recently, a pilot clinical trial testing a personalized vaccine created by autologous DCs pulsed with oxidized autologous whole tumor lysate found personalized vaccination to induce T-cell response to autologous tumor antigen and increase survival.[37]

SUMMARY

In conclusion, personalized medicine in gynecologic oncology remains an evolving science. In recent years, the rapid advances in identification of the molecular drivers of gynecologic malignancies and the promise of targeted therapies have led to great enthusiasm. Although some of these therapies have been shown to have significant impact on outcomes (ie, PARP inhibitors in BRCA-mutated patients), others are still in need of additional research to identify when pathways may be most vulnerable to specific treatments (ie, PI3K in endometrial cancer). Tumor heterogeneity and tumor resistance contribute to the complexity of developing effective personalized therapies, as several studies have highlighted that tumor sampling may vary even among the same patient. We must continue to dedicate clinical research efforts to understanding how targeted therapies will be most applicable to patient care, especially as genetic testing becomes more available to patients through DTC markets.

REFERENCES

1. Barroilhet L, Matulonis U. The NCI-MATCH trial and precision medicine in gynecologic malignancy. Gynecol Oncol 2018;148(3):585–90.
2. Wiener C. Harrison's principles of internal medicine. New York: McGraw-Hill, Medical Pub. Division; 2008.
3. Coyne GO, Takebe N, Chen AP. Defining precision: the precision medicine initiative trials NCI-IMPACT and NCI-match. Curr Probl Cancer 2017;41(3):182–93.
4. Horwitz N, Matulonis U. New biologic agents for the treatment of gynecologic cancers. Hematol Oncol Clin North Am 2012;26:133–56.
5. McFarland CD, Korolev KS, Kryukov GV, et al. Impact of deleterious passenger mutations on cancer progression. Proc Natl Acad Sci U S A 2013;110(8):2910–5.
6. Druker BJ. Translation of the Philadelphia chromosome into therapy for CML. Blood 2008;112(13):4808–17.
7. Zhang J, Liu J, Sun J, et al. Identifying driver mutations from sequencing data of heterogeneous tumors in the era of personalized genome sequencing. Brief Bioinform 2014;15(2):244–55.
8. Michael S. The cancer genome. Nature 2009;458:719–24.

9. Getz G, Gabriel SB, Cibulskis K, et al. Integrated genomic characterization of endometrial carcinoma. Nature 2013;497(7447):67–73.

10. Integrated genomic analysis of ovarian carcinoma. Nature 2011;474(7573): 609–15.

11. Bashashati A, Ha G, Tone A. Distinct evolutionary trajectories of primary high-grade serous ovarian cancers revealed through spatial mutational profiling. J Pathol 2013;231(1):21–34.

12. Rodda E, Chapman J. Genomic insights in gynecologic cancer. Curr Probl Cancer 2017;41:8–36.

13. Testa U, Petrucci E, Pasquinin L, et al. Ovarian cancers: genetic abnormalities, tumor heterogeneity and progression, clonal evolution and cancer stem cells. Medicines (Basel) 2018;5(1) [pii:E16].

14. Berek J, Hacker N. Gynecologic oncology. 6th edition. Philadelphia: Lippincott Williams & Wilkins; 2014.

15. Liu J, Matulonis U. New strategies in ovarian cancer: translating the molecular complexity of ovarian cancer into treatment advances. Clin Cancer Res 2014; 20(20):5150–6.

16. Aghajanian C, Blank SV, Goff B, et al. OCEANS: a randomized, double blind, placebo-controlled phase III trial of chemotherapy with or without bevacizumab in patients with platinum sensitive recurrent epithelial ovarian, primary peritoneal or fallopian tube cancer. J Clin Oncol 2012;30(17):2039–45.

17. Pujade-Lauraine E, Hilpert F, Weber N, et al. Bevacizumab combined with chemotherapy for platinum resistant recurrent ovarian cancer: the AURELIA open-label randomized phase III trial. J Clin Oncol 2014;32(13):1302–8.

18. Coleman R, Brady M, Herzog T. Bevacizumab and paclitaxel-carboplatin chemotherapy and secondary cytoreduction in recurrent, platinum-sensitive ovarian cancer (MRG Oncology/Gynecologic Oncology Group study GOG-0213): a multicentre, open label randomized phase 3 trial. Lancet Oncol 2017;18(6):779–91.

19. Tewari K, Sill M, Long H, et al. Improved survival with bevacizumab in advanced cervical cancer. N Engl J Med 2014;370(8):734–43.

20. Liu J, Westin S. Rational selection of biomarker driver therapies for gynecologic cancers: the more we know, the more we know we don't know. Gyncol Oncol 2016;141:65–71.

21. Audeh M, Carmichael K, Penson R, et al. Oral poly(ADP-ribose) polymerase inhibitor olaparib in patients with BRCA 1 or BRCA2 mutations and recurrent ovarian cancer: a proof of concept trial. Lancet 2010;376(9737):245–51.

22. Coleman R, sill M, Bell K, et al. A phase II evaluation of the potent highly selective PARP inhibitor veliparib in the treatment of persistent or recurrent epithelial ovarian, fallopian tube or primary peritoneal cancer in patients who carry germline BRCA 1 or 2 mutation. An NRG Oncology/Gynecologic Oncology Group study. Gynecol Oncol 2015;137(3):386–91.

23. Oza AM, Cibula D, Oaknin A, et al. Olaparib plus paclitaxel and carboplatin (P/C) followed by olaparib maintenance treatment in patients (pts) with platinum-sensitive recurrent serous ovarian cancer (PSR SOC): a randomized, open-label phase II study [abstract]. J Clin Oncol 2012;30(Suppl):a5001.

24. Mabuchi S. The PI3K/AKT/mTOR pathway as a therapeutic target in ovarian cancer. Gynecol Oncol 2015;137(1):173–9.

25. Haddadi N, Lin Y, Travis G, et al. PTEN/PTENP1: 'regulating the regulator of the RTK-dependent PI3K/Akt signalling', new targets for cancer therapy. Mol Cancer 2018;17(1):37.

26. Patrinos GP, Baker DJ, Al-Mulla F, et al. Genetic tests obtainable through pharmacies: the good, the bad, and the ugly. Hum Genomics 2013;7(1):17.
27. Storrs C. Patients armed with their own genetic data raise tough questions. Health Aff 2018;37:690–3.
28. Schnipper LE, Abel GA. Direct-to-consumer drug advertising in oncology is not beneficial to patients or public health. JAMA Oncol 2016;2(11):1397–8.
29. Kim H. Trouble spots in online direct-to-consumer prescription drug promotion: a content analysis of FDA warning letters. Int J Health Policy Manag 2015;4(12): 813–21.
30. Zhang L, Conejo-Garcia JR, Katsaros D, et al. Intratumoral T cells, recurrence, and survival in epithelial ovarian cancer. N Engl J Med 2003;348:203–13.
31. Adams SF, Levine DA, Cadungog MG, et al. Intraepithelial T cells and tumor proliferation: impact on the benefit from surgical cytoreduction in advanced serous ovarian cancer. Cancer 2009;115:2891–902.
32. Chu CS, Kim SH, June CH, et al. Immunotherapy opportunities in ovarian cancer. Expert Rev Anticancer Ther 2008;8:243–57.
33. Mantia-Smaldone G, Corr B, Chu CS, et al. Immunotherapy in ovarian cancer. Hum Vaccin Immunother 2012;8(9):1179–91.
34. Odunsi K, Qian F, Matsuzaki J, et al. Vaccination with an NY-ESO-1 peptide of HLA class I/II specificities induces integrated humoral and T cell responses in ovarian cancer. Proc Natl Acad Sci U S A 2007;104:12837–42.
35. Chiang CL, Kandalaft LE, Coukos G. Adjuvants for enhancing the immunogenicity of whole tumor cell vaccines. Int Rev Immunol 2011;30:150–82.
36. Santin AD, Hermonat PL, Ravaggi A, et al. In vitro induction of tumor-specific human lymphocyte antigen class I-restricted CD8 cytotoxic T lymphocytes by ovarian tumor antigen-pulsed autologous dendritic cells from patients with advanced ovarian cancer. Am J Obstet Gynecol 2000;183:601–9.
37. Tanyi JL, Bobisse S, Ophir E, et al. Personal cancer vaccine effectively mobilizes antitumor T cell immunity in ovarian cancer. Sci Transl Med 2018;10(436) [pii: eaao5931].

Precision Medicine in Rheumatoid Arthritis

James Bluett, MBBS, PhD[a],*, Anne Barton, FRCP, PhD[a,b]

KEYWORDS

- Methotrexate • Anti-TNF • Anti-TNF response • Genetic • Genomic
- Rheumatoid arthritis • Pharmacogenomics

KEY POINTS

- Treatment of rheumatoid arthritis (RA) has improved in recent years but response is not universal.
- Clinical predictors of response alone are not sufficiently predictive to aid treatment decisions.
- Understanding the pharmacogenomics of RA would allow more personalized health care.

INTRODUCTION

Rheumatoid arthritis (RA) is a heterogenous disease and can range from a mild, self-limiting arthritis to rapidly progressive joint damage. Treatment is based on controlling inflammation, and early effective therapy reduces disability, joint damage, and mortality.[1] A range of treatment options are available but none are universally effective, so treatment selection is based on a "trial-and-error" approach, trying different therapies until a drug that induces low disease activity or remission is identified.[2] Time on multiple ineffective medications affects the patient's quality of life, may lead to irreversible joint damage,[3] exposes the patient to potential adverse events, and is a waste of health care resources. Therefore, considerable research effort has been applied to identifying predictors of drug response to allow more rational prescribing of the drug most likely to be effective in individual patients, an approach known as precision (or stratified) medicine.

Methotrexate (MTX) is the first-line therapy for RA,[2] whereas biologic therapies target specific molecular pathways, including the tumor necrosis factor (TNF),

This article originally appeared in *Rheumatic Disease Clinics*, Volume 43, Issue 3, August 2017.
Disclosure Statement: The authors have nothing to disclose.
[a] Division of Musculoskeletal and Dermal Sciences, Arthritis Research UK Centre for Genetics and Genomics, Centre for Musculoskeletal Research, Manchester Academic Health Science Centre, The University of Manchester, Room 2.607, Stopford Building, Oxford Road, Manchester M13 9PT, UK; [b] NIHR Manchester Biomedical Research Centre, Central Manchester University Hospitals NHS Foundation Trust, Manchester Academic Health Science Centre, Manchester M139WU, UK
* Corresponding author.
E-mail address: james.bluett@manchester.ac.uk

interleukin-6, B-cell and T-cell costimulation pathways. The biologic drugs are typically reserved for those with an inadequate response to nonbiologic disease-modifying antirheumatic drugs,[2] but there is currently no guidance on which biologic agent to use first.[4] Each drug has a significant failure rate; for example, TNF inhibitors (TNFi) are ineffective in up to 30% patients,[5] yet remain the most commonly prescribed first-line biologic. As most research has investigated biomarkers predictive of response to MTX and TNFi biologics, the current review limits the focus to these drug classes.

Treatment response is likely to be multifactorial and influenced by clinical, psychological, and biological factors. For example, robust clinical predictors of TNFi response include disease severity, smoking status, concomitant MTX, and patient disability, but account for a small proportion ($r^2 = 0.17$) of the variance in response and so, alone, are not useful in informing therapy selection decisions.[6] There is, therefore, a need for accurate predictors (biomarkers) of response to RA therapies to enable precision medicine, defined by National Academy of Sciences as the use of genomic, epigenomic, exposure, and other data to define individual patterns of disease, potentially leading to better individual treatment.[7]

The use of genomic variants as predictors of response has several theoretic advantages. Genetic variants are stable and will not change because of the environment, unlike epigenetics or expression profiling. Genetic variants that are associated with response are likely to be involved in key molecular pathways and can therefore provide insight into the mechanisms of nonresponse. Whole-genome genotyping is now economically viable, and the assays are standardized, enabling their use in the clinical setting. Indeed, genetic biomarkers are already being used to personalize health care. In cystic fibrosis, for example, ivacaftor, a drug that targets the CFTR molecule, is recommended in the 4% of patients with the G551D mutation[8] whereas in rheumatology, screening for the enzyme TPMT, responsible for the metabolism of 6-mercaptopurine and related compounds, is recommended to identify the 13% of the population with reduced activity and who are at increased risk of toxicity to azathioprine.[9] There are currently more than 200 examples of US Food and Drug Administration–approved drugs that contain information on genomic biomarkers that may be used to inform treatment decisions.[10] Although many of these are not commonly used in clinical practice, TPMT screening is frequently in the United Kingdom.

STUDIES INVESTIGATING GENOMIC PREDICTORS OF METHOTREXATE

Given that MTX remains the treatment of choice for patients with newly diagnosed RA, several studies have investigated genes involved in the key molecular pathways affecting MTX absorption, metabolism, or its target enzymes as predictive biomarkers of response (**Fig. 1**).

The most consistent evidence for association is for the solute carrier family 19 member 1 (SLC19A1) gene, one of several transport carriers that allow MTX to enter cells. Studies have reported that the rs1051266 variant associates with intracellular MTX-polyglutamate levels and a recent meta-analysis of 12 studies (n = 2049) reported an association with MTX treatment response (odds ratio [OR] = 1.49 of AA genotype, $P = .001$).[11,12] Methylene tetrahydrofolate reductase is another key enzyme in the MTX pathway and has also been extensively investigated with several studies reporting associations with efficacy and toxicity. However, a meta-analysis including 17 previous studies revealed no association with either outcome,[13] and this finding has been replicated in 2 subsequent meta-analyses.[14,15] MTX is thought to exert an anti-

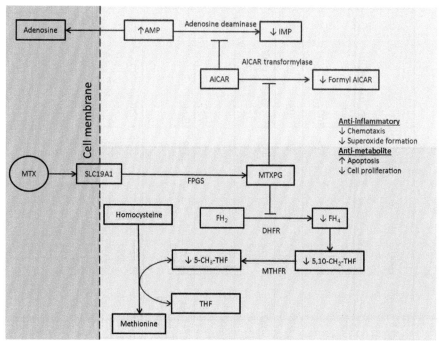

Fig. 1. The MTX metabolic pathway. 5-CH$_3$-THF, 5-methyltetrahydrofolate; 5,10-CH$_2$-THF, 5,10-methyltetrahydrofolate; AMP, adenosine monophosphate; DHFR, dihydrofolate reductase; FH$_2$, dihydrofolate; FH$_4$, tetrahydrofolate; FPGS, folylpolyglutamate synthetase; IMP, inosine monophosphate; MTHRF, methylene tetrahydrofolate reductase; MTXPG, methotrexate polyglutamate; SLC19A1, solute carrier family 19 member 1; THF, tetrahydrofolate.

inflammatory effect through inhibiting aminoimidazole carboxamido tibo nucleotide (AICAR) transformylase (ATIC) leading to an increase in AICAR levels and the anti-inflammatory agent adenosine.[16] Several studies have associated the (ATIC 347 C > G single nucleotide polymorphism [SNP] rs2372536) with toxicity,[17–19] but this finding has not been consistently replicated.[20–22]

As well as investigating MTX pathway genes, the major RA susceptibility gene, HLA-DRB1, has also been studied. As the gene is associated with more severe disease,[23] it was hypothesized that carriers of the risk allele would be less likely to respond to MTX monotherapy. In a study of 309 patients from an early inflammatory polyarthritis inception cohort, the presence of the HLA-DRB1 allele was associated with MTX monotherapy inefficacy at 2 years (OR = 3.04, P = .02), but this finding requires replication in other data sets.[24]

STUDIES INVESTIGATING GENOMIC PREDICTORS OF RESPONSE TO TUMOR NECROSIS FACTOR INHIBITOR

Early candidate gene studies investigating the pharmacogenomics of TNFi therapy revealed inconsistent findings, none of which have been robustly replicated. This review focuses on genome-wide association studies (GWAS): candidate gene studies where findings have been replicated by at least one group and candidate gene studies performed in sample sizes exceeding 1500 individuals (**Table 1**).

Table 1
Summary of pharmacogenomic studies investigating response to tumor necrosis factor inhibitors reported to date

Study	N	Study Design	Platform	SNPs for Analysis	Results	Validation Study	n	SNPs Validated
Liu et al,[25] 2008	89	GWAS	Illumina Beadstation and Hap300 chips	283,348	16 SNPs of suggestive association	Suarez-Gestal et al,[26] 2010 Krintel et al,[27] 2012	151 196	None None
Plant et al,[28] 2011	566	GWAS	Affymetrix GeneChip 500K	459,446	7 SNPs of suggestive association	Krintel et al,[27] 2012	196	None
Krintel et al,[27] 2012	196	GWAS	Illumina HumanHap550K duo array	561,466	10 SNPs of suggestive association	Acosta et al,[29] 2013	315	$PDEA3A\text{-}SLCO1C1$ (OR = 2.63, $P = 1.74 \times 10^{-5}$)
Mirkov et al,[30] 2013	882	GWAS	HumanHap550-Duo/Human660W-Quad BeadChips	2,557,253	No SNP of suggestive association			
Cui et al,[31] 2013	2706	GWAS	Various	>2,000,000	1 SNP of suggestive association in etanercept-treated cohort	Cui et al,[31] 2013	139	None
Cui et al,[32] 2010	1283	Candidate gene study	Various	31	1 SNP of suggestive association	Plant et al,[33] 2012 Ferreiro-Iglesias et al,[34] 2016 Pappas et al,[35] 2013 Zervou et al,[36] 2013	1115 755 233 183	$PTPRC$ ($\beta = 0.19$, $P = .04$) $PTPRC$ ($\beta = 0.33$, $P = .006$) Not validated Not validated

WHOLE-GENOME STUDIES

To date, 5 GWAS have been undertaken with the first including just 89 patients.[25] Sixteen SNPs showed suggestive association ($P < 5 \times 10^{-5}$), but none exceeded genome-wide significance thresholds and none have been replicated in subsequent, larger studies.[26]

A second GWAS undertaken by Plant and colleagues[28] in 2011 included a 3-stage design with an initial GWAS investigating change in Disease Activity Score on 28 joints (DAS-28) over 6 months (n = 566); variants with $P < 10^{-3}$ were subsequently genotyped in an independent cohort with a subsequent meta-analysis. In stage 3, variants whereby the signal was strengthened were investigated in a third independent cohort, and finally, a second meta-analysis of the data was performed. The results demonstrated 7 loci associated with response, but 3 SNPs showed an opposite effect in the meta-analysis compared with the first stage and no SNP reached genome-wide significance ($P < 5 \times 10^{-8}$). Neither the Liu[25] or Plant[28] and colleagues results have been replicated subsequently.

In 2012, Krintel and colleagues[27] performed a GWAS of 196 Danish RA patients treated with TNFi, most of whom were treated with infliximab, and performed a subsequent meta-analysis with the Liu and colleagues and Plant and colleagues datasets. Response was defined as the change in DAS-28 over 14 weeks. Suggestive association was detected at the PDE3A-SLC01C1 locus, where a C > T polymorphism at rs3794271 was associated with reduced efficacy according to the European League Against Rheumatism (EULAR) criteria (OR = 3.2, $P = 3.5 \times 10^{-6}$).[37] A Spanish study by Acosta-Colman and colleagues[29] tested the same variant in 315 RA patients and replicated the association (OR = 2.63, $P = 1.74 \times 10^{-5}$). The variant was associated with response to infliximab and etanercept but not adalimumab. A subsequent meta-analysis strengthened the association (OR = 2.91, $P = 3.34 \times 10^{-10}$). The PDE3A gene encodes a phosphodiesterase, inhibition of which suppresses TNF production in lipopolysaccharide-stimulated monocytes.[38] The association was not reported in previous GWA studies, but the variant was not tested by the Plant and colleagues study. However, a subsequent study in a UK population found no evidence for association.[39]

A multistage GWAS in 2013 recruited 882 Dutch patients and 2 further validation cohorts (n = 954 and 867, respectively)[30] through international collaboration. Response was defined as 3-month change in DAS-28, a shorter time period than previous studies, but no variants were associated even at suggestive association thresholds ($P < 5 \times 10^{-5}$).

In 2013, Cui and colleagues[31] performed the largest GWAS to date. Following international collaboration, 2706 RA patients from 13 different cohorts treated with etanercept, infliximab, or adalimumab were investigated. Response was defined as the change in DAS-28 at 3 to 12 months. No association reaching genome-wide significance was detected. A subset analysis revealed SNP rs6427528 nearing genome-wide significance ($P = 8 \times 10^{-8}$) in the etanercept-treated group. rs6427528 is thought to disrupt transcription binding site motifs of CD84 and is associated with higher CD84 expression in peripheral blood mononuclear cells. CD84 is involved in T-cell activation and maturation[40] and acts as a costimulatory molecule for interferon-γ secretion.[41] Despite the strong initial association, the SNP failed to replicate in Portuguese and Japanese cohorts (n = 290).

Recently, a rigorous community-based assessment of the utility of SNP data for predicting anti-TNF treatment efficacy in RA patients was performed in the context of a DREAM Challenge (http://www.synapse.org/RA_Challenge).[42] This approach enabled the comparative evaluation of treatment response predictions developed by 73 research groups using the most comprehensive available data on TNFi response and genome-wide data. Unfortunately, no significant genetic contribution to prediction accuracy was observed.

PROTEIN TYROSINE PHOSPHATASE RECEPTOR TYPE C, HUMAN LEUKOCYTE ANTIGEN-DRB1, AND RESPONSE TO TUMOR NECROSIS FACTOR INHIBITOR

In 2010, Cui and colleagues[32] hypothesized that genetic factors associated with RA susceptibility and severity may also be important in predicting treatment response. The investigators investigated Caucasian individuals (n = 1283) receiving infliximab, etanercept, or adalimumab. Response was defined according to the EULAR criteria at 3 to 12 months posttreatment. An association within the *PTPRC* gene was reported (rs10919563; OR = 0.55, $P = 10^{-5}$) with the strongest effect in the seropositive cohort. Subgroup analysis revealed *PTPRC* was associated with infliximab and etanercept response but not adalimumab. PTPRC is a transmembrane receptor-like molecule that regulates T- and B-cell antigen receptor signaling[43] and is a mediator of TNF secretion from monocytes.[44] The *PTPRC* association has been replicated by 2 independent studies,[33,34] but 2 other studies failed to replicate the association,[35,36] possibly because of lack of power as the 2 negative studies had smaller sample sizes (see **Table 1**). The *PTPRC* variant accounted for only 0.5% of the variance in response to TNFi and will therefore not be clinically useful at the individual patient level.

The shared epitope HLA-DRB1 amino acid at positions 11, 71, and 74 confer the largest susceptibility risk of RA and are associated with disease progression.[45] In a candidate gene study investigating the association between loci within the *HLA DRB1* gene and EULAR response in 1846 RA patients treated with TNFi, a VKA haplotype at the 3 amino acid positions was also significantly associated with improved EULAR response (OR = 1.23, $P = .007$).[23] The work suggests that the same variants may be associated with susceptibility, severity, and treatment response but with a sequential reduction in effect size, meaning that larger sample sizes are required for treatment response studies.

DISCUSSION

Despite the large number of studies investigating the pharmacogenetics and genomics of RA, results to date have been disappointing and have not yielded a change in clinical practice. There are several possible reasons for this. It could be argued that there is no genetic heritability for treatment response in RA, and the results to date are false positives, but 2 studies have reported that there is detectable heritability.[46,47] These observations, therefore, begs the question of where the missing heritability is (see Vincent A. Laufer and colleagues' article, "Integrative Approaches to Understanding the Pathogenic Role of Genetic Variation in Rheumatic Diseases", in this issue), and there are several explanations for the failure to consistently detect genetic predictors of response.

First, most studies have investigated common variants, with limited power to detect the effect of rare variants on treatment response. Technology is advancing at a staggering pace, and with the reducing cost of whole genome sequencing, it is now economically viable to evaluate the effect of rare variants; however, a recent exon sequencing study of candidate genes found no evidence for association with TNFi response in ~1000 individuals.[48]

Second, RA is not a simple monogenic disease, but a polygenic disease whereby environmental and multiple genetic loci increase the individuals risk of developing disease. It is therefore likely that treatment response is in part due to the multiple effects of many genetic variants, each of small effect size. A recent study used simulations to show that successful application of common polygenic modeling approaches would require sample sizes greater than 1000 individuals for traits with less than 50% heritability,[49] yet few studies, to date, have included such numbers.

Third, response in RA is difficult to capture, and several composite scores are used in clinical practice. Many research studies also use these measures, including DAS-28, American College of Rheumatology, or EULAR response criteria, which include subjective measures of disease and are known to have a placebo effect.[50] Previous research has reported that the swollen joint count and erythrocyte sedimentation rate are response markers that are associated with the greatest genetic influence and that psychological factors correlate with the subjective visual analogue score.[47,51] Some investigators have used imaging to objectively assess disease activity (synovitis) and to re-weight the DAS-28[52] score to more accurately reflect that feature as biologic drugs target that aspect of disease, but routine MR imaging remains impractical in the clinical setting.

Fourth, adherence to therapy is a potential confounder of predictive studies that is rarely accounted for; it has been shown, for example, that up to 20% of RA patients self-report nonadherence to TNFi therapy when asked and that nonadherence is associated with poorer clinical outcome.[53] Thus, a patient who is genetically predisposed to respond to treatment may be classified as a nonresponder because they are not taking the drug but, to date, no study has adjusted for inadequate adherence to treatment.

Finally, RA may not be one disease, but different diseases, with different molecular mechanisms that present as a similar, if heterogeneous, phenotype. For example, it is known that there are significant clinical and genetic differences between anticyclic citrullinated peptide (CCP) -positive and anti-CCP-negative patients.[54] Including all patients who fulfill classification criteria for RA may cause admixture of RA subsets, reducing the power of a study to detect genetic association. Furthermore, although response to TNFi therapies is broadly similar, there are differences illustrated by the fact that patients may experience inefficacy with one but subsequently respond to another.[55] Differences in the mechanism of action are recognized; for example, infliximab and adalimumab are licensed for Crohn disease, whereas etanercept is ineffective,[56] is associated with a lower risk of development of tuberculosis,[57] and appears to be the least immunogenic, with a reported incidence of 1% to 18% of antidrug antibodies without an effect on response.[58] Despite this, most studies investigate response by grouping together all TNFis, potentially reducing the power to detect association in subgroups.

THE FUTURE

Pharmacogenetic and genomic studies have the potential to enable precision medicine by providing biomarkers to target the right drug to the right patients. Current guidelines offer little advice as to which biologic therapy to offer patients first, but stratifying patients according to increased probability of response to a particular drug would be of major benefit.[4] However, studies to date have illustrated that it is unlikely that a single genetic variant will be highly and confidently predictive of an individual's response to drug treatment in RA. Progress in this area will require larger sample sizes with well-described patient cohorts to allow for adjustment of confounding clinical factors such as nonadherence, antidrug antibodies, disease severity, and smoking status. These study design changes would facilitate adequately powered studies to evaluate the effect of genetic variants on different TNFi therapies and gene-gene interactions. Alternative measures of response that are able to objectively characterize true responders are also required.

Patients are currently treated in a trial-and-error approach until an effective therapy is identified, but each cycle of trying a drug destined to be ineffective increases the probability of adverse events, cost to the state, patient dissatisfaction, and the development of disability. It is therefore vital that further research is conducted to develop precision medicine approaches, moving medicine into the twenty-first century.

REFERENCES

1. Scire CA, Lunt M, Marshall T, et al. Early remission is associated with improved survival in patients with inflammatory polyarthritis: results from the Norfolk Arthritis Register. Ann Rheum Dis 2014;73(9):1677–82.
2. Smolen JS, Landewe R, Breedveld FC, et al. EULAR recommendations for the management of rheumatoid arthritis with synthetic and biological disease-modifying antirheumatic drugs: 2013 update. Ann Rheum Dis 2014;73(3): 492–509.
3. Finckh A, Liang MH, van Herckenrode CM, et al. Long-term impact of early treatment on radiographic progression in rheumatoid arthritis: a meta-analysis. Arthritis Rheum 2006;55(6):864–72.
4. National Institute for Health and Care Excellence. TA375: adalimumab, etanercept, infliximab, certolizumab pegol, golimumab, tocilizumab and abatacept for rheumatoid arthritis not previously treated with DMARDs or after conventional DMARDs only have failed. 2016. Available at: https://www.nice.org.uk/guidance/ta375. Accessed August 9, 2016.
5. Gibbons LJ, Hyrich KL. Biologic therapy for rheumatoid arthritis: clinical efficacy and predictors of response. BioDrugs 2009;23(2):111–24.
6. Hyrich KL, Watson KD, Silman AJ, et al. Predictors of response to anti-TNF-alpha therapy among patients with rheumatoid arthritis: results from the British Society for Rheumatology Biologics register. Rheumatology (Oxford) 2006;45(12): 1558–65.
7. National Academy of Sciences. Toward precision medicine: building a knowledge network for biomedical research and a new taxonomy of disease. Washington, DC: National Academy of Sciences; 2011.
8. North of England Specialised Commissioning Group. Clinical commissioning policy: ivacaftor for cystic fibrosis. 2013. Available at: https://www.england.nhs.uk/wp-content/uploads/2013/04/a01-p-b.pdf. Accessed August 9, 2016.
9. Reuther LO, Vainer B, Sonne J, et al. Thiopurine methyltransferase (TPMT) genotype distribution in azathioprine-tolerant and -intolerant patients with various disorders. The impact of TPMT genotyping in predicting toxicity. Eur J Clin Pharmacol 2004;59(11):797–801.
10. US Food and Drug Administration. Table of pharmacogenomic biomarkers in drug labeling. 2016. Available at: http://www.fda.gov/drugs/scienceresearch/researchareas/pharmacogenetics/ucm083378.htm. Accessed August 9, 2016.
11. Li X, Hu M, Li W, et al. The association between reduced folate carrier-1 gene 80G/A polymorphism and methotrexate efficacy or methotrexate related-toxicity in rheumatoid arthritis: a meta-analysis. Int Immunopharmacol 2016;38:8–15.
12. Dervieux T, Kremer J, Lein DO, et al. Contribution of common polymorphisms in reduced folate carrier and gamma-glutamylhydrolase to methotrexate polyglutamate levels in patients with rheumatoid arthritis. Pharmacogenetics 2004;14(11): 733–9.

13. Owen SA, Lunt M, Bowes J, et al. MTHFR gene polymorphisms and outcome of methotrexate treatment in patients with rheumatoid arthritis: analysis of key polymorphisms and meta-analysis of C677T and A1298C polymorphisms. Pharmacogenomics J 2013;13(2):137–47.

14. Spyridopoulou KP, Dimou NL, Hamodrakas SJ, et al. Methylene tetrahydrofolate reductase gene polymorphisms and their association with methotrexate toxicity: a meta-analysis. Pharmacogenet Genomics 2012;22(2):117–33.

15. Lee YH, Song GG. Associations between the C677T and A1298C polymorphisms of MTHFR and the efficacy and toxicity of methotrexate in rheumatoid arthritis: a meta-analysis. Clin Drug Investig 2010;30(2):101–8.

16. Cronstein BN, Naime D, Ostad E. The antiinflammatory mechanism of methotrexate. Increased adenosine release at inflamed sites diminishes leukocyte accumulation in an in vivo model of inflammation. J Clin Invest 1993;92(6): 2675–82.

17. Dervieux T, Greenstein N, Kremer J. Pharmacogenomic and metabolic biomarkers in the folate pathway and their association with methotrexate effects during dosage escalation in rheumatoid arthritis. Arthritis Rheum 2006;54(10): 3095–103.

18. Weisman MH, Furst DE, Park GS, et al. Risk genotypes in folate-dependent enzymes and their association with methotrexate-related side effects in rheumatoid arthritis. Arthritis Rheum 2006;54(2):607–12.

19. Grabar PB, Rojko S, Logar D, et al. Genetic determinants of methotrexate treatment in rheumatoid arthritis patients: a study of polymorphisms in the adenosine pathway. Ann Rheum Dis 2010;69(5):931–2.

20. Takatori R, Takahashi KA, Tokunaga D, et al. ABCB1 C3435T polymorphism influences methotrexate sensitivity in rheumatoid arthritis patients. Clin Exp Rheumatol 2006;24(5):546–54.

21. Stamp LK, Chapman PT, O'Donnell JL, et al. Polymorphisms within the folate pathway predict folate concentrations but are not associated with disease activity in rheumatoid arthritis patients on methotrexate. Pharmacogenet Genomics 2010; 20(6):367–76.

22. Owen SA, Hider SL, Martin P, et al. Genetic polymorphisms in key methotrexate pathway genes are associated with response to treatment in rheumatoid arthritis patients. Pharmacogenomics J 2013;13(3):227–34.

23. Viatte S, Plant D, Han B, et al. Association of HLA-DRB1 haplotypes with rheumatoid arthritis severity, mortality, and treatment response. JAMA 2015;313(16): 1645–56.

24. Hider SL, Silman AJ, Thomson W, et al. Can clinical factors at presentation be used to predict outcome of treatment with methotrexate in patients with early inflammatory polyarthritis? Ann Rheum Dis 2009;68(1):57–62.

25. Liu C, Batliwalla F, Li W, et al. Genome-wide association scan identifies candidate polymorphisms associated with differential response to anti-TNF treatment in rheumatoid arthritis. Mol Med 2008;14(9–10):575–81.

26. Suarez-Gestal M, Perez-Pampin E, Calaza M, et al. Lack of replication of genetic predictors for the rheumatoid arthritis response to anti-TNF treatments: a prospective case-only study. Arthritis Res Ther 2010;12(2):R72.

27. Krintel SB, Palermo G, Johansen JS, et al. Investigation of single nucleotide polymorphisms and biological pathways associated with response to TNFalpha inhibitors in patients with rheumatoid arthritis. Pharmacogenet Genomics 2012;22(8): 577–89.

28. Plant D, Bowes J, Potter C, et al. Genome-wide association study of genetic predictors of anti-tumor necrosis factor treatment efficacy in rheumatoid arthritis identifies associations with polymorphisms at seven loci. Arthritis Rheum 2011; 63(3):645–53.

29. Acosta-Colman I, Palau N, Tornero J, et al. GWAS replication study confirms the association of PDE3A-SLCO1C1 with anti-TNF therapy response in rheumatoid arthritis. Pharmacogenomics 2013;14(7):727–34.

30. Umicevic Mirkov M, Cui J, Vermeulen SH, et al. Genome-wide association analysis of anti-TNF drug response in patients with rheumatoid arthritis. Ann Rheum Dis 2013;72(8):1375–81.

31. Cui J, Stahl EA, Saevarsdottir S, et al. Genome-wide association study and gene expression analysis identifies CD84 as a predictor of response to etanercept therapy in rheumatoid arthritis. PLoS Genet 2013;9(3):e1003394.

32. Cui J, Saevarsdottir S, Thomson B, et al. Rheumatoid arthritis risk allele PTPRC is also associated with response to anti-tumor necrosis factor alpha therapy. Arthritis Rheum 2010;62(7):1849–61.

33. Plant D, Prajapati R, Hyrich KL, et al. Replication of association of the PTPRC gene with response to anti-tumor necrosis factor therapy in a large UK cohort. Arthritis Rheum 2012;64(3):665–70.

34. Ferreiro-Iglesias A, Montes A, Perez-Pampin E, et al. Replication of PTPRC as genetic biomarker of response to TNF inhibitors in patients with rheumatoid arthritis. Pharmacogenomics J 2016;16(2):137–40.

35. Pappas DA, Oh C, Plenge RM, et al. Association of rheumatoid arthritis risk alleles with response to anti-TNF biologics: results from the CORRONA registry and meta-analysis. Inflammation 2013;36(2):279–84.

36. Zervou MI, Myrthianou E, Flouri I, et al. Lack of association of variants previously associated with anti-TNF medication response in rheumatoid arthritis patients: results from a homogeneous Greek population. PLoS One 2013;8(9):e74375.

37. van Gestel AM, Prevoo ML, van 't Hof MA, et al. Development and validation of the European League Against Rheumatism response criteria for rheumatoid arthritis. Comparison with the preliminary American College of Rheumatology and the World Health Organization/International league against rheumatism criteria. Arthritis Rheum 1996;39(1):34–40.

38. Prabhakar U, Lipshutz D, Bartus JO, et al. Characterization of cAMP-dependent inhibition of LPS-induced TNF alpha production by rolipram, a specific phosphodiesterase IV (PDE IV) inhibitor. Int J Immunopharmacol 1994;16(10):805–16.

39. Smith SL, Plant D, Lee XH, et al. Previously reported PDE3A-SLCO1C1 genetic variant does not correlate with anti-TNF response in a large UK rheumatoid arthritis cohort. Pharmacogenomics 2016;17(7):715–20.

40. Tangye SG, Nichols KE, Hare NJ, et al. Functional requirements for interactions between CD84 and Src homology 2 domain-containing proteins and their contribution to human T cell activation. J Immunol 2003;171(5):2485–95.

41. Martin M, Romero X, de la Fuente MA, et al. CD84 functions as a homophilic adhesion molecule and enhances IFN-gamma secretion: adhesion is mediated by Ig-like domain 1. J Immunol 2001;167(7):3668–76.

42. Sieberts SK, Zhu F, Garcia-Garcia J, et al. Crowdsourced assessment of common genetic contribution to predicting anti-TNF treatment response in rheumatoid arthritis. Nat Commun 2016;7:12460.

43. Hermiston ML, Xu Z, Weiss A. CD45: a critical regulator of signaling thresholds in immune cells. Annu Rev Immunol 2003;21:107–37.

44. Hayes AL, Smith C, Foxwell BM, et al. CD45-induced tumor necrosis factor alpha production in monocytes is phosphatidylinositol 3-kinase-dependent and nuclear factor-kappaB-independent. J Biol Chem 1999;274(47):33455–61.

45. Plant D, Thomson W, Lunt M, et al. The role of rheumatoid arthritis genetic susceptibility markers in the prediction of erosive disease in patients with early inflammatory polyarthritis: results from the Norfolk arthritis register. Rheumatology (Oxford, England) 2011;50(1):78–84.

46. Umicevic Mirkov M, Janss L, Vermeulen SH, et al. Estimation of heritability of different outcomes for genetic studies of TNFi response in patients with rheumatoid arthritis. Ann Rheum Dis 2015;74(12):2183–7.

47. Plant D, Bowes J, Orozco G, et al. Estimating heritability of response to treatment with anti-TNF biologic agents using linear mixed models. Ann Rheum Dis 2013; 71(Suppl 3):474–5.

48. Cui J, Diogo D, Stahl EA, et al. The role of rare protein-coding variants to anti-TNF treatment response in rheumatoid arthritis. Arthritis Rheumatol 2017;69(4): 735–41.

49. Marshall SL, Guennel T, Kohler J, et al. Estimating heritability in pharmacogenetic studies. Pharmacogenomics 2013;14(4):369–77.

50. Strand V, Cohen S, Crawford B, et al. Patient-reported outcomes better discriminate active treatment from placebo in randomized controlled trials in rheumatoid arthritis. Rheumatology (Oxford, England) 2004;43(5):640–7.

51. Cordingley L, Prajapati R, Plant D, et al. Impact of psychological factors on subjective disease activity assessments in patients with severe rheumatoid arthritis. Arthritis Care Res 2014;66(6):861–8.

52. Baker JF, Conaghan PG, Smolen JS, et al. Development and validation of modified disease activity scores in rheumatoid arthritis: superior correlation with magnetic resonance imaging-detected synovitis and radiographic progression. Arthritis Rheumatol 2014;66(4):794–802.

53. Bluett J, Morgan C, Thurston L, et al. Impact of inadequate adherence on response to subcutaneously administered anti-tumour necrosis factor drugs: results from the Biologics in Rheumatoid Arthritis Genetics and Genomics Study Syndicate cohort. Rheumatology (Oxford, England) 2015;54(3):494–9.

54. van der Helm-van Mil AH, Verpoort KN, Breedveld FC, et al. Antibodies to citrullinated proteins and differences in clinical progression of rheumatoid arthritis. Arthritis Res Ther 2005;7(5):R949–58.

55. Soliman MM, Hyrich KL, Lunt M, et al. Rituximab or a second anti-tumor necrosis factor therapy for rheumatoid arthritis patients who have failed their first anti-tumor necrosis factor therapy? Comparative analysis from the British Society for rheumatology biologics register. Arthritis Care Res 2012;64(8):1108–15.

56. Sandborn WJ, Hanauer SB, Katz S, et al. Etanercept for active Crohn's disease: a randomized, double-blind, placebo-controlled trial. Gastroenterology 2001; 121(5):1088–94.

57. Dixon WG, Hyrich KL, Watson KD, et al. Drug-specific risk of tuberculosis in patients with rheumatoid arthritis treated with anti-TNF therapy: results from the British Society for Rheumatology Biologics Register (BSRBR). Ann Rheum Dis 2010;69(3):522–8.

58. Emi Aikawa N, de Carvalho JF, Artur Almeida Silva C, et al. Immunogenicity of Anti-TNF-alpha agents in autoimmune diseases. Clin Rev Allergy Immunol 2010;38(2–3):82–9.

Precision Medicine for Sleep Loss and Fatigue Management

Luis E. Pichard, MHS, PhD[a],*, Guido Simonelli, MD[b],
Lindsay Schwartz, PhD[c], Thomas J. Balkin, PhD[b],
Steven Hursh, PhD[c]

KEYWORDS

- Sleep • Insufficiency • Loss • Fatigue • Performance • Management • Modeling

KEY POINTS

- Sleep loss and/or sleep insufficiency has many causes, it is a widespread phenomenon, and has short- and long-term consequences.
- Consequences to sleep loss are not homogenous across populations and many individual traits have been linked to resiliency and/or susceptibility to sleep loss.
- There are no quantifiable biomarkers for sleep loss. As such, mitigations are aimed at restoring daytime function.
- Decrements in cognitive performance have led the way to objectively assess sleep sufficiency.
- Maintenance of cognitive performance, a day-to-day necessary function, is the primary outcome used in predictive models aimed at fatigue management caused by sleep insufficiency.

This article originally appeared in *Sleep Medicine Clinics*, Volume 14, Issue 3, September 2019.
Conflicts of Interest: S. Hursh is the inventor of the SAFTE model and SleepTank and the Institutes for Behavior Resources, Inc, sells products using the models.
Disclaimer: Material has been reviewed by the Walter Reed Army Institute of Research. There is no objection to its presentation and/or publication. The opinions or assertions contained herein are the private views of the authors, and are not to be construed as official, or as reflecting true views of the Department of the Army or the Department of Defense. The investigators have adhered to the policies for protection of human subjects as prescribed in AR 70–25.

[a] Division of Pulmonary and Critical Care Medicine, Department of Medicine, The Johns Hopkins University School of Medicine, 5501 Hopkins Bayview Circle, Baltimore, MD 21224, USA; [b] Behavioral Biology Branch, Walter Reed Army Institute of Research, 503 Robert Grant Avenue, Silver Spring, MD 20910, USA; [c] Institutes for Behavior Resources, Inc, 2104 Maryland Avenue, Baltimore, MD 21218, USA
* Corresponding author. Shush Performance Technologies, Inc., 626C Admiral Drive, #528, Annapolis, Maryland 21401, USA.
E-mail addresses: Luis.E.Pichard@gmail.com; Luis.Pichard@ShushPerformance.com

Clinics Collections 8 (2020) 229–238
https://doi.org/10.1016/j.ccol.2020.07.018
2352-7986/20/© 2020 Elsevier Inc. All rights reserved.

CAUSE OF SLEEP LOSS

Despite a growing body of scientific literature describing an ever-widening array of short-term behavioral deficits and long-term pathologies that are associated with sleep loss, and despite public health campaigns and the continuing efforts of such groups as the National Sleep Foundation, the American Academy of Sleep Medicine, and the National Institutes of Health, acute and chronic sleep loss remains an expanding widespread phenomenon.[1] Insufficient sleep is common, with approximately 25% of adults reporting sleep-related complaints at any given time.[2] The causes of insufficient sleep may result from a variety of factors, including medical conditions, sleep disorders, and occupation.[3] Sleep disorders, such as sleep disordered breathing, insomnia, and restless legs syndrome, can lead to insufficient sleep.[4] Medical conditions, such as musculoskeletal disorders including arthritis, fibromyalgia, or chronic back pain, can also disrupt sleep and lead to insufficient sleep.[5–7] The underlying mechanisms by which these disorders and medical conditions curtail sleep have been described elsewhere in this series. Lifestyle and occupational factors include shift work, long work hours, jet lag, and irregular schedules. Other lifestyle factors, such as sleep habits, timing of exercise, and diet, can also lead to insufficient sleep by diminishing sleep's restorative value (ie, worsening sleep quality). The underlying mechanisms by which lifestyle and occupational factors may lead to insufficient sleep include shortened sleep duration, increased sleep fragmentation, and circadian misalignment. Short sleep duration occurs when individuals reduce quantitatively or qualitatively their sleep opportunity. From a lifestyle/occupational standpoint, this is common in individuals with early shifts, long work hours, and long commutes. For instance, data on 6338 working adults from the National Health and Nutrition Examination Survey indicated that the prevalence of short sleep duration was twice as high in night shift workers.[8] Another study showed that those who worked an average of 55 hours per week or more are 2.5 times more likely to be short sleepers than those who work standard work weeks (35–40 hours).[9] In adults and adolescents it has also been shown that longer commutes are associated with shorter sleep.[10,11] A precision sleep medicine approach for sleep loss takes into consideration that consequences of sleep loss, sleep need, and efficacy of mitigation strategies to cope with insufficient sleep vary among individuals.

CONSEQUENCES OF SLEEP LOSS

Regardless of the underlying cause, accumulated chronic sleep loss is thought to have widespread and variegated consequences, including increased risk of atherosclerosis and cardiovascular disease[12,13]; increased rate of weight gain; and associated health risks, such as diabetes and cancer,[14] increased likelihood of Alzheimer disease,[15] impaired immune function,[16–21] and increased mortality[22,23] (to name but a few). Furthermore, individuals who obtain sufficient sleep have better cognitive functioning than those whose sleep is insufficient.[24] Findings from studies where the effects of sleep loss were assessed invariably show that it results in impaired performance on a wide variety of cognitive measures.[24] Additionally, because the spectrum of cognitive abilities impacted is broad, it is logical to hypothesize that one or more of the brain functions impacted by sleep loss are common to most types of cognitive performance (or are at least commonly reflected on tests of cognitive performance). For example, slowed response speed, difficulty concentrating, and reductions in vigilance and alertness[25,26] underlie, or are a critical component of, performance on virtually all cognitive tasks. Functional neuroimaging studies have revealed that sleep loss results in relative deactivation of the brain, with heteromodal-associated areas, such as the prefrontal cortex (ie, those cortical regions that mediate the highest-order executive functions) especially impacted.[24,27] Consistent with these findings, sleep loss has been shown to degrade higher-order cognitive functions, such as creativity, divergent reasoning, and innovation, and planning, decision-making, and rule-based or convergent reasoning.[26,28] In general, measures of cognitive performance for which attention/vigilance are critical seem to be especially sensitive to sleep loss.[24]

INTERINDIVIDUAL RESPONSIVITY TO SLEEP LOSS

Healthy adults typically carry some level of "sleep debt"[29] that is paid down if they are afforded the opportunity and/or the proper motivation to do so. Paying down sleep debt ostensibly results in a nightly total sleep time that reflects the optimal homeostatic balance between the restorative properties of nighttime sleep and the daytime expenditure of sleep-produced resources (with, of course, sleep duration and timing also mediated by the circadian rhythm of alertness).[30] Even at equal levels of sleep debt, individuals respond differently to sleep loss, which may have implications for precision-based sleep medicine. In fact, there seems to be a normal distribution of neurobehavioral responsivity to lack of sleep.[31] Although there are considerable interindividual differences, the extent to which sleep loss impacts performance within individuals is fairly stable. Several studies have documented traitlike individual differences in terms of the magnitude of sleep need, the extent to which fatigue and sleepiness manifest, and neurobiologic vulnerability to lack of sleep.[32–36] That interindividual neurobiologic differences are not uniquely explained by sleep history suggests a genetic basis, a supposition that is supported by findings from several studies.[33,35,36] For example, Kuna and colleagues[37] showed that performance during sleep deprivation is highly heritable. When comparing monozygotic and dizygotic twins, monozygotic twins showed a significantly higher concordance following 38-hour sleep deprivation period, and concordance rates were similar to those expected for repeated intraindividual trials. Other studies have revealed several polymorphisms of clock genes that are determinants of interindividual variability in performance and recovery sleep.[38–40] Furthermore, polymorphisms that alter molecular pathways, such as the adenosine pathway, have been shown to determine interindividual response variability to caffeine intake and to modulate performance during sleep deprivation.[41]

Age is another important factor determining individual responsivity to sleep loss. Younger individuals are more susceptible to sleep loss. Profound differences in sleep architecture have been demonstrated in humans and animals across life spans. Several hypotheses have been proposed to explain the greater susceptibility to sleep loss of younger individuals.[42,43] These hypotheses have been described in Zitting and colleagues,[42] and are outside of the scope of this review.

Finally, personality traits have also been identified as potential determinants of vulnerability/resilience to sleep loss. For example, there is a small body of literature that shows differences between introverts and extroverts.[44,45] In this study, extroverts demonstrated increased vulnerability to the effects of sleep loss after social interaction.[45] However, the extent to which phenotypic variability is mediated by the aforementioned putative predictors is unknown.

ASSESSMENT TOOLS FOR SLEEP LOSS

Taking into consideration the existence of large interindividual differences described previously, an ideal assessment tool would include sleep duration obtained by each individual relative to the duration of nightly sleep needed by each individual. Because an accurate, quantifiable biomarker of sleep debt level is yet to be discovered, in this section we describe some of the existing tools to measure and monitor sleep sufficiency. The examples of assessment tools for sleep loss described in this section are listed in **Table 1**, and the impacted cognitive abilities following sleep loss.

Both sleepiness and fatigue are impacted by insufficient sleep. Sleepiness varies systematically as a function of the daily sleep/wake cycle, but it is also a physiologic state that is mediated by circadian, homeostatic, rhythmic, and behavioral factors.[19] The Multiple Sleep Latency Test and the Maintenance of Wakefulness Test are generally considered the gold standard measures of sleepiness. Self-reported sleepiness measures, such as the Stanford Sleepiness Scale or the Karolinska Sleepiness Scale, quantify extant subjective sleepiness state.[46,47] In contrast, the Epworth Sleepiness Scale is a validated measure of chronic sleepiness level (ie, traitlike sleepiness).[48] Fatigue, however, which is less clearly defined, has been described as "weariness" related to a lack of motivation, weakness, or depleted energy,[20] or, alternatively, a failure to initiate or sustain tasks requiring motivation.[21] The most common measure of fatigue, the Fatigue Severity Scale, has been validated for the assessment and quantification of fatigue in healthy and clinical populations,[47] as has the Fatigue Assessment Scale.[49,50] Additionally, work-related fatigue is assessed with such measures as the Occupational Fatigue Exhaustion/Recovery Scale, which measure chronic and acute fatigue, and fatigue recovery.[51]

Monitoring sleep sufficiency is critical for operational performance. It has been argued that carrying a mild level of sleep debt is not necessarily a liability. In this view, there are progressively diminishing returns for extending sleep, and on a normal day-to-day basis there is a point at which it becomes more beneficial to remain awake and productive than to obtain additional sleep.[52] However, two recent studies showed that although sleep extension does little to improve alertness or performance on the next day, its benefits do manifest under subsequent challenge of extended wakefulness.[53,54] Therefore, sleep extension clearly enhances resilience to decrements in alertness and performance resulting from sleep loss. As such, models based on sleep history may help with fatigue-related decision making. These models are based on self-reported sleep and/or actigraphic sleep measures, and can vary substantially in terms of complexity. One example of a model based on self-reported sleep history

---

Table 1
Summary of examples of tools to assess sleep loss and examples of cognitive impairments associated with sleep loss

	Self-Reported	Objective	Cognitive Impaired Ability
Tool	Karolinska Sleepiness Scale	PSG	Ability to recognize failed solutions
	Stanford Sleepiness Scale	MWT	Ability to generate novel solutions
	Fatigue Severity Scale	Actigraphy	Anticipating problems
	Epworth Sleepiness Scale	PVT	Planning and prioritizing
			Risk assessments
			Problem-solving
			Vigilance
			Attention to detail
			Ability to multitask
			Concentration/focus
			Emotional stability
			Motivation

Abbreviations: MWT, maintenance of wakefulness task; PSG, polysomnography; PVT, psychomotor vigilance task.

is a simple rule of thumb approach that aims to identify fitness for work, the Prior Sleep Wake Model.[55] The Prior Sleep Wake Model is comprised of three simple calculations: prior sleep in the last 24 and 48 hours, and length of the wakefulness period from awakening to end of work. An individual is unfit for work if any of the following criteria is met: less than 5 hours sleep in prior 24 hours; less than 12 hours sleep in prior 48 hours; current time awake exceeds amount of sleep in prior 48 hours. The US Army's sleep management software (2B-Alert), which is under development, is another tool that provides real-time feedback based on sleep history and also provides intervention recommendations (ie, caffeine usage) for maintaining alertness.[56] An interesting feature of this tool, which applies the Unified Model of Performance (UMP), is its capability to learn and predict at an individualized level. The software learns from the individual and is able to provide personalized feedback that fits that individual's need, independently of the source of the potential interindividual variability (eg, genetic, age, personality).[57] Another example of a fatigue management tool is SleepTank, a model in which wakefulness drains, and sleep refills, a sleep reservoir in much the same way that a gas tank is emptied and refilled on an automobile.[58] A final example that monitors sleep sufficiency is Fatigue Science's Readiband, which determines sleep/wake history from wrist actigraphy and inputs this information into the US Army's Sleep, Activity, Fatigue, and Task Effectiveness (SAFTE) model.[59] The model then produces a nonindividualized performance prediction (ie, based on group sleep/performance data) that equates to sleep sufficiency (ie, considers sleep history relative to an average 8-hour sleep need[60]).

MITIGATING STRATEGIES

The causes of insufficient sleep may be related to an untreated sleep disorder. In those cases, there are different precision sleep medicine approaches that have been described in this series. When the underlying cause of insufficient sleep relates to lifestyle and occupational factors, there are several mitigating strategies that can be used, especially when the sleep loss responds to operational demands that have inherently inflexible schedules.[3] For example, using the tools described previously, at an individualized level, it is possible to recommend interventions to sustain neurobehavioral performance based on the current sleep reservoir.[56] These interventions could be aimed at (1) increasing sleep opportunities, (2) improving sleep quality, and (3) mitigating the consequences of sleep loss.

Quantitatively, nonpharmacologic interventions aimed at increasing restorative sleep quantity and quality include: scheduling sufficient recovery sleep following a long workday, prophylactic naps in the operational environment, and/or extending sleep with the goal of banking/storing sleep in anticipation of a long workday.[53] Nonpharmacologic interventions include interventions aimed at maximizing the recuperative value of the sleep period. These interventions lead to increased sleep efficiency and promote a less fragmented sleep. Nonpharmacologic interventions are a heterogeneous category that encompasses interventions related to lifestyle factors (diet and exercise), the sleep environment, and to sleep per se (eg, auditory stimulation during sleep[61]). For example, there is growing evidence that sleep quality is impacted by the timing of meals, and the types of food consumed during those meals.[62] When comparing a high-fat diet with a high-carbohydrate diet, those with a high carbohydrate consumption had significantly less slow wave sleep, which is strongly associated with restorative processes, in the first sleep cycle.[63] Meal timing has long been identified as a zeitgeber, and may help synchronize the circadian rhythm of alertness.[64] Furthermore, there is some evidence that food choice may interact with the timing of the food intake.[65] Physical activity has also been linked to improved sleep quality[66]; it has been suggested that in the context of high cognitive demand, maintaining an exercise routine improves sleep quality.[66] Providing a comfortable sleep environment that mitigates environmental disruptors (light, noise, temperature, and air quality) improves sleep quality.[67] Finally, interventions that use auditory closed-loop stimulation to augment restorative sleep show some promise.[61] In terms of pharmacologic interventions, the next 2B-Alert version will include individualized recommendations for caffeine intake that are based on the individual's sensitivity to sleep loss and his/her responsivity to caffeine.[68] However, it should be noted that interventions aimed at mitigating the consequences of sleep loss are self-limiting and not sustainable. For example, a recent study suggests waning effectiveness of daytime caffeine administration over several consecutive days of sleep restriction.[69]

FUTURE DIRECTIONS: INDIVIDUALIZED SLEEP, FATIGUE MANAGEMENT, AND PREDICTIVE MODELING

An accruing sleep debt unquestionably leads to fatigue and detriments in neurobehavioral performance.[31,70] As previously suggested by Dawson and colleagues,[71] perhaps the most important question in fatigue management is an individual's sleep debt, which determines not only their fitness-for-duty but also dictates their ability to sustain performance throughout their work shift. Unfortunately, as described in this article and others,[56] individual susceptibilities to sleep loss, and thus fitness-for-duty, needs treatment plans to be individualized. Although they are informative and useful for such tasks as work/rest schedule making, population-based models are of limited utility for predicting (and thus managing) operational performance at the level of the individual.

Data models, some with their proprietary sleep predictors, that proactively address fatigue based on planned sleep opportunities have clear advantages in preventing incidents and are key for fatigue risk management systems (FRMS). These are widely used in air, ground, and rail transportation industries. Models include Boeing Alertness Model, InterDynamics fatigue evaluation model, System for Aircrew Fatigue Evaluation (SAFE), McCauley and colleagues[72] model, Pulsar's Fatigue evaluation model, and the SAFTE and UMP models,[73] but to name a few. However, individual susceptibilities and/or sleep needs are not accounted for in most of these models. At present, only the UMP model has been individualized via the 2B-Alert application.[57] The operational metric for predicting performance is the psychomotor vigilance test (PVT), and although the PVT has been validated and correlated with some aspects of operational performance,[73,74] it may not necessarily be appropriate for predicting all of operational performance. Yet, studies have shown that predictions based on PVT metrics do provide statistically significant predictions of railroad accident risk and accident cost in an operational environment.[75,76]

The recent, massive expansion of wearable technology is creating unprecedented possibilities in terms of the measurement, monitoring, and prediction of operational performance at the individual level. Currently the relevant technologies (eg, Optalert and LifeBand/SmartCap systems) function in a primarily reactive fashion. That is, they are designed to identify signs of extant fatigue, but they do not predict future fatigue (eg, whether an individual operator's fatigue level will remain at an acceptable level for the remainder of his/her 8-hour shift). Obviously, this approach may be less than ideal because, for example, a pilot that is already flying the plane cannot stop flying because of excessive fatigue.

Individualized sleep assessments, sleep loss, and fatigue management remains a work in progress. An ideal FRMS would include individualized predictive modeling based on sleep opportunity, sleep history, and individual differences in sensitivity/resilience to sleep loss; and would accordingly provide individualized countermeasure recommendations. At present, no fully functioning individualized FRMS exists, but progress is being made rapidly. But the 2B-Alert app, which proactively predicts performance at the individual level based on sleep history and individual sensitivity/resilience to sleep loss, and makes recommendations regarding optimal dosing and timing of caffeine to sustain performance, constitutes a significant step forward in the right direction.

REFERENCES

1. Colten HR, Altevogt BM, editors. Sleep disorders and sleep deprivation: an unmet public health problem. The National Academies Collection: Reports funded by National Institutes of Health; 2006.
2. Morin CM, Benca RM. Insomnia nature, diagnosis, and treatment. Handb Clin Neurol 2011;99:723–46.
3. Akerstedt T. Shift work and disturbed sleep/wakefulness. Sleep Med Rev 1998;2: 117–28.
4. Young T, Peppard PE, Gottlieb DJ. Epidemiology of obstructive sleep apnea: a population health perspective. Am J Respir Crit Care Med 2002;165:1217–39.
5. Diaz-Piedra C, Di Stasi LL, Baldwin CM, et al. Sleep disturbances of adult women suffering from fibromyalgia: a systematic review of observational studies. Sleep Med Rev 2015;21:86–99.
6. Kim JH, Park EC, Lee KS, et al. Association of sleep duration with rheumatoid arthritis in Korean adults: analysis of seven years of aggregated data from the Korea National Health and Nutrition Examination Survey (KNHANES). BMJ Open 2016;6:e011420.
7. Marin R, Cyhan T, Miklos W. Sleep disturbance in patients with chronic low back pain. Am J Phys Med Rehabil 2006;85:430–5.
8. Yong LC, Li J, Calvert GM. Sleep-related problems in the US working population: prevalence and association with shiftwork status. Occup Environ Med 2017;74: 93–104.
9. Virtanen M, Ferrie JE, Gimeno D, et al. Long working hours and sleep disturbances: the Whitehall II prospective cohort study. Sleep 2009;32:737–45.
10. Petrov ME, Weng J, Reid KJ, et al. Commuting and sleep: results from the Hispanic community health study/study of Latinos Sueno ancillary study. Am J Prev Med 2018;54:e49–57.
11. Pereira EF, Moreno C, Louzada FM. Increased commuting to school time reduces sleep duration in adolescents. Chronobiol Int 2014;31:87–94.
12. Knutsson A, Boggild H. Shiftwork and cardiovascular disease: review of disease mechanisms. Rev Environ Health 2000;15:359–72.
13. Knutsson A, Hallquist J, Reuterwall C, et al. Shiftwork and myocardial infarction: a case-control study. Occup Environ Med 1999;56:46–50.
14. Cappuccio FP, D'Elia L, Strazzullo P, et al. Quantity and quality of sleep and incidence of type 2 diabetes: a systematic review and meta-analysis. Diabetes Care 2010;33:414–20.
15. Musiek ES, Xiong DD, Holtzman DM. Sleep, circadian rhythms, and the pathogenesis of Alzheimer disease. Exp Mol Med 2015;47:e148.

16. Spiegel K, Sheridan JF, Van Cauter E. Effect of sleep deprivation on response to immunization. JAMA 2002;288:1471–2.
17. Lange T, Dimitrov S, Bollinger T, et al. Sleep after vaccination boosts immunological memory. J Immunol 2011;187:283–90.
18. Lange T, Perras B, Fehm HL, et al. Sleep enhances the human antibody response to hepatitis A vaccination. Psychosom Med 2003;65:831–5.
19. Patel SR, Malhotra A, Gao X, et al. A prospective study of sleep duration and pneumonia risk in women. Sleep 2012;35:97–101.
20. Prather AA, Hall M, Fury JM, et al. Sleep and antibody response to hepatitis B vaccination. Sleep 2012;35:1063–9.
21. Cohen S, Doyle WJ, Alper CM, et al. Sleep habits and susceptibility to the common cold. Arch Intern Med 2009;169:62–7.
22. Cappuccio FP, Cooper D, D'Elia L, et al. Sleep duration predicts cardiovascular outcomes: a systematic review and meta-analysis of prospective studies. Eur Heart J 2011;32:1484–92.
23. Cappuccio FP, D'Elia L, Strazzullo P, et al. Sleep duration and all-cause mortality: a systematic review and meta-analysis of prospective studies. Sleep 2010;33:585–92.
24. Killgore WD. Effects of sleep deprivation on cognition. Prog Brain Res 2010;185:105–29.
25. Lim J, Dinges DF. Sleep deprivation and vigilant attention. Ann N Y Acad Sci 2008;1129:305–22.
26. Lim J, Dinges DF. A meta-analysis of the impact of short-term sleep deprivation on cognitive variables. Psychol Bull 2010;136:375–89.
27. Harrison Y, Horne JA, Rothwell A. Prefrontal neuropsychological effects of sleep deprivation in young adults: a model for healthy aging? Sleep 2000;23:1067–73.
28. Harrison Y, Horne JA. The impact of sleep deprivation on decision making: a review. J Exp Psychol Appl 2000;6:236–49.
29. Basner M, Fomberstein KM, Razavi FM, et al. American time use survey: sleep time and its relationship to waking activities. Sleep 2007;30:1085–95.
30. Schwartz JR, Roth T. Neurophysiology of sleep and wakefulness: basic science and clinical implications. Curr Neuropharmacol 2008;6:367–78.
31. Goel N, Rao H, Durmer JS, et al. Neurocognitive consequences of sleep deprivation. Semin Neurol 2009;29:320–39.
32. Van Dongen HP, Bender AM, Dinges DF. Systematic individual differences in sleep homeostatic and circadian rhythm contributions to neurobehavioral impairment during sleep deprivation. Accid Anal Prev 2012;45(Suppl):11–6.
33. Van Dongen HP, Baynard MD, Maislin G, et al. Systematic interindividual differences in neurobehavioral impairment from sleep loss: evidence of trait-like differential vulnerability. Sleep 2004;27:423–33.
34. Van Dongen HP, Maislin G, Dinges DF. Dealing with inter-individual differences in the temporal dynamics of fatigue and performance: importance and techniques. Aviat Space Environ Med 2004;75:A147–54.
35. Goel N, Banks S, Lin L, et al. Catechol-O-methyltransferase Val158Met polymorphism associates with individual differences in sleep physiologic responses to chronic sleep loss. PLoS One 2011;6:e29283.
36. Goel N, Banks S, Mignot E, et al. DQB1*0602 predicts interindividual differences in physiologic sleep, sleepiness, and fatigue. Neurology 2010;75:1509–19.
37. Kuna ST, Maislin G, Pack FM, et al. Heritability of performance deficit accumulation during acute sleep deprivation in twins. Sleep 2012;35:1223–33.

38. Viola AU, Archer SN, James LM, et al. PER3 polymorphism predicts sleep structure and waking performance. Curr Biol 2007;17:613–8.
39. Groeger JA, Viola AU, Lo JC, et al. Early morning executive functioning during sleep deprivation is compromised by a PERIOD3 polymorphism. Sleep 2008; 31:1159–67.
40. Maire M, Reichert CF, Gabel V, et al. Time-on-task decrement in vigilance is modulated by inter-individual vulnerability to homeostatic sleep pressure manipulation. Front Behav Neurosci 2014;8:59.
41. Bodenmann S, Hohoff C, Freitag C, et al. Polymorphisms of ADORA2A modulate psychomotor vigilance and the effects of caffeine on neurobehavioural performance and sleep EEG after sleep deprivation. Br J Pharmacol 2012;165: 1904–13.
42. Zitting KM, Munch MY, Cain SW, et al. Young adults are more vulnerable to chronic sleep deficiency and recurrent circadian disruption than older adults. Sci Rep 2018;8:11052.
43. Bliese PD, Wesensten NJ, Balkin TJ. Age and individual variability in performance during sleep restriction. J Sleep Res 2006;15:376–85.
44. Killgore WD, Richards JM, Killgore DB, et al. The trait of introversion-extraversion predicts vulnerability to sleep deprivation. J Sleep Res 2007;16:354–63.
45. Rupp TL, Killgore WD, Balkin TJ. Socializing by day may affect performance by night: vulnerability to sleep deprivation is differentially mediated by social exposure in extraverts vs introverts. Sleep 2010;33:1475–85.
46. Kaida K, Takahashi M, Akerstedt T, et al. Validation of the Karolinska sleepiness scale against performance and EEG variables. Clin Neurophysiol 2006;117: 1574–81.
47. MacLean AW, Fekken GC, Saskin P, et al. Psychometric evaluation of the Stanford sleepiness scale. J Sleep Res 1992;1:35–9.
48. Lapin BR, Bena JF, Walia HK, et al. The Epworth sleepiness scale: validation of one-dimensional factor structure in a large clinical sample. J Clin Sleep Med 2018;14:1293–301.
49. De Vries J, Michelson H, Van Heck GL, et al. Measuring fatigue in sarcoidosis: the fatigue assessment scale (FAS). Br J Health Psychol 2004;9:279–91.
50. Michelson HJ, De Vries J, Van Heck GL. Psychometric qualities of a brief self-rated fatigue measure: the fatigue assessment scale. J Psychosom Res 2003; 54:345–52.
51. Winwood PC, Winefield AH, Dawson D, et al. Development and validation of a scale to measure work-related fatigue and recovery: the occupational fatigue exhaustion/recovery scale (OFER). J Occup Environ Med 2005;47:594–606.
52. Horne J. The end of sleep: 'sleep debt' versus biological adaptation of human sleep to waking needs. Biol Psychol 2011;87:1–14.
53. Rupp TL, Wesensten NJ, Bliese PD, et al. Banking sleep: realization of benefits during subsequent sleep restriction and recovery. Sleep 2009;32:311–21.
54. Arnal PJ, Sauvet F, Leger D, et al. Benefits of sleep extension on sustained attention and sleep pressure before and during total sleep deprivation and recovery. Sleep 2015;38:1935–43.
55. Darwent D, Dawson D, Paterson JL, et al. Managing fatigue: it really is about sleep. Accid Anal Prev 2015;82:20–6.
56. Capaldi VF, Balkin TJ, Mysliwiec V. Optimizing sleep in the military: challenges and opportunities. Chest 2019;155:215–26.
57. Reifman J, Ramakrishnan S, Liu J, et al. 2B-alert app: a mobile application for real-time individualized prediction of alertness. J Sleep Res 2018;28(2):e12725.

58. Dorrian J, Hursh S, Waggoner L, et al. How much is left in your "sleep tank"? Proof of concept for a simple model for sleep history feedback. Accid Anal Prev 2019; 126:177–83.

59. Mallis MM, Mejdal S, Nguyen TT, et al. Summary of the key features of seven biomathematical models of human fatigue and performance. Aviat Space Environ Med 2004;75:A4–14.

60. Hursh SR, Balkin TJ, Van Dongen HPA. Sleep and performance modeling. In: Kryger M, Roth T, Dement WC, editors. Principles and practice of sleep medicine. Philadelphia: Elsevier; 2017. p. 689–96.

61. Ngo HV, Miedema A, Faude I, et al. Driving sleep slow oscillations by auditory closed-loop stimulation-a self-limiting process. J Neurosci 2015;35:6630–8.

62. St-Onge MP, Mikic A, Pietrolungo CE. Effects of diet on sleep quality. Adv Nutr 2016;7:938–49.

63. Yajima K, Seya T, Iwayama K, et al. Effects of nutrient composition of dinner on sleep architecture and energy metabolism during sleep. J Nutr Sci Vitaminol (Tokyo) 2014;60:114–21.

64. Asher G, Sassone-Corsi P. Time for food: the intimate interplay between nutrition, metabolism, and the circadian clock. Cell 2015;161:84–92.

65. Afaghi A, O'Connor H, Chow CM. High-glycemic-index carbohydrate meals shorten sleep onset. Am J Clin Nutr 2007;85:426–30.

66. Wunsch K, Kasten N, Fuchs R. The effect of physical activity on sleep quality, well-being, and affect in academic stress periods. Nat Sci Sleep 2017;9:117–26.

67. Caddick ZA, Gregory K, Arsintescu L, et al. A review of the environmental parameters necessary for an optimal sleep environment. Build Environ 2018;132:11–20.

68. Reifman J, Kumar K, Wesensten NJ, et al. 2B-Alert web: an open-access tool for predicting the effects of sleep/wake schedules and caffeine consumption on neurobehavioral performance. Sleep 2016;39:2157–9.

69. Doty TJ, So CJ, Bergman EM, et al. Limited efficacy of caffeine and recovery costs during and following 5 days of chronic sleep restriction. Sleep 2017;40.

70. Dinges DF, Pack F, Williams K, et al. Cumulative sleepiness, mood disturbance, and psychomotor vigilance performance decrements during a week of sleep restricted to 4-5 hours per night. Sleep 1997;20:267–77.

71. Dawson, McCulloch K. Managing fatigue: It's about sleep. Sleep Medicine Reviews 2005;9(5):365–80.

72. McCauley P, Kalachev LV, Mollicone DJ, et al. Dynamic circadian modulation in a biomathematical model for the effects of sleep and sleep loss on waking neurobehavioral performance. Sleep 2013;36:1987–97.

73. Lieberman HR, Bathalon GP, Falco CM, et al. The fog of war: decrements in cognitive performance and mood associated with combat-like stress. Aviat Space Environ Med 2005;76:C7–14.

74. Caldwell JA. Fatigue in aviation. Travel Med Infect Dis 2005;3:85–96.

75. Hursh SR, Raslear TG, Kaye AS, et al. Validation and calibration of a fatigue assessment tool for railroad work schedules, final report. Washington, DC: U.S. Department of Transportation; 2008.

76. Hursh SR, Fanzone JF, Raslear TG. Analysis of the relationship between operator effectiveness measures and economic impacts of rail accidents. Washington, DC: U.S. Department of Transportation; 2011.

Sleep Pharmacogenetics
The Promise of Precision Medicine

Andrew D. Krystal, MD, MS[a,b],*, Aric A. Prather, PhD[a,1]

KEYWORDS

- Pharmacogenetics • Genetic polymorphism • Sleep disorder

KEY POINTS

- Pharmacogenetics is the branch of personalized medicine concerned with the variability in drug response occurring because of heredity.
- In recent years, advances in genetics research, including the mapping of the human genome and the increasing availability and decreasing costs of gene sequencing, have promoted tremendous growth in pharmacogenetics.
- There are several studies indicating that there are genetic influences on the outcomes of pharmacologic treatment of sleep disorders that seem ripe for application to clinical practice.
- Clinical implementation faces several challenges, including small effect sizes, perceived lack of clinical utility, the absence of effective guidelines for clinical application, and limited insurance reimbursement.
- The increasing availability and continued decreasing costs of genome sequencing and rapid development of research methods designed to improve the capacity to predict drug response fuel optimism that the existing limitations will be overcome and lead to an increasing capacity to apply pharmacogenetics to improve the treatment of individuals with sleep disorders.

INTRODUCTION

The concept of personalized or precision medicine is based on the observation that there is great variation among individuals in their clinical presentation, course of illness, and response to treatment.[1] Pharmacogenetics is the branch of personalized medicine concerned with the variability in drug response occurring because of

This article originally appeared in *Sleep Medicine Clinics*, Volume 14, Issue 3, September 2019.
Disclosure: A. Krystal has received grants/research support from NIH, Janssen, Jazz, Axsome, Reveal Biosensors, and is a consultant for Adare, Eisai, Ferring, Galderma, Harmony Biosciences, Idorsia, Jazz, Janssen, Takeda, Merck, Neurocrine, Pernix, Physician's Seal. A. Prather has received grants/research support from NIH, Headspace Inc.
[a] University of California San Francisco, San Francisco, CA, USA; [b] Duke University School of Medicine, Durham, NC, USA
[1] Present address: 3333 California Street, San Francisco CA 94118.
* Corresponding author. 401 Parnassus Avenue, San Francisco, CA 94143.
E-mail address: andrew.krystal@ucsf.edu

heredity.[2] Pharmacogenetics goes back at least to Pythagoras who, in 510 BC, is credited with the observation that only some individuals died when eating fava beans.[3] The modern era of pharmacogenetics is reported to have begun in 1959 when an article was published using this term, which reported that drug-induced porphyria occurred only in a small subset of the population and that phenylthiourea is tasteless to some individuals and perceived as extremely bitter by others.[4] The aim of pharmacogenetics is to identify genetic variations that affect the response to pharmacotherapies so as to improve the capacity to predict who will have a favorable therapeutic response and who is predisposed to having adverse effects so that treatment can be tailored to each patient as a means of optimizing outcomes. Such genetic variations (**Table 1**) include (1) single nucleotide polymorphisms (SNPs), in which individuals vary in a single nucleotide at a specific position in the genome; (2) variable number tandem repeat (VNTR) polymorphisms, in which individuals vary in the number of times a short sequence of nucleotides is repeated at a specific location in the genome; (3) copy number variants, in which specific sections of the genome are repeated a variable number of times in individuals; (4) deletions, in which a sequence of DNA is lost during replication and absent from the genome, and; (5) insertions, in which 1 or more nucleotide base pairs is added into the DNA sequence.[5–8] These variations can affect drug response in a variety of ways, including by altering the function of drug receptors; ion channels affected by drug binding; a variety of enzymes, including enzymes that metabolize drugs; immune molecules; drug transporters; plasma protein binding of drugs; or proteins that synthesize, clear, or degrade the neurotransmitters that bind to the receptors that drugs bind to.[5]

In recent years, advances in genetics research, including the mapping of the human genome and the increasing availability and decreasing costs of gene sequencing, have promoted tremendous growth in pharmacogenetics. This growth has affected all areas of medicine, including sleep medicine, in which a growing body of research points to genetic factors that modulate the therapeutic and adverse responses to pharmacotherapy. This article reviews this body of work. It begins by providing a brief overview of sleep disorders and then identifies sleep disorders for which studies have been performed that have reported genetic variations that affect the therapeutic actions of agents or for which there is reason to believe that such an effect is likely and may have implications for a personalized medicine approach in caring for patients with sleep disorders.

OVERVIEW OF THE MAJOR SLEEP DISORDERS AND THEIR PRIMARY PHARMACOTHERAPIES

The Third Edition of the International Classification of Sleep Disorders (ICSD-3) identified 7 major categories of sleep disorders: insomnia, sleep-related breathing

Table 1 Potential genetic variations	
Genetic Variation	**Definition**
SNPs	Variation in a single nucleotide at a specific position in the genome
VNTR polymorphisms	Variation in the number of times a short sequence of nucleotides is repeated at a specific location in the genome
Copy number variants	Specific sections of the genome are repeated a variable number of times
Deletions	A sequence of DNA is absent from the genome
Insertions	One or more nucleotide base pairs is added into the genome

Abbreviations: SNPs, single nucleotide polymorphisms; VNTR, variable number tandem repeat.

disorders, central disorders of hypersomnolence, circadian rhythm sleep-wake disorders, parasomnias, sleep-related movement disorders, and other sleep disorders.[9] With the exception of sleep-related breathing disorders, existing literature suggests that there are genetic variants that affect or are likely to affect the response to treatments for these sleep disorders. A brief overview of these sleep disorders are provided here.

Insomnia

The ICSD-3 defines 1 overarching condition, chronic insomnia disorder, which is defined as a report of persistent (at least 3 times per week for at least 3 months) difficulty falling or staying asleep in the context of the affected individual having an adequate opportunity and circumstances for sleep and associated daytime consequences.[9] There are a variety of pharmacologic treatments that are used to treat chronic insomnia disorder (**Table 2**).[10–14] These treatments include benzodiazepines, mechanistically related agents referred to as nonbenzodiazepines, selective histamine H1 receptor antagonists, hypocretin/orexin receptor antagonists, melatonin receptor agonists, nonselective histamine H1 receptor antagonists, antidepressants, antipsychotics, and anticonvulsants.

Benzodiazepines

The benzodiazepines are a group of chemically related compounds that are positive allosteric modulators (PAMs) at the benzodiazepine binding site on the gamma-aminobutyric acid (GABA) type A receptor complex.[11–14] They exert a sleep-enhancing effect by potentiating GABA-A receptor–mediated inhibition. Benzodiazepines most commonly used to treat insomnia include triazolam, temazepam, flurazepam, alprazolam, clonazepam, and lorazepam.[14,15] Placebo-controlled trials indicate the efficacy of triazolam, temazepam, flurazepam, quazepam, and estazolam for sleep onset and maintenance difficulties.[14] These agents vary in their affinity to different types of GABA-A receptors in the brain.[16–18] As a result, they have differing clinical effects, which can include cognitive impairment, myorelaxant effects, antiseizure effects, and anxiolytic effects in addition to their sleep-enhancing effects.

Nonbenzodiazepines

Nonbenzodiazepines is a term used to refer to a group of medications that, like the benzodiazepines, are GABA-A receptor PAMs acting at the benzodiazepine binding site but are unrelated chemically to the benzodiazepines.[11–14] These agents include zolpidem, zolpidem CR (controlled release), zolpidem tartrate (sublingual), zaleplon, and eszopiclone. Their clinical effects are mediated by the same mechanism as the benzodiazepines and also vary in their clinical effects like the benzodiazepines because of variable binding to GABA-A receptors in the brain.[11–14,16–18] A sizable number of placebo-controlled trials have been performed that establish the efficacy and safety profiles of these agents in treating insomnia. Sleep onset effects have been documented for zolpidem and zaleplon, whereas sleep onset and maintenance therapeutic effects have been reported for zolpidem CR and eszopiclone.[14,19–24] Zolpidem tartrate and zaleplon have also been shown to have a favorable risk-benefit profile for middle-of-the-night administration.[25,26]

Selective histamine H1 receptor antagonists

The histamine H1 receptor exerts a wake-promoting effect when activated.[27] As a result, drugs that block this receptor can promote sleep.[27] Although many agents have H1 antagonist effects, nearly all of them do so nonselectively. The exceptions to this are doxepin in the 3-gm to 6-mg range of dosing and esmirtazapine (the

Table 2
Medications used to treat sleep disorders

Medication Type	Mechanism of Action	Agents Most Commonly Used
Insomnia		
Benzodiazepines	GABA-A receptor positive allosteric modulation	Triazolam, temazepam, flurazepam, alprazolam, clonazepam, lorazepam
Nonbenzodiazepines	GABA-A receptor positive allosteric modulation	Zolpidem, zolpidem CR, transoral zolpidem, zaleplon, eszopiclone
Selective H1 antagonists	Antagonism of H1 histamine receptors	Doxepin 3–6 mg
Nonselective H1 antagonists	Antagonism of H1 histamine and acetylcholine receptors	Diphenhydramine, doxylamine
Hypocretin/orexin receptor antagonists	Antagonism of hypocretin/orexin receptors	Suvorexant
Melatonin receptor agonists	Agonists at MT1 and MT2 melatonin receptors	Ramelteon, melatonin
Antidepressants	Antagonism of serotonin transporter and a variety of other receptors	Trazodone, mirtazapine, amitriptyline, doxepin (in doses >6 mg), and trimipramine
Antipsychotics	Antagonism of dopamine D2 receptors and variety of other receptors	Quetiapine, olanzapine
N-type voltage-gated calcium channel modulators	Inhibiting N-type voltage-gated calcium channels by binding to alpha-2 subunit	Pregabalin, gabapentin
Central Disorders of Hypersomnolence		
Amphetamines	Stimulating release and inhibiting reuptake of norepinephrine and dopamine	Amphetamine/D-amphetamine and methamphetamine
Methylphenidate	Increases release of norepinephrine and dopamine	Methylphenidate
Modafinil	Mechanism of action thought to be inhibition of reuptake of norepinephrine and dopamine	Modafinil, R-modafinil
GABA-B agonists	Mechanism of wake promotion unknown	Sodium oxybate
Circadian Rhythm Sleep Disorders		
Melatonin receptor agonists	Agonists at MT1 and MT2 receptors, possibly intracellular melatonin receptors	Melatonin

(continued on next page)

Table 2
(continued)

Medication Type	Mechanism of Action	Agents Most Commonly Used
Modafinil	Mechanism of action thought to be inhibition of reuptake of norepinephrine and dopamine	Modafinil, R-modafinil
Parasomnias		
Benzodiazepines	GABA-A receptor positive allosteric modulators	Clonazepam
Sleep-related Movement Disorders		
Dopamine agonists	Agonists at dopamine D2, D3, and D4 receptors	Pramipexole, ropinirole
Dopamine precursors	Increase synthesis of dopamine	L-Dopa
N-type voltage-gated calcium channel modulators	Inhibiting N-type voltage-gated calcium channels by binding to alpha-2 subunit	Pregabalin, gabapentin

Abbreviations: CR, controlled release; GABA, gamma-aminobutyric acid.

S-isomer of mirtazapine) in a dose of 3 to 4.5 mg.[27–30] These two agents have H1 antagonism as by far their most potent effect. In higher doses used to treat depression (doxepin, $\geq$75 mg; mirtazapine, $\geq$15 mg) they have broad pharmacologic effects but, if the dose is low enough, they can have clinical effects only at the H1 receptor.[27] Studies with these medications in the range in which they have H1 selectivity show that H1 antagonism is associated with a unique set of effects, including greater effects on sleep maintenance than sleep onset, greatest effect size at the end of the night despite peak blood level occurring in the middle of the night, and a shortening of the time it takes to return to sleep without decreasing number of awakenings.[28–30]

Nonselective H1 antagonists

Several medications, are referred to as antihistamines, were developed to treat allergy problems but are frequently used to treat insomnia. As described earlier, these agents are not selective H1 antagonists in that they also block acetylcholine receptors with comparable potency as their H1 antagonist effects and this affects their sleep profile and also can lead to side effects.[27] Such agents include diphenhydramine and doxylamine, which are obtainable over the counter in the United States.[27] Double-blind placebo-controlled trials have only been performed with diphenhydramine, and these are limited. These studies provide an indication that the effects may be more potent on maintenance than at onset.[27] One study of daytime dosing of diphenhydramine suggests that benefits versus placebo do not sustain beyond a few days; however, it remains unknown whether this is also true when diphenhydramine is taken at bedtime.[27]

Hypocretin/orexin receptor antagonists

Hypocretin/orexin receptor antagonists enhance sleep by blocking the wake-promoting effects of the peptide hypocretin/orexin.[31] One such agent, suvorexant, is U. Food and Drug Administration (FDA) approved for the treatment of insomnia and available in the United States. This agent has been shown to have robust efficacy and a favorable adverse effects profile in several double-blind, randomized, placebo-controlled studies.[31–36] The profile is somewhat reminiscent of doxepin in the 3-mg to 6-mg range in that the effects on sleep maintenance are more pronounced than on sleep onset (onset effects of suvorexant are dose dependent), are greatest in the last third of the night, and decrease wake time without preventing awakenings.[31–36]

Melatonin receptor agonists

Melatonin is a hormone produced by the pineal gland that seems to have several physiologic effects, including that it seems to be related to circadian rhythmicity.[13] Melatonin agonists are thought to exert their therapeutic effects on sleep by binding to MT1 and MT2 melatonin receptors, which has been hypothesized to lead to a diminution of arousal systems emerging from the suprachiasmatic nucleus of the thalamus.[13,37] There are 2 melatonin agonists available for use in the United States: melatonin and ramelteon.[38] Melatonin is best established as a modulator of the circadian rhythm.[13] A large number of controlled studies have been performed on the effects of melatonin on insomnia symptoms in a variety of dosages and when given at various times with respect to sleep onset.[37,39,40] The studies do not generally provide robust evidence of a therapeutic effect on insomnia symptoms.[37,39–41] However, it does seem to have a consistent therapeutic effect in some populations, including those with neurodevelopmental disorders.[42–45] Ramelteon has been shown to have robust therapeutic effects in patients with insomnia but only for sleep onset problems, and the therapeutic effect is larger when measured with polysomnography than self-report assessment.[46] It does not seem to have abuse potential and has a favorable side effect profile.

Agents used off label to treat insomnia

A large number of agents of different types are not indicated for the treatment of insomnia but are used clinically for this purpose. These agents include antidepressants such as trazodone, mirtazapine, amitriptyline, doxepin (in doses >6 mg), and trimipramine; antipsychotics such as quetiapine and olanzapine; and anticonvulsants, including gabapentin and pregabalin.[12] The antidepressants and antipsychotics differ in their mechanisms of action but tend to have broad pharmacologic effects, including varying degrees of antagonism of histamine H1 receptors, α_1-adrenergic receptors, muscarinic cholinergic receptors, serotonin type 2 (5HT2) receptors, dopamine D2 receptors, and the serotonin transporter.[12] Gabapentin and pregabalin are thought to exert their primary effects by binding to the alpha-2-delta subunit of N-type voltage-gated calcium channels, thereby diminishing the level of activity of wake-promoting neurotransmitter systems, including glutamate and norepinephrine.[12] Although some of these agents are widely used to treat insomnia, most notably trazodone, the evidence base supporting their use in treating insomnia is limited. Double-blind placebo-controlled trials showing efficacy for the treatment of insomnia exist for the antidepressants trimipramine (50–200 mg; improved sleep quality and efficiency but not onset latency vs placebo) and doxepin (25–50 mg; improved sleep quality and onset and maintenance difficulties).[10,47–51]

Central Disorders of Hypersomnolence

This group of disorders consists of a set of conditions associated with excessive daytime sleepiness that is not caused by another sleep disorder, such as a breathing-related sleep disorder or a circadian rhythm disorder.[9] This group of disorders consists of narcolepsy, idiopathic hypersomnia, Kleine-Levin Syndrome, hypersomnia caused by a medical disorder, hypersomnia caused by a medication or substance, hypersomnia associated with a psychiatric disorder, and insufficient sleep syndrome.[9]

Of these conditions, only 1 is associated with FDA-approved pharmacotherapies: narcolepsy. Although others of these conditions are sometimes treated with pharmacotherapy off label, those treatments are generally the same medications used to treat narcolepsy. As a result, this article discusses only treatments for narcolepsy, with the understanding that they are sometimes used to treat other hypersomnia disorders. In addition to excessive sleepiness, narcolepsy is also frequently associated with hypnogogic (occurring at sleep onset) or hypnopompic (occurring on waking) hallucinations and/or paralysis and cataplexy, a condition defined by episodes of sudden short-lived loss of muscle tone that are triggered by strong emotions, including fear, excitement, and laughter.[9]

Treatment of narcolepsy may include prescribing wake-promoting medications for the sleepiness and medications to target the other symptoms of narcolepsy.[52] Medications that are used to enhance wakefulness include amphetamine/D-amphetamine, methamphetamine, methylphenidate, modafinil, R-modafinil, and sodium oxybate. Amphetamine/D-amphetamine and methamphetamine are thought to enhance waking by stimulating release of norepinephrine and dopamine, and inhibiting the reuptake of these neurotransmitters.[52] Methylphenidate increases norepinephrine and dopamine release and has a lower risk of decreasing appetite and cardiovascular side effects than amphetamines but shares their abuse liability.[52] Although the mechanism of modafinil and R-modafinil are less well established, the available evidence suggests that they inhibit the reuptake of norepinephrine and serotonin.[52] Sodium oxybate is also used to treat sleepiness in patients with narcolepsy, although it works in a different way than the other wake-promoting medications. Its primary pharmacologic effect is binding to GABA-B receptors.[52] Notably, it is a sedating medication that is dosed at bedtime and has such a short half-life (0.5–1 hour) that it is redosed in the middle of the night. However, by unknown mechanism, it stimulates wakefulness the next day after nighttime dosing. It is hypothesized that this occurs via enhancing dopamine and norepinephrine release after it is eliminated.[52] This medication has also been shown to have a significant therapeutic effect on cataplexy during the day with nighttime dosing and is approved by the FDA for this purpose. Other medications used off label to treat cataplexy and other symptoms of narcolepsy other than sleepiness include antidepressants, including tricyclic antidepressants, selective serotonin reuptake inhibitors, and serotonin-norepinephrine reuptake inhibitors.[52]

Circadian Rhythm Sleep Disorders

This set of conditions includes delayed sleep-wake phase disorder, advanced sleep-wake phase disorder, irregular sleep-wake rhythm disorder, non–24-hour sleep-wake rhythm disorder, shift-work disorder, jet lag disorder, and circadian sleep-wake disorder not otherwise specified.[9] These disorders are defined as the presence of at least 3 months of difficulty (for all but jet lag disorder) consisting of a chronic or recurrent pattern of sleep-wake rhythm disruption primarily caused by an alteration in the endogenous circadian timing system or misalignment between the endogenous circadian rhythm and the sleep-wake schedule desired or required, occurring in conjunction with insomnia or excessive sleepiness and associated with distress or impairment.[9] Treatments of these conditions include timed light exposure; timed melatonin administration; and, for shift-work sleep disorder, modafinil and R-modafinil.[53]

Parasomnias

Parasomnias consist of a group of recurrent, episodic phenomena that occur during sleep. Some of these occur as partial arousals out of non–rapid eye movement

(REM) sleep and are defined by incomplete awakening, alteration in responsiveness, diminished cognition (including no report of a dream experience), and some degree of amnesia for what occurred.[9] These include confusional arousals, sleepwalking, sleep terrors, and sleep-related eating disorder. Some individuals experience events during REM sleep, the most important of which are REM sleep behavior disorder, in which dream enactment occurs because of a loss of the usual paralysis that occurs during REM sleep, and nightmare disorder. The best-established and most commonly used treatment of both non-REM and REM parasomnias is the benzodiazepine clonazepam.[54]

Sleep-related Movement Disorders

The sleep-related movement disorders include stereotyped movements occurring during sleep as well as a dysesthesia that occurs during waking that prevents sleep from occurring (eg, restless legs syndrome).[9] The most important of these for the purposes of this article are restless legs syndrome (RLS), also known as Willis-Ekbom disease, and periodic limb movement disorder (PLMD). RLS is characterized by an urge to move the legs, sometimes accompanied by an uncomfortable sensation that occurs primarily with rest/inactivity and that is partially relieved by movement, for as long as the movement occurs; it occurs primarily in the evening or night and is associated with disturbance of sleep, distress, or daytime impairment.[55] PLMD is defined by repetitive dorsal flexion of the foot or flexion of the knee or hip occurring at least 15 times per hour in adults and associated with sleep disturbance or functional impairment.[9,55] Periodic limb movements occur in most patients with RLS. Therefore, it is not surprising that there is significant overlap in pharmacotherapy for these conditions. Dopamine agonists, including pramipexole, and ropinirole, and the dopamine precursor L-dopa are considered first-line therapy for both conditions.[55,56] The alpha-2-delta calcium channel blockers gabapentin and pregabalin can also be used to treat these conditions and preliminary data support the use of clonazepam and melatonin for PLMD.[56]

GENETIC POLYMORPHISMS WITH POTENTIAL TO AFFECT ACTION OF TREATMENTS FOR SLEEP DISORDERS
Insomnia Therapies

There is some evidence that polymorphisms of liver cytochrome P450 (CYP) isoenzymes involved in the metabolism of some insomnia therapies affect optimal dosing in terms of achieving an optimal therapeutic effect and avoiding adverse effects, including daytime impairment (**Table 3**). Although some animal data indicate that there are genetic variations in GABA-A receptor constituent peptide among individuals that have been reported to affect the responsivity of mice to benzodiazepines and nonbenzodiazepines, there is no evidence that this is the case in humans.[57–59]

Zolpidem

Zolpidem is among the best examples of a drug with clinically important differences in subgroups of the population. Women have been noted to have a higher incidence of adverse effects with zolpidem than men, including greater morning sedation and higher rates of abuse, dependence, and withdrawal.[60–65] Further, women have been found to show greater impairment in automobile driving after receiving zolpidem during the day and in the morning after receiving zolpidem in the middle of the night.[63] Based on such observations, the FDA recommended halving the initial dose of zolpidem in all forms for women.[66]

The sex difference in zolpidem adverse effects is grounded in differences in pharmacokinetics. Zolpidem absorption seems to be greater in women and clearance is slower, such that women experience significantly higher blood levels (area under the curve is approximately 50% higher in women vs men receiving the same dose); an effect that is not explained by differences in body weight.[64,65,67,68]

There has been some debate about the mechanism responsible for the sex difference in zolpidem pharmacokinetics. The key steps in the metabolism of zolpidem are thought to be its hydroxylation by CYP3A4, its oxidation to an aldehyde by alcohol dehydrogenases (ADHs), and its conversion into a carboxylic acid by aldehyde dehydrogenases (ALDHs).[69,70] Some clinicians have argued for a role of sex differences in CYP3A4 activity; however, this is implausible because several drugs primarily metabolized by this liver enzyme do not manifest sex differences in pharmacokinetics and, if anything, CYP3A4 activity is greater in women than in men.[71] Instead, the evidence suggests that lesser activity of ADHs and ALDHs in women is responsible for the greater absorption and slower elimination of zolpidem.[72] ADHs and ALDHs are well known to have double the activity in male versus female humans and rats.[73,74] More direct evidence for the role of ADHs and ALDHs is that the absorption and elimination of zolpidem in male rats became comparable with that in female rats following both castration and administration of a blocker of ADHs/ALDHs (Peer and colleagues,[72] 2016).

Clonazepam

Clonazepam is metabolized primarily by CYP3A4 into 7-amonoclonazepam, which undergoes a second stage of metabolism via acetylation by NAT2 (N-acetyl transferase 2).[75] There are polymorphisms in the population of NAT2 that lead to decreased efficacy of this acetylation and results in greater blood levels and, therefore, greater risks for side effects, such as daytime sedation/impairment for a given dose of clonazepam.[75]

Lorazepam

Similar to clonazepam, lorazepam undergoes a second stage of metabolism by UGT (UDP-glucuronosyltransferase). Polymorphisms of UGT genes in the population include some forms of UGT that are less effective in eliminating lorazepam, thereby increasing the likelihood of adverse effects in affected individuals, as documented in a recent case report.[76]

Diphenhydramine

Multiple CYP450 isoenzymes are involved in metabolizing diphenhydramine, including CPY2D6, CYP1A2, CYP2C9, and CYP2C19.[77] Polymorphisms of CYP2D6 have been reported to affect the clinical effects of this medication and are thought to be responsible, at least to a degree, for observed variability in clinical treatment outcomes.[5] Those with more effective CYP2D6 metabolize diphenhydramine very rapidly and have been reported to experience a countertherapeutic excitation when treated with this medication.[78] A CYP2D6 polymorphism that is associated with less effective metabolism (CYP2D6*10) is associated with an increased risk for daytime sleepiness.[5,79]

Doxepin

There are variants in the population in 2 of the main enzymes involved in the metabolism of doxepin, CYP2D6, CYP2D9, and CYP2C19, which lead to variability in both therapeutic and adverse effects among treated individuals.[5,80]

Trazodone

Trazodone has long been established to be associated with significant interindividual variation in metabolism, with a half-life ranging from 2.6 to 6.1 hours.[81–86] Key factors

Table 3
Genetic polymorphisms with potential to affect action of treatments for sleep disorders

Medication	Polymorphism	Potential Clinical Effect
Insomnia		
Zolpidem	Not a polymorphism; sex hormone-related enhancement of activity of ADHs/ALDHs (involved in degradation of zolpidem) in men	Higher blood levels in women vs men at the same dose. Potential for increased side effects in women and lack of efficacy in men
Clonazepam	Loss-of-function polymorphism of NAT2 (N-acetyl transferase 2) involved in metabolism of clonazepam	Increases blood levels in affected individuals with potential for adverse effects
Lorazepam	Loss-of-function polymorphism of UGT involved in metabolism of lorazepam	Increases blood levels in affected individuals with potential for adverse effects
Diphenhydramine	Polymorphisms of CYP2D6 (involved in metabolism of diphenhydramine) exist that increase and decrease efficacy of metabolism	Affected individuals may have increased risk of side effects or loss of efficacy depending on type of polymorphism
Doxepin	Polymorphisms exist of 2 main enzymes in metabolism: CYP2D6 and CYP2D9, associated with increased and decreased efficacy of metabolism	Affected individuals may have increased risk of side effects or loss of efficacy depending on type of polymorphism
Trazodone	Polymorphisms exist in the 3 main enzymes involved in the degradation of this trazodone: CYP3A4, CYP2D6, and CYP1A2	Those with more effective CYP1A2 and CYP3A4 may experience inadequate therapeutic effects at a dosage at which benefit often occurs and those with less effective activity of these isoenzymes are likely to experience increased risk of adverse effects. Those with relatively effective CYP3A4 but relative inactivity of CYP2D6 experience buildup of mCPP and can experience stimulantlike effects, anxiety, shivering, dizziness, and heightened sensitivity toward light and noise
Central Disorders of Hypersomnolence		
Amphetamines, methylphenidate, modafinil	VNTR polymorphism exists in the SLC6A3 gene coding for the dopamine transporter, which affects clinical effects occurring with agents that	Dopamine transporter polymorphisms associated with greater clinical effects in a subset of the population associated with greater risks

(continued on next page)

Table 3 *(continued)*		
Medication	**Polymorphism**	**Potential Clinical Effect**
	block this transporter (amphetamines, modafinil); common SNP exists in the gene for an enzyme that breaks down dopamine (catechol O-methyl transferase COMT), which leads to variation in dopamine levels and cortical dopamine tone	of side effects such as psychosis COMT polymorphisms lead some individuals to experience lack of efficacy with these agents and others to be prone to adverse effects
Circadian Rhythm Sleep Disorders		
Melatonin	An SNP of a key enzyme involved in metabolism of melatonin (CYP1A2) leads some individuals to have significantly lower melatonin blood levels	Affected individuals have a lessened therapeutic response to melatonin
Parasomnias		
Clonazepam	Loss-of-function polymorphism of NAT2, involved in metabolism of clonazepam	Increases blood levels in affected individuals, with potential for adverse effects
Sleep-related Movement Disorders		
L-Dopa	SNPS affecting COMT activity exist; there are also variations in the gene for the MAO -B, which is also involved in breakdown of dopamine	Individuals with low COMT activity are at risk for L-dopa–induced dyskinesia; those with high COMT activity require higher doses to achieve a therapeutic effects Similar to COMT, those with low MAO-B activity are at risk for dyskinesia; Those with high MAO-B activity require higher doses to achieve a therapeutic effects
Dopamine agonists	Polymorphisms in CYP1A2, primary enzyme involved in ropinirole metabolism lead to variations in ropinirole blood levels Polymorphisms of the gene for SLC22A1 (involved in pramipexole metabolism) affect pramipexole blood levels DRD3 polymorphisms alter the effects of pramipexole	Those with more effective CYP1A2 are prone to adverse effects with ropinirole Those with more effective SLC22A1 require higher pramipexole dosage Individuals with particular DRD3 polymorphisms require a higher dosage of pramipexole

Abbreviations: ADH, alcohol dehydrogenase; ALDH, aldehyde dehydrogenase; COMT, catechol O-methyl transferase; DRD3, dopamine receptor type 3; MAO, monoamine oxidase; mCPP, methyl-chlorophenylpiperazine; NAT2, N-acetyl transferase 2; UGT, UDP-glucuronosyltransferase.

responsible for this are polymorphisms in the population of the enzymes involved in the degradation of this molecule: CYP3A4, CYP2D6, and CYP1A2.[81,82,85,86] Trazodone is cleaved into methyl-chlorophenylpiperazine (mCPP), an active metabolite, and an inactive metabolite by CYP3A4.[86] Trazodone is also metabolized by CYP1A2 into another inactive metabolite.[85] As a result, polymorphisms in either of these enzymes can affect blood levels of trazodone. Those with more effective CYP1A2 and CYP3A4 may experience inadequate therapeutic effects at a dosage at which benefit often occurs, and those with less effective activity of these isoenzymes are likely to experience increased risk of adverse effects.[87] Speaking to the clinical relevance of such effects, CYP3A4 levels vary 5-fold to 20-fold in the population.

The fact that trazodone has an active metabolite, mCPP, adds significant complexity to clinical management because mCPP has effects that are in some ways the opposite of what the patients are hoping to experience when taking trazodone for treating their insomnia. mCPP is a serotonergic postsynaptic receptor agonist (5-HT1 and 5-HT2) and is a drug of abuse that is closely related to ecstasy (methylenedioxymethamphetamine [MDMA]).[82,88,89] The effects of mCPP, which include stimulantlike effects, anxiety, shivering, dizziness, heightened sensitivity toward light and noise, are highly unexpected by patients with insomnia receiving this medication and can be extremely upsetting.[82,88,89]

Because CYP3A4 is responsible for the production of mCPP from trazodone, individuals with polymorphisms of this isoenzyme that are more effective are at increased risk for experiencing mCPP effects with treatment. This risk is particularly heightened in those with relatively effective CYP3A4 but relative inactivity of CYP2D6, the isoenzyme responsible for inactivating mCPP.[86] The available data suggest that 1% of the population are CYP2D6 ultrarapid metabolizers, 7% to 10% of white people are poor metabolizers, whereas Asians and Africans are less likely to have a low level of CYP2D6 activity.[90]

It should be clear from the considerations discussed earlier that the optimal use of trazodone involves a higher degree of complexity than most other medications. Achieving optimal clinical outcomes with trazodone requires starting with the lowest possible dose, titrating the dose slowly as needed, and warning patients of the possibility of mCPP-mediated effects, including activation and anxiety.

Hypocretin/orexin receptor antagonists

Genetic polymorphisms have been identified that affect the synthesis of hypocretin/orexin and hypocretin/orexin type 1 and 2 receptors.[91] However, it is currently unclear whether these variants affect the clinical effects of antagonists of hypocretin/orexin receptors used to treat insomnia.[5]

Therapies for Central Disorders of Hypersomnolence

Stimulants

Clinically relevant polymorphisms exist for 2 mechanisms related to the effects of stimulants: the dopamine (DAT) transporter, which is inhibited by some of these agents, and the enzyme catechol-O-methyltransferase (COMT), responsible for breaking down central dopamine, levels of which are increased by several stimulant agents.[5] The relevant DAT transporter polymorphisms have a VNTR in the SLC6A3 gene coding for the DAT; the most common and clinically important of these are 10-repeat (*10R) and 9-repeat (*9R) polymorphisms.[92] Observations of the clinical effects of these polymorphisms suggest greater clinical effects in the *9R compared with

*10R allele and include a greater likelihood of psychosis occurring with methamphetamine,[93] and a greater functional MRI neural response during a go-no-go task.[94]

The relevant COMT polymorphism is a common SNP occurring at codon 158 in the COMT gene.[95] The *met* allele of the val158met SNP, which causes a substitution of the amino acid methionine for valine, is associated with a significant reduction in COMT activity compared with the val allele and results in significantly increased cortical dopamine tone.[95] Observations of greater clinical effects of stimulants in val compared with met individuals include that modafinil given during sleep deprivation led to maintenance of baseline performance on several cognitive tests throughout sleep deprivation in val/val homozygotes, whereas minimal effects of modafinil were noted in met/met homozygotes[96]; and D-amphetamine was found to improve attention and processing speed performance in both val/val and val/met individuals, but not in met/met homozygotes.[97] An additional observation that seems to suggest that there is complexity to understanding the clinical effects of these alleles is that the treatment of daytime sleepiness in those with narcolepsy required a significantly greater daily dose of modafinil in val/val homozygotes compared with met/met individuals.[98]

Based on these observations, it should be expected that some individuals in the population will be prone to adverse effects with D-amphetamine such that lower dosages would be indicated, modafinil and D-amphetamine will fail to have therapeutic effects on sleepiness in some individuals, and modafinil doses in narcolepsy will need to be higher in some individuals than others.

Circadian Rhythm Disorders

Melatonin

Melatonin metabolism is primarily driven by CYP1A2.[99] An SNP of CYP1A2 has been found to affect CYP1A2 activity such that individuals who are homozygous for the *1A allele, which is associated with lesser CYP1A2 activity, have higher blood levels of melatonin than *1F homozygotes.[99] Clinically, *1F homozygotes have been reported to have fewer therapeutic sleep effects from melatonin than *1A homozygotes and heterozygotes.[100]

Parasomnias

Clonazepam

As described earlier related to insomnia, polymorphisms of NAT2, which is responsible for the second stage of metabolism of clonazepam, vary in their effectiveness such that the less effective polymorphism is associated with increased clonazepam blood levels and greater risks of adverse effects.[75]

Sleep-related Movement Disorders

L-Dopa

There is no direct evidence indicating whether genetic polymorphisms affect the clinical effects of L-dopa when used to treat sleep-related movement disorders. However, there is some evidence that there are polymorphisms affecting clinical effects when this agent is used to treat Parkinson disease (PD).[101–104] Given that L-dopa is broken down by COMT, it is not surprising that the effective dose of L-dopa when used to treat PD differs as a function of SNPs altering the effectiveness of this enzyme.[101,104] Patients with PD with SNPs associated with high COMT activity have been found to require higher doses of L-dopa to achieve therapeutic effects.[101,104] Genetic variations in COMT also affect the risk of L-dopa–induced dyskinesia. Individuals who are LL homozygotes for the COMT rs4680 gene were more likely to experience this adverse effect, whereas the C allele of the rs393795 gene was associated with a greater time until the onset of dyskinesia.[103] The activity of monoamine oxidase enzymes also affects the clinical effects of L-dopa. The basis for this is that the clinical effects of L-dopa are thought to be mediated by increasing dopamine synthesis and dopamine is degraded by monoamine oxidase enzymes. Greater doses of L-dopa seem to be required for the treatment of patients with PD who carry the monoamine oxidase (MAO)-B G allele and who have high MAO-A enzyme activity, and a greater risk of dyskinesia with L-dopa was reported for individuals with A and AA genotypes of the MAO-B rs1799836 gene.[103,104]

Dopamine agonists

There are no studies rigorously assessing whether polymorphisms of genes encoding for key enzymes degrading dopamine agonists have clinical effects. However, because the enzyme primarily involved in ropinirole metabolism is CYP1A2, which varies in effectiveness because of polymorphisms in the population, it seems likely that individuals with less effective CYP1A2 will be prone to adverse effects and be best treated with a lower dosage than those with more effective CP1A2.[5,105,106]

It has reported that there are clinical effects of polymorphisms of the SLC22A1 gene, which encodes for the organic cation transporter 1, for which pramipexole is a substrate.[107] The rs622342 A polymorphism is associated with higher prescribed dosages of pramipexole and possibly other medications used to treat PD than the C polymorphism.[107]

Polymorphisms of dopamine receptor genes have also been studied to determine whether they influence the clinical effects of dopamine agonists. Two studies suggested that dopamine receptor type 3 (DRD3) Ser9Gly polymorphisms influence the effects of pramipexole such that Gly/Gly homozygotes required higher pramipexole doses than Ser/Gly and Ser/Ser individuals.[108,109]

SUMMARY

The genetic influences on the treatment of sleep disorders described earlier seem ripe for application to clinical practice. However, clinical implementation faces several challenges in the clinical application of pharmacogenetic findings in all areas of medicine (Scott,[1] 2011). These challenges include small effect sizes, perceived lack of clinical utility, the absence of effective guidelines for clinical application, and limited insurance reimbursement (Scott,[1] 2011). Several trials have been performed and are in progress attempting to define/establish clinical utility, but these have so far had limited impact. However, the increasing availability and continued decreasing costs of genome sequencing and rapid development of research methods designed to improve the capacity to predict drug response fuel optimism that the existing limitations will be overcome and lead to an increasing capacity to apply pharmacogenetics to tailor the treatment of sleep disorders in individuals.

REFERENCES

1. Scott SA. Personalizing medicine with clinical pharmacogenetics. Genet Med 2011;13(12):987–95.
2. Pirmohamed M. Pharmacogenetics and pharmacogenomics. Br J Clin Pharmacol 2001;52:345–7.
3. Nebert DW. Pharmacogenetics and pharmacogenomics: why is this relevant to the clinical geneticist? Clin Genet 1999;56:247–58.
4. Vogel F. Moderne Probleme der Humangenetik. In: Heilmeyer L, Schoen R, de Rudder B, editors. Ergebnisse der Inneren Medizin und Kinderheilkunde.

Ergebnisse der Inneren Medizin und Kinderheilkunde, vol 12. Heidelberg: Springer, Berlin; 1959.

5. Landolt HP, Holst SC, Valomon A. Clinical and experimental human sleep-wake pharmacogenetics. Handb Exp Pharmacol 2018. [Epub ahead of print].

6. Sadee W, Dai Z. Pharmacogenetics/genomics and personalized medicine. Hum Mol Genet 2005;14:R207–14.

7. Roden DM, Wilke RA, Kroemer HK, et al. Pharmacogenomics the genetics of variable drug responses. Circulation 2011;123:1661–70.

8. Holst SC, Valomon A, Landolt HP. Sleep pharmacogenetics: personalized sleep-wake therapy. Annu Rev Pharmacol Toxicol 2016;56:577–603.

9. American Academy of Sleep Medicine. International classification of sleep disorders. 3rd edition. Darien (IL): American Academy of Sleep Medicine; 2014.

10. Sateia MJ, Buysse DJ, Krystal AD, et al. Clinical practice guideline for the pharmacologic treatment of chronic insomnia in adults: an American Academy of Sleep Medicine Clinical Practice Guideline. J Clin Sleep Med 2017;13(2): 307–49.

11. Krystal AD. Current, emerging, and newly available insomnia medications. J Clin Psychiatry 2015;76(8):e1045.

12. Minkel J, Krystal AD. Optimizing the pharmacologic treatment of insomnia: current status and future horizons. Sleep Med Clin 2013;8(3):333–50.

13. Richey SM, Krystal AD. Pharmacological advances in the treatment of insomnia. Curr Pharm Des 2011;17(15):1471–5.

14. Krystal AD. A compendium of placebo-controlled trials of the risks/benefits of pharmacological treatments for insomnia: the empirical basis for US clinical practice. Sleep Med Rev 2009;13(4):265–74.

15. Walsh JK. Drugs used to treat insomnia in 2002: regulatory-based rather than evidence-based medicine. Sleep 2004;27(8):14441–2.

16. Sieghart W, Sperk G. Subunit composition, distribution and function of GABA(A) receptor subtypes. Curr Top Med Chem 2002;2:795–816.

17. Sanna E, Busonero F, Talani G, et al. Comparison of the effects of zaleplon, zolpidem, and triazolam at various GABA(A) receptor subtypes. Eur J Pharmacol 2002;451(2):103–10.

18. Jia F, Goldstein PA, Harrison NL. The modulation of synaptic GABA(A) receptors in the thalamus by eszopiclone and zolpidem. J Pharmacol Exp Ther 2009; 328(3):1000–6.

19. Krystal AD, Walsh JK, Laska E, et al. Sustained efficacy of eszopiclone over six months of nightly treatment: results of a randomized, double-blind, placebo controlled study in adults with chronic insomnia. Sleep 2003;26:793–9.

20. Walsh J, Krystal AD, Amato DA. Nightly treatment of primary insomnia with eszopiclone for six months: effect on sleep, quality of life and work limitations. Sleep 2007;30(8):959–68.

21. Krystal AD, Erman M, Zammit GK, et al. Long-term efficacy and safety of zolpidem extended-release 12.5 mg, administered 3 to 7 nights per week for 24 weeks, in patients with chronic primary insomnia: a 6-month, randomized, double-blind, placebo-controlled, parallel-group, multicenter study. Sleep 2008;31(1):79–90.

22. Fava M, McCall WV, Krystal A, et al. Eszopiclone Co-administered with fluoxetine in patents with insomnia Co-existing with major depressive disorder. Biol Psychiatry 2006;59:1052–60.

23. Pollack M, Kinrys G, Krystal A, et al. Eszopiclone co-administered with escitalo-pram in patients with insomnia and comorbid generalized anxiety disorder. Arch Gen Psychiatry 2008;65(5):551–62.

24. Goforth HW, Preud'homme XA, Krystal AD. A randomized, double-blind, pla-cebo-controlled trial of eszopiclone for the treatment of insomnia in patients with chronic low back pain. Sleep 2014;37(6):1053–60.

25. Roth T, Krystal A, Steinberg FJ, et al. Novel sublingual low-dose zolpidem tablet reduces latency to sleep onset following spontaneous middle-of-the-night awak-ening in insomnia in a randomized, double-blind, placebo-controlled, outpatient study. Sleep 2013;36(2):189–96.

26. Zammit GK, Corser B, Doghramji K, et al. Sleep and residual sedation after administration of zaleplon, zolpidem, and placebo during experimental middle-of-the-night awakening. J Clin Sleep Med 2006;2(4):417–23.

27. Krystal AD, Richelson E, Roth T. Review of the histamine system and the clinical effects of H1 antagonists: basis for a new model for understanding the effects of insomnia medications. Sleep Med Rev 2013;17(4):263–72.

28. Krystal AD, Durrence HH, Scharf M, et al. Efficacy and safety of doxepin 1 mg and 3 mg in a 12-week sleep laboratory and outpatient trial of elderly subjects with chronic primary insomnia. Sleep 2010;33(11):1553–61.

29. Krystal AD, Lankford A, Durrence HH, et al. Efficacy and safety of doxepin 3 and 6 mg in a 35-day sleep laboratory trial in adults with chronic primary insomnia. Sleep 2011;34(10):1433.

30. Ivgy-May N, Ruwe F, Krystal A, et al. Esmirtazapine in non-elderly adult patients with primary insomnia: efficacy and safety from a randomized, 6-week sleep laboratory trial. Sleep Med 2015;16(7):838–44.

31. Herring WJ, Connor KM, Ivgy-May N, et al. Suvorexant in patients with insomnia: results from two 3-month randomized controlled clinical trials. Biol Psychiatry 2016;79(2):136–48.

32. Michelson D, Snyder E, Paradis E, et al. Safety and efficacy of suvorexant dur-ing 1-year treatment of insomnia with subsequent abrupt treatment discontinu-ation: a phase 3 randomised, double-blind, placebo-controlled trial. Lancet Neurol 2014;13(5):461–71.

33. Herring WJ, Connor KM, Snyder E, et al. Suvorexant in patients with insomnia: pooled analyses of three-month data from phase-3 randomized controlled clin-ical trials. J Clin Sleep Med 2016;12(9):1215–25.

34. Herring WJ, Connor KM, Snyder E, et al. Clinical profile of suvorexant for the treatment of insomnia over 3 months in women and men: subgroup analysis of pooled phase-3 data. Psychopharmacology (Berl) 2017;234(11):1703–11.

35. Herring WJ, Connor KM, Snyder E, et al. Suvorexant in elderly patients with insomnia: pooled analyses of data from phase III randomized controlled clinical trials. Am J Geriatr Psychiatry 2017;25(7):791–802.

36. Herring WJ, Roth T, Krystal AD, et al. Orexin receptor antagonists for the treat-ment of insomnia and potential treatment of other neuropsychiatric indications. J Sleep Res 2018;28:e12782.

37. Sack R, Hughes RJ, Edgar DM, et al. Sleep-promoting effects of melatonin: at what dose, in whom, under what conditions, and by what mechanisms? Sleep 1997;20(10):908–15.

38. Morin CM, Drake C, Harvey AG, et al. Insomnia disorder. Nat Rev Dis Primers 2015;1:15026.

39. Ferracioli-Oda E, Qawasmi A, Bloch MH. Meta-analysis: melatonin for the treat-ment of primary sleep disorders. PLoS One 2013;8:e63773.

40. Buscemi N, Vandermeer B, Hooton N, et al. The efficacy and safety of exoge-nous melatonin for primary sleep disorders. A meta-analysis. J Gen Intern Med 2005;20(12):1151–8.
41. Mendelson WB. Efficacy of melatonin as a hypnotic agent. J Biol Rhythms 1997; 12(6):651–6.
42. Zhdanova I, Wurtman RJ, Wagstaff J. Effects of a low dose of melatonin on sleep in children with Angelman syndrome. J Pediatr Endocrinol 1999;12(1):57–67.
43. Van der Heijden K, Smits MG, Van Someren EJ, et al. Effect of melatonin on sleep, behavior, and cognition in ADHD and chronic sleep-onset insomnia. J Am Acad Child Adolesc Psychiatry 2007;46(2):233–41.
44. Wasdell M, Jan JE, Bomben MM, et al. A randomized, placebo-controlled trial of controlled release melatonin treatment of delayed sleep phase syndrome and impaired sleep maintenance in children with neurodevelopmental disabilities. J Pineal Res 2008;44(1):57–64.
45. Braam W, Didden R, Smits M, et al. Melatonin treatment in individuals with intel-lectual disability and chronic insomnia: a randomized placebo-controlled study. J Intellect Disabil Res 2008;52(3):256–64.
46. Mayer G, Wang-Weigand S, Roth-Schechter B, et al. Efficacy and safety of 6-month nightly ramelteon administration in adults with chronic primary insomnia. Sleep 2009;32(3):351.
47. Riemann D, Voderholzer U, Cohrs S, et al. Trimipramine in primary insomnia: re-sults of a polysomnographic double-blind controlled study. Pharmacopsychiatry 2002;35(5):165–74.
48. Hohagen F, Montero RF, Weiss E. Treatment of primary insomnia with trimipr-amine: an alternative to benzodiazepine hypnotics? Eur Arch Psychiatry Clin Neurosci 1994;244(2):65–72.
49. Rodenbeck A, Cohrs S, Jordan W, et al. The sleep-improving effects of doxepin are paralleled by a normalized plasma cortisol secretion in primary insomnia. Psychopharmacology (Berl) 2003;170:423–8.
50. Hajak G, Rodenbeck A, Adler L, et al. Nocturnal melatonin secretion and sleep after doxepin administration in chronic primary insomnia. Pharmacopsychiatry 1996;29(5):187–92.
51. Hajak G, Rodenbeck A, Voderholzer U, et al. Doxepin in the treatment of primary insomnia: a placebo-controlled, double-blind, polysomnographic study. J Clin Psychiatry 2001;62(6):453–63.
52. Szabo ST, Thorpy MJ, Mayer G, et al. Neurobiological and immunogenetic as-pects of narcolepsy: implications for pharmacotherapy. Sleep Med Rev 2018; 43:23–36.
53. Morgenthaler TI, Lee-Chiong T, Alessi C, et al. Standards of Practice Committee of the American Academy of Sleep Medicine. Practice parameters for the clin-ical evaluation and treatment of circadian rhythm sleep disorders. An American Academy of Sleep Medicine report. Sleep 2007;30(11):1445–59.
54. Proserpio P, Terzaghi M, Manni R, et al. Drugs used in parasomnia. Sleep Med Clin 2018;13(2):191–202.
55. Iranzo A. Parasomnias and sleep-related movement disorders in Older adults. Sleep Med Clin 2018;13(1):51–61.
56. Aurora RN, Kristo DA, Bista SR, et al, American Academy of Sleep Medicine. The treatment of restless legs syndrome and periodic limb movement disorder in adults–an update for 2012: practice parameters with an evidence-based sys-tematic review and meta-analyses: an American Academy of Sleep Medicine Clinical Practice Guideline. Sleep 2012;35(8):1039–62.

57. Tobler I, Kopp C, Deboer T, et al. Diazepam-induced changes in sleep: role of the α1 GABAA receptor subtype. Proc Natl Acad Sci U S A 2001;98(11):6464–9.

58. Kopp C, Rudolph U, Low K, et al. Modulation of rhythmic brain activity by diazepam: GABAA receptor subtype and state specificity. Proc Natl Acad Sci U S A 2004;101(10):3674–9.

59. Cope DW, Wulff P, Oberto A, et al. Abolition of zolpidem sensitivity in mice with a point mutation in the GABAA receptor γ2 subunit. Neuropharmacology 2004; 47(1):17–34.

60. Huang MC, Lin HY, Chen CH. Dependence on zolpidem. Psychiatry Clin Neurosci 2007;61:207–8.

61. Cubala WJ, Landowski J. Seizure following sudden zolpidem withdrawal. Prog Neuropsychopharmacol Biol Psychiatry 2007;31:539–40.

62. Hajak G, Müller WE, Wittchen HU, et al. Abuse and dependence potential for the non-benzodiazepine hypnotics zolpidem and zopiclone: a review of case reports and epidemiological data. Addiction 2003;98:1371–8.

63. Verster JC, van de Loo AJ, Moline ML, et al. Middle-of-the-night administration of sleep medication: a critical review of the effects of next morning ability. Curr Drug Saf 2014;9:205–11.

64. Greenblatt DJ, Harmatz JS, Singh NN, et al. Gender differences in pharmacokinetics and pharmacodynamics of zolpidem following sublingual administration. J Clin Pharmacol 2014;54:282–90.

65. Greenblatt DJ, Harmatz JS, von Moltke LL, et al. Comparative kinetics and response to the benzodiazepine agonists triazolam and zolpidem: evaluation of sex-dependent differences. J Pharmacol Exp Ther 2000;293:435–43.

66. Farkas RH, Unger EF, Temple R. Zolpidem and driving impairment–identifying persons at risk. N Engl J Med 2013;369(8):689–91.

67. Greenblatt DJ, Harmatz JS, Roth T, et al. Comparison of pharmacokinetic profiles of zolpidem buffered sublingual tablet and zolpidem oral immediate-release tablet: results from a single-center, single-dose, randomized, open-label crossover study in healthy adults. Clin Ther 2013;35:604–11.

68. Olubodun JO, Ochs HR, von Moltke LL, et al. Pharmacokinetic properties of zolpidem in elderly and young adults: possible modulation by testosterone in men. Br J Clin Pharmacol 2003;56:297–304.

69. Pichard L, Gillet G, Bonfils C, et al. Oxidative metabolism of zolpidem by human liver cytochrome P450S. Drug Metab Dispos 1995;23:1253–62.

70. Gillet G. In vitro and in vivo metabolism of zolpidem in three animal species and in man, in Proceedings of the Third International ISSX Meeting Amsterdam.1991.

71. Wolbold R, Klein K, Burk O, et al. Sex is a major determinant of CYP3A4 expression in human liver. Hepatology 2003;38:978–88.

72. Peer CJ, Strope JD, Beedie S, et al. Alcohol and aldehyde dehydrogenases contribute to sex-related differences in clearance of zolpidem in rats. Front Pharmacol 2016;7:260.

73. Aasmoe L, Aarbakke J. Sex-dependent induction of alcohol dehydrogenase activity in rats. Biochem Pharmacol 1999;57:1067–72.

74. Parlesak A, Billinger MH, Bode C, et al. Gastric alcohol dehydrogenase activity in man: influence of gender, age, alcohol consumption and smoking in a caucasian population. Alcohol 2002;37:388–93.

75. Olivera M, Martınez C, Gervasini G, et al. Effect of common NAT2 variant alleles in the acetylation of the major clonazepam metabolite, 7-aminoclonazepam. Drug Metab Lett 2007;1(1):3–5.

76. Siller N, Egerer G, Weiss J, et al. Prolonged sedation of lorazepam due to absent UGT2B4/2B7 glucuronidation. Arch Toxicol 2014;88(1):179–80.
77. Akutsu T, Kobayashi K, Sakurada K, et al. Identification of human cytochrome p450 isozymes involved in diphenhydramine N-demethylation. Drug Metab Dispos 2007;35(1):72–8.
78. de Leon J, Nikoloff DM. Paradoxical excitation on diphenhydramine may be associated with being a CYP2D6 ultrarapid metabolizer: three case reports. CNS Spectr 2008;13(2):133–5.
79. Saruwatari J, Matsunaga M, Ikeda K, et al. Impact of CYP2D6*10 on H1-antihistamine-induced hypersomnia. Eur J Clin Pharmacol 2006;62(12): 995–1001.
80. Kirchheiner J, Meineke I, Müller G, et al. Contributions of CYP2D6, CYP2C9 and CYP2C19 to the biotransformation of E- and Z-doxepin in healthy volunteers. Pharmacogenetics 2002;12(7):571–80.
81. Mihara K, Kondo T, Suzuki A, et al. Effects of genetic polymorphism of CYP1A2 inductibility on the steady-state plasma concentrations of trazodone and its active metabolite m-chlorophenylpiperazine in depressed Japanese patients. Pharmacol Toxicol 2001;88(5):267–70.
82. Mihara K, Yasui-Furukori N, Kondo T, et al. Relationship between plasma concentrations of trazodone and its active metabolite, m-chlorophenylpiperazine, and its clinical effect in depressed patients. Ther Drug Monit 2002;24(4):563–6.
83. Feuchtl A, Bagli M, Stephan R, et al. Pharmacokinetics of m-chlorophenylpiperazine after intravenous and oral administration in healthy male volunteers: implication for the pharmacodynamic profile. Pharmacopsychiatry 2004;37(4):180–8.
84. Greenblatt DJ, Friedman H, Burstein ES, et al. Trazodone kinetics: effect of age, gender, and obesity. Clin Pharmacol Ther 1987;42(2):193–200.
85. Ishida M, Otani K, Kaneko S, et al. Effects of various factors on steady state plasma concentrations of trazodone and its active metabolite m-chlorophenylpiperazine. Int Clin Psychopharmacol 1995;10(3):143–6.
86. Rotzinger S, Fang J, Coutts RT, et al. Human CYP2D6 and metabolism of m-Chlorophenylpiperazine. Biol Psychiatry 1998;44:1185–91.
87. Zalma A, von Moltke LL, Granda BW, et al. In vitro metabolism of trazodone by CYP3A: inhibition by ketoconazole and human immunodeficiency viral protease inhibitors. Biol Psychiatry 2000;47(7):655–61.
88. Staack RF, Maurer HH. Piperazine-derived designer drug 1-3-chlorophenyl) piperazine (mCPP): GC-MS studies on its metabolism and its toxicological detection in rat urine including analytical differentiation from its precursor drugs trazodone and nefazodone. J Anal Toxicol 2003;27:561–8.
89. Tancer ME, Johanson C-E. The subjective effects of MDMA and mCPP amongst moderate MDMA users. Drug Alcohol Depend 2001;65:97–101.
90. Bertilsson L, Dahl ML, Dalén P, et al. Molecular genetics of CYP2D6: clinical relevance with focus on psychotropic drugs. Br J Clin Pharmacol 2002;53(2): 111–22.
91. Thompson MD, Xhaard H, Sakurai T, et al. OX1 and OX2 orexin/hypocretin receptor pharmacogenetics. Front Neurosci 2014;8:57.
92. van Dyck CH, Malison RT, Jacobsen LK, et al. Increased dopamine transporter availability associated with the 9-repeat allele of the SLC6A3 gene. J Nucl Med 2005;46(5):745–51.
93. Ujike H, Harano M, Inada T, et al. Nine- or fewer repeat alleles in VNTR polymorphism of the dopamine transporter gene is a strong risk factor for prolonged methamphetamine psychosis. Pharmacogenomics J 2003;3(4):242–7.

94. Kasparbauer AM, Rujescu D, Riedel M, et al. Methylphenidate effects on brain activity as a function of SLC6A3 genotype and striatal dopamine transporter availability. Neuropsychopharmacology 2015;40(3):736–45.

95. Schacht JP. COMT val158met moderation of dopaminergic drug effects on cognitive function: a critical review. Pharmacogenomics J 2016;16(5):430–8.

96. Bodenmann S, Xu S, Luhmann UF, et al. Pharmacogenetics of modafinil after sleep loss: catechol-O-methyltransferase genotype modulates waking functions but not recovery sleep. Clin Pharmacol Ther 2009;85(3):296–304.

97. Hamidovic A, Dlugos A, Palmer AA, et al. Catechol-O-methyltransferase val158-met genotype modulates sustained attention in both the drug-free state and in response to amphetamine. Psychiatr Genet 2010;20(3):85–92.

98. Dauvilliers Y, Neidhart E, Tafti M. Sexual dimorphism of the catechol-O-methyltransferase gene in narcolepsy is associated with response to modafinil. Pharmacogenomics J 2002;2(1):65–8.

99. Hartter S, Korhonen T, Lundgren S, et al. Effect of caffeine intake 12 or 24 hours prior to melatonin intake and CYP1A2*1F polymorphism on CYP1A2 phenotyping by melatonin. Basic Clin Pharmacol Toxicol 2006;99(4):300–4.

100. Braam W, Keijzer H, Struijker Boudier H, et al. CYP1A2 polymorphisms in slow melatonin metabolisers: a possible relationship with autism spectrum disorder? J Intellect Disabil Res 2013;57(11):993–1000.

101. Bialecka M, Kurzawski M, Klodowska-Duda G, et al. The association of functional catechol-O-methyltransferase haplotypes with risk of Parkinson's disease, levodopa treatment response, and complications. Pharmacogenet Genomics 2008;18(9):815–21.

102. Kaplan N, Vituri A, Korczyn AD, et al. Sequence variants in SLC6A3, DRD2, and BDNF genes and time to levodopa-induced dyskinesias in Parkinson's disease. J Mol Neurosci 2014;53(2):183–8.

103. Sampaio TF, Dos Santos EUD, de Lima GDC, et al. MAO-B and COMT genetic variations associated with levodopa treatment response in patients with Parkinson's disease. J Clin Pharmacol 2018;58(7):920–6.

104. Cheshire P, Bertram K, Ling H, et al. Influence of single nucleotide polymorphisms in COMT, MAO-A and BDNF genes on dyskinesias and levodopa use in Parkinson's disease. Neurodegener Dis 2014;13(1):24–8.

105. Kaye CM, Nicholls B. Clinical pharmacokinetics of ropinirole. Clin Pharmacokinet 2000;39(4):243–54.

106. Agundez JAG, García-Martín E, Alonso-Navarro H, et al. Anti-Parkinson's disease drugs and pharmacogenetic considerations. Expert Opin Drug Metab Toxicol 2013;9(7):859–74.

107. Becker ML, Visser LE, van Schaik RH, et al. OCT1 polymorphism is associated with response and survival time in anti-Parkinsonian drug users. Neurogenetics 2011;12(1):79–82.

108. Liu Y-Z, Tang B-S, Yan X-X, et al. Association of the DRD2 and DRD3 polymorphisms with response to pramipexole in Parkinson's disease patients. Eur J Clin Pharmacol 2009;65(7):679–83.

109. Xu S, Liu J, Yang X, et al. Association of the DRD2 CAn-STR and DRD3 Ser9Gly polymorphisms with Parkinson's disease and response to dopamine agonists. J Neurol Sci 2017;372:433–8.

Genomics Testing and Personalized Medicine in the Preoperative Setting

Rodney A. Gabriel, MD, MAS[a,b,]*, Brittany N. Burton, MHS[c],
Richard D. Urman, MD, MBA[d], Ruth S. Waterman, MD, MSc[e]

KEYWORDS

- Pharmacogenomics • Preoperative • Genetics • Outcomes • Opioids

KEY POINTS

- The application of pharmacogenomics principles in perioperative medicine is fairly novel and only a limited number of studies have shown its potential benefit in this clinical setting.
- Many enzymes are involved with the metabolism of various analgesic medications, leading to genetic variability, and consequently play a role in drug toxicity and efficacy. It seems logical that having pharmacogenomics information on patients before surgery would be a valuable tool to anesthesiologists because it would allow tailored and effective analgesic use in each patient.
- Challenges in executing pharmacogenomics programs into health care systems include physician buy-in and integration into usual clinical workflow, including the electronic health record.
- The preoperative testing clinic, a facility usually run by anesthesiologists and designed to screen patients for appropriateness of surgery, is an ideal location to perform pharmacogenomics screening.

INTRODUCTION

Pharmacogenomics (PGx) is the study of how individuals' personal genotypes may affect their responses (phenotype) to various pharmacologic agents. The application

This article originally appeared in *Anesthesiology Clinics*, Volume 36, Issue 4, December 2018.
Disclosure: R.A. Gabriel, R.S. Waterman, and R.D. Urman use CQuentia (Fort Worth, TX) for pharmacogenomics screening at their respective institutions.
[a] Division of Regional Anesthesia and Acute Pain, Department of Anesthesiology, University of California, San Diego, 200 W Arbor Dr, San Diego, CA 92103, USA; [b] Department of Medicine, Division of Biomedical Informatics, University of California, San Diego, 9500 Gilman Dr, La Jolla, CA 92093, USA; [c] School of Medicine, University of California, San Diego, 9500 Gilman Dr, La Jolla, CA 92093, USA; [d] Department of Anesthesiology, Perioperative and Pain Medicine, Harvard Medical School, Brigham and Women's Hospital, 75 Francis St, Boston, MA 02115, USA; [e] Department of Anesthesiology, University of California, San Diego, 200 W Arbor Dr, San Diego, CA 92103, USA
* Corresponding author. Department of Anesthesiology, University of California, San Diego, 9500 Gilman Drive, MC 0881, La Jolla, CA 92093-0881.
E-mail address: ragabriel@ucsd.edu

of PGx principles in perioperative medicine is fairly novel and only a limited number of studies have shown its potential benefit in this clinical setting.[1–3] During a patient's perioperative experience, anesthesiology providers are tasked with the management of multimodal pharmacotherapy; these involve medications that are used to manage pain, prevent nausea and vomiting, induce and maintain anesthesia, provide muscle relaxation, and manage hemodynamics. Although the mechanisms of action of the many medications anesthesiologists use are to some degree understood, the precise effect a given dose will have on an individual may not be known until it is given. These inherent variations in response to medications are partly caused by PGx, a profile that is unique to each individual. Thus, in theory, having this personalized information for every patient planned to undergo surgery may aid in fine-tuning precision medicine when it comes to optimizing perioperative care.

Enhanced recovery after surgery (ERAS) pathways and perioperative surgical home (PSH) models are being widely adopted in an effort to protocolize evidence-based medicine systematically.[4] The goal is therefore to improve outcomes. Integration of PGx into such pathways may provide a huge step in optimizing care even further by having available additional information on patient-specific response to medications. Enhanced recovery pathways involve integral steps at all stages in a patient's perioperative journey, including:

1. Preadmission (ie, surgery clinic and preoperative care clinic)
2. Preoperative (ie, day of surgery before operation)
3. Intraoperative
4. Immediate postoperative (ie, recovery, physical therapy, nutrition, pain management)
5. Long-term postoperative phase (**Fig. 1**)

There are a variety of pharmacologic agents that are used at each stage of this perioperative process. Integration of PGx early in this process (ie, preadmission) may help providers practice precision medicine at all subsequent stages.

This article discusses the current evidence highlighting the potential of PGx with various drug categories used in the perioperative process and the challenges of integrating PGx into a health care system and relevant workflows.

PHARMACOGENOMICS AND PERIOPERATIVE MEDICATIONS

It is important to discuss the current evidence of PGx as it applies to various drug classes relevant to surgical patients; these include opioids, nonopioids, antiemetics, anticoagulants, and β-blockers. Much of anesthesiologists' clinical practice involves the titration of various drugs individualized to each patient.[2,3] Many enzymes are involved with the metabolism of various analgesic medications, leading to genetic variability, and consequently playing a role in drug toxicity and efficacy. It seems logical that having PGx information on patients before surgery would be a valuable tool to anesthesiologists because it would allow tailored and effective analgesic use in each patient. More studies are still needed to assess the effects of personalized dosing of anesthetics and analgesics during the perioperative process for various major surgeries.

Opioids

An individual's metabolism of opioids is largely determined by variations of cytochrome P (CYP) enzymes, including CYP2D6[5] and CYP3A4.[6,7] Studies have shown variations in metabolism based on CYP2D6 for codeine,[8,9] tramadol,[10] and

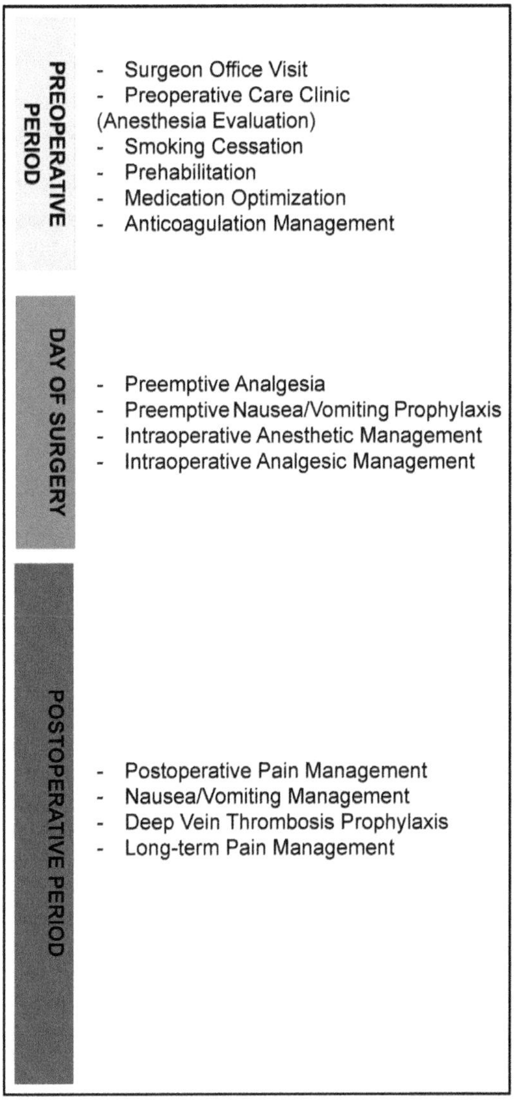

Fig. 1. Work flow of the perioperative process and how pharmacogenomics may be applied at each stage: preoperative, day of surgery, and postoperative phases.

hydrocodone.[11] Morphine metabolism has been shown to be affected by canalicular multispecific organic anion transporter 2 (ABCC3),[12] organic cation transporter,[12] CYP2D6,[5] and P-glycoprotein transporter (encoded by ABCB1).[13] Adverse events related to morphine may also be affected by mu-receptor genotype (OPRM1).[14] Fentanyl metabolism can be affected by the CYP3A4 enzyme.[6,7] Furthermore, postoperative requirements for fentanyl have been associated with genotypes for catechol-O-methyltransferase (COMT) enzymes.[15] Tramadol metabolism may be affected by variations in CYP3A4, CYP2B6, CYP2D6, and various other transporter and receptor genes.[10] Hydromorphone metabolism is related to several types of

CYP genes.[16] In addition, methadone has been associated with several genes, including ABCB1, CYP2B6, CYP3A4, OPRM1, and UGT1A.[8,17–20]

Nonopioid Analgesics

The World Health Organization developed the so-called pain ladder to guide treatment of mild to moderate acute pain, advocating for the administration of nonopioid analgesics as the first step.[21] Nonopioid analgesics comprise a diverse class of medications that have antiinflammatory properties. For example, animal studies have shown that metabolism of acetaminophen is mediated by CYP2E1 oxidation.[22] Acetaminophen overdose represents more than 50% of drug-related acute liver failure, and studies have identified polymorphisms associated with hepatotoxicity.[23] In their investigation of 15 adults with thalassemia/hemoglobin E, Tankanitlert and colleagues[24] showed that the UGT1A6*2/UGT1A1*28 haplotype was associated with increased paracetamol concentrations. Another study found decreased acetaminophen glucuronide concentrations in urine samples in patients expressing the UGT2B15*2 variant.[25] Acetaminophen glucuronidation partial clearance and increased plasma concentration of acetaminophen plasma protein complexes are largely determined by UGT2B15*2 polymorphism.[26] Moreover, sulfotransferase (SULT) enzymes are involved in the sulfate conjugation of acetaminophen. A systematic meta-analysis identified SULT1A1, SULT1A2, and SULT1A3 as determinants of sulfation of acetaminophen.[27] Several studies have shown that UGT1A6 and UGT1A9 are the primary human allele variants mediating acetaminophen glucuronidation. Compared with the UGT1A6*1 allele variant, UGT1A6*2 had 60% higher acetaminophen glucuronidation activity.[28] However, for select human populations, a reduction in glucuronidation activity is observed with the UGTA1*28 isoform.[28] Ibuprofen is primarily metabolized by cytochrome enzymes and excreted into the urine. CYP2C9 plays a major role in ibuprofen clearance. Studies have shown that concomitant administration of ibuprofen and CYP2C9 inhibitors leads to drug-drug interactions and toxic effects. CY2C8 and CYP3A4 are also involved in ibuprofen clearance. Although the contribution of UDP-glucuronosyltransferases (UGTs) in vivo remains unclear, in vitro studies show that UGT1A3, UGT1A9, UGT2B7, and UGT2B17 glucuronidate ibuprofen to ibuprofen-acyl glucuronide.[29] Most studies have suggested a decrease in ibuprofen clearance with CYP2C9*3 polymorphism compared with individuals with the CYP2C9*1/*1 genotype.[29] Naproxen metabolism is mediated by UGT2B7 and CYP2C9 and interindividual genetic variations that lead to decreased metabolism of naproxen have been linked to higher risk of acute gastrointestinal hemorrhage.[30–32] Celecoxib is primarily metabolized by CYP2C9 and CYP3A4.[33,34] Prieto-Pérez and colleagues[33] investigated the association of CYP polymorphisms and pharmacokinetics and they found that individuals with CYP2C9*1/*3 and CYP2C9*3/*3 had lower celecoxib clearance compared with individuals with CYP2C9*1/*1. Chan and colleagues[35] evaluated cytochrome polymorphisms on colorectal adenoma recurrence in 1660 adult patients with colorectal cancer receiving celecoxib and found that patients who expressed CYP2C9*3 genotypes and received high-dose celecoxib had a lower risk of recurrence; however, this association was not found for patients with CYP2C9*2.

Benzodiazepines

It is well established that benzodiazepines primarily act on the central nervous system and are clinically used as sedative-anxiolytics and antiepileptics. In nerve cells, benzodiazepines facilitate ionotropic γ-aminobutyric acid (GABA) action by increasing the frequency of chloride channel opening. Metabolism of benzodiazepines is determined largely by oxidative metabolizing cytochrome enzymes, such as CYP3A4 and CYP3A5, which are expressed primarily in the liver and intestine.[36] One study showed that CYP3A activity reflected clearance of urinary ratios of endogenous steroids, which was positively correlated with midazolam clearance.[36] Several studies have shown interindividual variability in CYP3A expression and activity, which influences the adverse effect profile.[37] It has been shown that midazolam is largely metabolized by CY3A4 and CYP3B to its active metabolite, 1'-hydroxymidazolam.[38] Miao and colleagues[37] found that CYP3A5*3, the most prevalent variant, was expressed in 85% to 95% of white people, 27% to 50% of African Americans, and 60% to 73% in Asian people. Further studies have shown that CYP3A4 290 A>G and CYP3Ab 22893 A>G allelic variants lead to reduced drug clearance.[39] In European and African American adults, CYP3A*5 was associated with 50% increase in enzyme induction.[39] The average population clearance of midazolam was shown to be 22% lower in patients with cancer expressing CYP3A5*3.[40] Increased midazolam concentrations and decreased metabolite ratios were observed in patients with cancer expressing CYP3A4*22, which is associated with decreased CYP3A4 activity.[41] Studies have shown that UGT1A4, UGT2B4, and UGT2B7 isoforms are primarily involved in glucuronide conjugation of midazolam metabolites.[42] After midazolam undergoes oxidative phosphorylation to its metabolite (ie, hydroxymidazolam) by CYP3A4, glucuronidated metabolites are produced by UDP-glucuronosyltransferases (UGTs) and ultimately excreted into the urine.[42] Studies have shown that variation in the response to lorazepam is determined largely by UGT2B15. In in vitro studies, ketoconazole was associated with inhibition of UGT2B7 glucuronidation of lorazepam.[43] The UGT1A1*28 variant has been shown to be associated with reduced elimination and consequently increased toxicity of lorazepam.[44]

Antiemetics

Ondansetron is a 5-hydroxytryptamine (5-HT3) serotonin antagonist and is used to prevent postoperative and chemotherapy-induced nausea and vomiting. Ondansetron has been shown to be metabolized by CYP3A4, CYP2D6, and CYP1A2.[45] The most common CYP2D6 variants of ondansetron metabolism may be divided into groups such as normal function (ie, CYP2D6*1 and *2), decreased function (ie, CYP2D6*9, *10, and *41), and no function (eg, CYP2D6*3–*6).[46] Individuals who express CYP2D6*2 are ultrametabolizers who experience treatment failure and therefore have increased risk of nausea and vomiting.[47] ATP-binding cassette (ABC) proteins are important in transport of ondansetron across cellular membranes. He and colleagues[48] evaluated 215 patients with acute myeloid leukemia with clinical resistance to ondansetron and found that the ABC subfamily B member 1 (ABCB1) transporter C3435T polymorphisms were associated with grade 3/4 vomiting. Moreover, ondansetron metabolism has been shown to be associated with hepatic organic cation transporter 1 (OCT1).[49] Although metoclopramide is partially metabolized by cytochromes, CYP2D6 is the primary determinant of metoclopramide metabolism. Parkman and colleagues[50] investigated the metoclopramide adverse effect profile in 100 adult patients with gastroparesis and found that patients with polymorphisms in CYP2D6 (ie, rs1080985, rs16947, rs3892097) and potassium voltage-gated channel subfamily H member 2 (KCNH2; ie, rs3815459) were more likely to experience side effects, however KCNH2 (ie, rs1805123) and ADRA1D (ie, rs2236554) polymorphisms were associated with a favorable clinical response. Although the exact antiemetic mechanism of action of dexamethasone is unclear, studies show that dexamethasone is involved in reduction in prostaglandin synthesis in the nervous system.[51] Expression of CYP2D6*3/*4/*5/*6 results in poor metabolism of haloperidol. As such, these individuals are at risk of increased risk for QT prolongation and arrhythmias.[47] In their evaluation of novel loci associated with the response to antipsychotic medication, Yu and colleagues[52] found several polymorphisms associated with an increased risk of psychotic disorders and response to antipsychotic medications. CYP2D6 has been shown to be associated with metabolism of promethazine.[53] Moreover, CYP2D6 polymorphisms have been shown to be associated with H1 antihistamine–induced sedation.[54]

Anticoagulants

Anticoagulation is prescribed for a wide range of conditions, including, but not limited to, atrial fibrillation, acute coronary syndrome, pulmonary embolism, deep venous thrombosis, and cerebrovascular accident. It is well established that warfarin, which is most widely used in the prevention of venous thromboembolism and cerebrovascular accident in patients with atrial fibrillation, is metabolized by CYP2C9 and vitamin K epoxide reductase complex (VKORC1).[55] Studies have shown that CYP 2C9*2, CYP 2C9*3, and VKORC1 A haplotype warfarin polymorphisms are associated with slower metabolism.[55] The antiplatelet activity of clopidogrel has been shown to reduce the risk of vascular disease.[56] Roughly 25% of individuals treated with clopidogrel experience treatment failure, and studies have shown that CYP2C9 and CYP2C19 are involved in the metabolism of clopidogrel.[56] Polymorphism in ATP-Binding Cassette Subfamily B Member 1 (ABCB1), Paraoxonase-1 (PON1), Carboxyl Esterase 1 (CES1), and P2Y12 receptors are associated with clopidogrel metabolism.[56]

β-Blockers

Metoprolol is a β_1-adrenoreceptor antagonist and is often prescribed to manage myocardial infarction, supraventricular tachycardia, hypertension, and heart failure. Blocking adrenergic receptors reduces heart rate and contractility. Although there are more than 100 identified polymorphisms of CYP2D6, studies have shown that CYP2D6 is responsible for 70% to 80% of metoprolol metabolism. The wide genetic variation in CYP2D6 for metoprolol and carvedilol has been shown to lead to variation in clinical response. Individuals may be classified as poor, intermediate, extensive, and ultrarapid metoprolol or carvedilol metabolizers.[57,58] Studies have shown that CYP2D6 nonexpressors have roughly a 5-fold increase in plasma concentrations of metoprolol and consequently decreased cardioselectivity and increased risk of adverse effects.[59,60] As such, ultrarapid metabolizers are at risk of treatment failure, whereas poor metabolizers may experience toxic adverse effects. Gao and colleagues[59] evaluated 319 patients who received metoprolol succinate for heart rate control following percutaneous coronary intervention and found that CYP2D6*10 polymorphisms were associated with a lower heart rate. As such, metoprolol guidelines have been published to recommend dosing adjustments and requirements based on CYP2D6 polymorphisms.[47] Carvedilol is also commonly prescribed to treat hypertension and heart failure.[58] Luzum and colleagues[57] assessed the relationship of CYP2D6 polymorphisms and maintenance does of metoprolol and carvedilol. Patients with CY2D6*4 had lower and higher maintenance dose requirements for metoprolol and carvedilol, respectively.

Local Anesthetics

Common local anesthetics used in the perioperative period include lidocaine, bupivacaine, ropivacaine, and mepivacaine. Their primary site of action is neuronal sodium channels. Few studies have shown any clinical correlation between genomics and response to local anesthetics. Lidocaine and bupivacaine are metabolized by

CYP3A4, whereas ropivacaine is metabolized by CYP1A2.[38] Furthermore, patients with MC1R variants have decreased response to lidocaine.[61]

Malignant Hyperthermia

Malignant hyperthermia (MH) is a rare and potentially life-threatening autosomal dominant inherited condition associated with inhaled anesthetics or succinylcholine. Roughly 50% of MH cases are associated with ryanodine receptors (RYRs) or calcium voltage-gated channels (CACNA1S).[62] RYR and CACNA1S polymorphisms have been identified in families with multiple cases of MH.[63] Genetics variations in RYR1 account for roughly 80% of all cases of MH, whereas polymorphisms of CACNA1S have been shown to account for less than 1% of MH cases.[64] Preoperative PGx information for RYRs would be useful in determining which patients should not receive succinylcholine or volatile anesthetics.

INTEGRATION INTO PERIOPERATIVE WORKFLOW

Although PGx is not new, its widespread implementation into perioperative care is still at its infancy. Challenges in executing such programs include physician buy-in and integration into usual clinical workflow, including the electronic health record (EHR).[1] To facilitate physician buy-in would require more published data reporting both the prevalence of genetic risk to various perioperative medications and definitive outcomes associated with tailoring medications based on PGx. Integration into clinical work flow is also key and would require a collaboration between health care providers and the informatics department to create useful and user-friendly interfaces and alerts that may lead to improved execution of PGx. In order to obtain more universal adoption of perioperative PGx, there needs to be:

1. More high-quality evidence that surgical outcomes improve with PGx
2. Easy-to-access and user-friendly interfaces integrated into electronic medical record systems
3. Protocols put into place that allow PGx to easily fit into regular clinical workflow

More High-Quality Evidence that Surgical Outcomes Improve with Pharmacogenomics

Integration of PGx-guided therapy for surgical patients has potential to improve outcomes; however, more large-scale definitive studies are required. To date, there have been some small-scale cohort studies reporting its impact.[2,3] In one cross-sectional study, approximately 150 patients with postoperative trauma were analyzed and genetic associations of OPRM1 and COMT and postoperative pain/opioid consumption were made. The investigators concluded that OPRM1 and COMT may contribute to the variability of opioid consumption.[65] Other studies have shown that there is no genetic association of various genes with fentanyl consumption in gynecologic patients[66] and obstetric patients.[67] Several studies, as described earlier, have shown associations between different genes and postoperative opioid use.[65–77] However, studies are now needed that focus on PGx interventions and postoperative outcomes. Senagore and colleagues[68] conducted a study whose methodology involved comparing results with historical controls in patients undergoing colorectal resections or ventral hernia repair and showed improvement in opioid consumption. The investigators produced a guided analgesic protocol based on the assessment of 6 CYP, COMT, OPRM1, and ABCB1 genes. Depending on the patients' genotypes,

A

Genetic Summary

Gene	Result	Activity
CYP2C19	*1/*17	Rapid metabolizer
CYP2C9	*1/*3	Intermediate metabolizer
CYP2D6	*1/*2	Extensive metabolizer
CYP3A4	*1/*1	Extensive metabolizer
CYP3A5	*3/*3	Poor metabolizer
DPYD	*1/*1	Extensive metabolizer
TPMT	*1/*1	Extensive metabolizer
Factor V Leiden (F5)	Normal	See Thrombosis Profile (Pg. 4)
Prothrombin (F2)	Normal	See Thrombosis Profile (Pg. 4)
MTHFR (A1298C)	Heterozygous	See Thrombosis Profile (Pg. 4)
MTHFR (C677T)	Heterozygous	See Thrombosis Profile (Pg. 4)

B

Thrombosis Profile

Tested Genes (Alleles)	Genotype	Predicted Phenotype	Clinical Guidance
Prothrombin (F2)	Normal	Normal risk expected based on the patient's genotype.	The absence of these variant alleles of Prothrombin (Factor 2) and Factor V Leiden suggests that the patient does not have the elevated risk of thrombosis associated with these genetic markers.
Factor V Leiden	Normal		
MTHFR (A1298C)	Heterozygous		
MTHFR (C677T)	Heterozygous		

C

Drug	Finding	Recommendation	Evidence
NSAIDs			
Celecoxib	⚠ Intermediate metabolizer CYP2C9 *1/*3	Patients with this CYP2C9 metabolism status who are treated with celecoxib may have an increased risk of gastrointestinal bleeding as compared to patients with the wild-type (*1/*1) genotype.	◓
	AGT rs699 A/A (WT)	Patients with this genotype may have increased likelihood of acute coronary syndrome when exposed to NSAIDs compared to patients with the homozygous genotype.	○
Diclofenac	⚠ Intermediate metabolizer CYP2C9 *1/*3	Patients with this CYP2C9 metabolism status who are treated with diclofenac may have an increased risk of gastrointestinal bleeding as compared to patients with the wild-type (*1/*1) genotype.	◓
	AGT rs699 A/A (WT)	Patients with this genotype may have increased likelihood of acute coronary syndrome when exposed to NSAIDs compared to patients with the homozygous genotype.	○
Opioids			
Codeine	✓ Extensive metabolizer CYP2D6 *1/*2	The genotype predicts that the patient is an Extensive Metabolizer for Codeine. Consider label recommended dosage of Codeine if no contraindication.	●
Hydrocodone	✓ Extensive metabolizer CYP2D6 *1/*2	The genotype predicts that the patient is an Extensive Metabolizer for Hydrocodone. Consider label recommended dosage of Hydrocodone if no contraindication.	●
Methadone	✓ CYP2B6 rs3745274 G/T (HET)	Consider label recommended dosage of Methadone if no contraindication.	◓
Oxycodone	✓ Extensive metabolizer CYP2D6 *1/*2	Consider label recommended dosage of Oxycodone if no contraindication.	◓

Fig. 2. Example screenshots of a pharmacogenomics tool integrated into the EHR. (*A*) A patients' metabolism status to various genes. (*B*) A patient's thrombosis profile based on pharmacogenomics. (*C*) A patient's response to various analgesics based on pharmacogenomics. (*Courtesy of* CQuentia, Fort Worth, TX.)

analgesics were dose adjusted or avoided as appropriate. Large-scale prospective randomized controlled trials are needed to prove its efficacy.

Easy-to-Access and Easy-to-Understand Interfaces Integrated into Electronic Medical Record Systems

Because there are several genes that have already been implicated in perioperative medication metabolism, a complete list of genetic interactions with pharmacologic agents may prove to be too long and complex for the average health care provider to review. Therefore, the interface presenting this information should be strategically designed. Specifically, integrating known PGx polymorphisms into ERAS protocols could prove to be the most useful for the health care provider.

Protocols Put into Place that Allow Pharmacogenomics to Easily Fit into Regular Clinical Workflow

The perioperative work flow needs to be an efficient process while maintaining patient safety. PGx screening results should be transferred directly into EHR systems and should contain some of these components: (1) customized report generation depending on provider and institution preferences; (2) data tracking and analytics; (3) easy-to-use provider-facing interface in the record explaining the key salient results for each patient as well as a separate section with more detailed information; and (4) EHR-integrated real-time alerts associated with genetic risks. On a daily operating room schedule integrated into the EHR, patients who have PGx screening available are identified by a unique icon next to their names. The presence of this icon alerts providers that results are available in the EHR. **Fig. 2**A is an example screenshot of 1 component of a patient's test results, listing each gene screened and the metabolism status of that gene. Based on the genes tested, providers are given information regarding potential drug responses to different pharmacologic categories, including anticoagulation, beta-blockade, sedatives, antiemetics, hypnotics, muscle relaxants, analgesics (opioid and nonopioids), and volatile anesthetics. **Fig. 2**B and C are example screenshots of a patient's thrombosis profile summary and response to analgesic medications, respectively.

WHEN TO PERFORM PHARMACOGENOMICS SCREENING

The time at which to perform PGx screening must take into consideration the time required to obtain the final results in relation to when the patient's surgery is scheduled. In addition, there must be an appropriate amount of allocated time to consent and educate the patient regarding PGx. The preoperative testing clinic (a facility usually run by anesthesiologists and designed to screen patients for appropriateness of surgery) is an ideal location to perform such tasks. At that time, health care providers can perform preoperative behavioral and medical risk assessments to determine appropriateness of PGx testing. Patients at risk for opioid dependence or pharmacologically associated adverse events can be recognized early and PGx may be used to potentially optimize perioperative care. Furthermore, genetics do not change and results may be used for multiple subsequent surgical encounters.

SUMMARY

The use of PGx to personalize perioperative care is promising, but there are several challenges that must be met before this becomes a widespread practice. This article discusses studies in the basic and clinical science showing the association of various genes and response to perioperative medications, both opioid and nonopioid medications. However, more evidence needs to be generated by high-quality large-scale randomized controlled trials to show efficacy and cost-effectiveness. Furthermore, protocols need to be developed that guide perioperative providers on how to interpret genetic testing findings in terms of medication dose adjustment. There is a plethora of results that may be generated from a single PGx screening (especially if there are hundreds/thousands of genes tested), but a detailed presentation of these results to a provider may prove to be useless given the fast-paced nature of the operating room. The presentation of results must be strategically designed so that it proves functional to the providers. In addition, clinical decision support could be integrated into such systems to help improve PGx implementation into the perioperative space. The centerpiece to meet these challenges involves EHR integration, because this is the key to minimally disturbing the clinical flow, easing the visualization and execution of the results to physicians (eg, automated alerts/notifications, clinical decision support, and data visualization), while contributing to the cost-effectiveness of PGx testing.

REFERENCES

1. Gabriel RA, Ehrenfeld JM, Urman RD. Preoperative genetic testing and personalized medicine: changing the care paradigm. J Med Syst 2017;41(12):185.

2. Saba R, Kaye AD, Urman RD. Pharmacogenomics in pain management. Anesthesiol Clin 2017;35(2):295–304.

3. Saba R, Kaye AD, Urman RD. Pharmacogenomics in anesthesia. Anesthesiol Clin 2017;35(2):285–94.

4. Beverly A, Kaye AD, Ljungqvist O, et al. Essential elements of multimodal analgesia in enhanced recovery after surgery (ERAS) guidelines. Anesthesiol Clin 2017;35(2):e115–43.

5. Linares OA, Fudin J, Schiesser WE, et al. CYP2D6 phenotype-specific codeine population pharmacokinetics. J Pain Palliat Care Pharmacother 2015;29(1):4–15.

6. Tateishi T, Krivoruk Y, Ueng YF, et al. Identification of human liver cytochrome P-450 3A4 as the enzyme responsible for fentanyl and sufentanil N-dealkylation. Anesth Analg 1996;82(1):167–72.

7. Feierman DE, Lasker JM. Metabolism of fentanyl, a synthetic opioid analgesic, by human liver microsomes. Role of CYP3A4. Drug Metab Dispos 1996;24(9):932–9.

8. Armstrong SC, Cozza KL. Pharmacokinetic drug interactions of morphine, codeine, and their derivatives: theory and clinical reality, part I. Psychosomatics 2003;44(2):167–71.

9. Crews KR, Gaedigk A, Dunnenberger HM, et al. Clinical pharmacogenetics implementation consortium (CPIC) guidelines for codeine therapy in the context of cytochrome P450 2D6 (CYP2D6) genotype. Clin Pharmacol Ther 2012;91(2):321–6.

10. Lassen D, Damkier P, Brosen K. The pharmacogenetics of tramadol. Clin Pharmacokinet 2015;54(8):825–36.

11. Hutchinson MR, Menelaou A, Foster DJ, et al. CYP2D6 and CYP3A4 involvement in the primary oxidative metabolism of hydrocodone by human liver microsomes. Br J Clin Pharmacol 2004;57(3):287–97.

12. Venkatasubramanian R, Fukuda T, Niu J, et al. ABCC3 and OCT1 genotypes influence pharmacokinetics of morphine in children. Pharmacogenomics 2014; 15(10):1297–309.

13. Sadhasivam S, Chidambaran V, Zhang X, et al. Opioid-induced respiratory depression: ABCB1 transporter pharmacogenetics. Pharmacogenomics J 2015;15(2):119–26.
14. Chidambaran V, Mavi J, Esslinger H, et al. Association of OPRM1 A118G variant with risk of morphine-induced respiratory depression following spine fusion in adolescents. Pharmacogenomics J 2015;15(3):255–62.
15. Zhang F, Tong J, Hu J, et al. COMT gene haplotypes are closely associated with postoperative fentanyl dose in patients. Anesth Analg 2015;120(4):933–40.
16. Benetton SA, Borges VM, Chang TK, et al. Role of individual human cytochrome P450 enzymes in the in vitro metabolism of hydromorphone. Xenobiotica 2004; 34(4):335–44.
17. Bunten H, Liang WJ, Pounder DJ, et al. OPRM1 and CYP2B6 gene variants as risk factors in methadone-related deaths. Clin Pharmacol Ther 2010;88(3):383–9.
18. Bunten H, Liang WJ, Pounder D, et al. CYP2B6 and OPRM1 gene variations predict methadone-related deaths. Addict Biol 2011;16(1):142–4.
19. Hodges LM, Markova SM, Chinn LW, et al. Very important pharmacogene summary: ABCB1 (MDR1, P-glycoprotein). Pharmacogenet Genomics 2011;21(3): 152–61.
20. Kharasch ED, Hoffer C, Whittington D, et al. Role of hepatic and intestinal cytochrome P450 3A and 2B6 in the metabolism, disposition, and miotic effects of methadone. Clin Pharmacol Ther 2004;76(3):250–69.
21. Carlson CL. Effectiveness of the World Health Organization cancer pain relief guidelines: an integrative review. J Pain Res 2016;9:515–34.
22. Lee SS, Buters JT, Pineau T, et al. Role of CYP2E1 in the hepatotoxicity of acetaminophen. J Biol Chem 1996;271(20):12063–7.
23. Yoon E, Babar A, Choudhary M, et al. Acetaminophen-induced hepatotoxicity: a comprehensive update. J Clin Transl Hepatol 2016;4(2):131–42.
24. Tankanitlert J, Morales NP, Howard TA, et al. Effects of combined UDP-glucuronosyltransferase (UGT) 1A1*28 and 1A6*2 on paracetamol pharmacokinetics in beta-thalassemia/HbE. Pharmacology 2007;79(2):97–103.
25. Navarro SL, Chen Y, Li L, et al. UGT1A6 and UGT2B15 polymorphisms and acetaminophen conjugation in response to a randomized, controlled diet of select fruits and vegetables. Drug Metab Dispos 2011;39(9):1650–7.
26. Court MH, Zhu Z, Masse G, et al. Race, gender, and genetic polymorphism contribute to variability in acetaminophen pharmacokinetics, metabolism, and protein-adduct concentrations in healthy African-American and European-American volunteers. J Pharmacol Exp Ther 2017;362(3):431–40.
27. Yamamoto A, Liu MY, Kurogi K, et al. Sulphation of acetaminophen by the human cytosolic sulfotransferases: a systematic analysis. J Biochem 2015;158(6): 497–504.
28. Mazaleuskaya LL, Sangkuhl K, Thorn CF, et al. PharmGKB summary: pathways of acetaminophen metabolism at the therapeutic versus toxic doses. Pharmacogenet Genomics 2015;25(8):416–26.
29. Mazaleuskaya LL, Theken KN, Gong L, et al. PharmGKB summary: ibuprofen pathways. Pharmacogenet Genomics 2015;25(2):96–106.
30. Sullivan-Klose TH, Ghanayem BI, Bell DA, et al. The role of the CYP2C9-Leu359 allelic variant in the tolbutamide polymorphism. Pharmacogenetics 1996;6(4): 341–9.
31. Bowalgaha K, Elliot DJ, Mackenzie PI, et al. S-Naproxen and desmethylnaproxen glucuronidation by human liver microsomes and recombinant human UDP-

glucuronosyltransferases (UGT): role of UGT2B7 in the elimination of naproxen. Br J Clin Pharmacol 2005;60(4):423–33.

32. Agundez JA, Garcia-Martin E, Martinez C. Genetically based impairment in CYP2C8- and CYP2C9-dependent NSAID metabolism as a risk factor for gastro-intestinal bleeding: is a combination of pharmacogenomics and metabolomics required to improve personalized medicine? Expert Opin Drug Metab Toxicol 2009;5(6):607–20.

33. Prieto-Pérez R, Ochoa D, Cabaleiro T, et al. Evaluation of the relationship between polymorphisms in CYP2C8 and CYP2C9 and the pharmacokinetics of celecoxib. J Clin Pharmacol 2013;53(12):1261–7.

34. Wang B, Wang J, Huang SQ, et al. Genetic polymorphism of the human cyto-chrome P450 2C9 gene and its clinical significance. Curr Drug Metab 2009; 10(7):781–834.

35. Chan AT, Zauber AG, Hsu M, et al. Cytochrome P450 2C9 variants influence response to celecoxib for prevention of colorectal adenoma. Gastroenterology 2009;136(7):2127–36.e1.

36. Shin KH, Choi MH, Lim KS, et al. Evaluation of endogenous metabolic markers of hepatic CYP3A activity using metabolic profiling and midazolam clearance. Clin Pharmacol Ther 2013;94(5):601–9.

37. Miao J, Jin Y, Marunde RL, et al. Association of genotypes of the CYP3A cluster with midazolam disposition in vivo. Pharmacogenomics J 2009;9(5):319–26.

38. Cohen M, Sadhasivam S, Vinks AA. Pharmacogenetics in perioperative medi-cine. Curr Opin Anaesthesiol 2012;25(4):419–27.

39. Floyd MD, Gervasini G, Masica AL, et al. Genotype-phenotype associations for common CYP3A4 and CYP3A5 variants in the basal and induced metabolism of midazolam in European- and African-American men and women. Pharmacoge-netics 2003;13(10):595–606.

40. Seng KY, Hee KH, Soon GH, et al. CYP3A5*3 and bilirubin predict midazolam population pharmacokinetics in Asian cancer patients. J Clin Pharmacol 2014; 54(2):215–24.

41. Elens L, Nieuweboer A, Clarke SJ, et al. CYP3A4 intron 6 C>T SNP (CYP3A4*22) encodes lower CYP3A4 activity in cancer patients, as measured with probes mid-azolam and erythromycin. Pharmacogenomics 2013;14(2):137–49.

42. Seo KA, Bae SK, Choi YK, et al. Metabolism of 1'- and 4-hydroxymidazolam by glucuronide conjugation is largely mediated by UDP-glucuronosyltransferases 1A4, 2B4, and 2B7. Drug Metab Dispos 2010;38(11):2007–13.

43. Sawamura R, Sato H, Kawakami J, et al. Inhibitory effect of azole antifungal agents on the glucuronidation of lorazepam using rabbit liver microsomes in vitro. Biol Pharm Bull 2000;23(5):669–71.

44. Herman RJ, Chaudhary A, Szakacs CB. Disposition of lorazepam in Gilbert's syn-drome: effects of fasting, feeding, and enterohepatic circulation. J Clin Pharma-col 1994;34(10):978–84.

45. Dixon CM, Colthup PV, Serabjit-Singh CJ, et al. Multiple forms of cytochrome P450 are involved in the metabolism of ondansetron in humans. Drug Metab Dis-pos 1995;23(11):1225–30.

46. Bell GC, Caudle KE, Whirl-Carrillo M, et al. Clinical Pharmacogenetics Implemen-tation Consortium (CPIC) guideline for CYP2D6 genotype and use of ondansetron and tropisetron. Clin Pharmacol Ther 2017;102(2):213–8.

47. MacKenzie M, Hall R. Pharmacogenomics and pharmacogenetics for the inten-sive care unit: a narrative review. Can J Anaesth 2017;64(1):45–64.

48. He H, Yin JY, Xu YJ, et al. Association of ABCB1 polymorphisms with the efficacy of ondansetron in chemotherapy-induced nausea and vomiting. Clin Ther 2014; 36(8):1242–52.e2.
49. Tzvetkov MV, Saadatmand AR, Bokelmann K, et al. Effects of OCT1 polymorphisms on the cellular uptake, plasma concentrations and efficacy of the 5-HT(3) antagonists tropisetron and ondansetron. Pharmacogenomics J 2012; 12(1):22–9.
50. Parkman HP, Mishra A, Jacobs M, et al. Clinical response and side effects of metoclopramide: associations with clinical, demographic, and pharmacogenetic parameters. J Clin Gastroenterol 2012;46(6):494–503.
51. Perwitasari DA, Gelderblom H, Atthobari J, et al. Anti-emetic drugs in oncology: pharmacology and individualization by pharmacogenetics. Int J Clin Pharm 2011; 33(1):33–43.
52. Yu H, Yan H, Wang L, et al. Five novel loci associated with antipsychotic treatment response in patients with schizophrenia: a genome-wide association study. Lancet Psychiatry 2018;5(4):327–38.
53. Nakamura K, Yokoi T, Inoue K, et al. CYP2D6 is the principal cytochrome P450 responsible for metabolism of the histamine H1 antagonist promethazine in human liver microsomes. Pharmacogenetics 1996;6(5):449–57.
54. Saruwatari J, Matsunaga M, Ikeda K, et al. Impact of CYP2D6*10 on H1-antihistamine-induced hypersomnia. Eur J Clin Pharmacol 2006;62(12): 995–1001.
55. Li J, Wang S, Barone J, et al. Warfarin pharmacogenomics. P T 2009;34(8):422–7.
56. Brown SA, Pereira N. Pharmacogenomic impact of CYP2C19 variation on clopidogrel therapy in precision cardiovascular medicine. J Pers Med 2018; 8(1) [pii:E8].
57. Luzum JA, Sweet KM, Binkley PF, et al. CYP2D6 genetic variation and beta-blocker maintenance dose in patients with heart failure. Pharm Res 2017;34(8): 1615–25.
58. Lymperopoulos A, McCrink KA, Brill A. Impact of CYP2D6 genetic variation on the response of the cardiovascular patient to carvedilol and metoprolol. Curr Drug Metab 2015;17(1):30–6.
59. Gao X, Wang H, Chen H. Impact of CYP2D6 and ADRB1 polymorphisms on heart rate of post-PCI patients treated with metoprolol. Pharmacogenomics 2017. https://doi.org/10.2217/pgs-2017-0203.
60. Dean L. Metoprolol therapy and CYP2D6 genotype. In: Pratt V, McLeod H, Dean L, et al, editors. Medical genetics summaries. Bethesda (MD): National Center for Biotechnology Information (US); 2012.
61. Liem EB, Joiner TV, Tsueda K, et al. Increased sensitivity to thermal pain and reduced subcutaneous lidocaine efficacy in redheads. Anesthesiology 2005; 102(3):509–14.
62. Kim JH, Jarvik GP, Browning BL, et al. Exome sequencing reveals novel rare variants in the ryanodine receptor and calcium channel genes in malignant hyperthermia families. Anesthesiology 2013;119(5):1054–65.
63. Muniz VP, Silva HC, Tsanaclis AM, et al. Screening for mutations in the RYR1 gene in families with malignant hyperthermia. J Mol Neurosci 2003;21(1):35–42.
64. Gonsalves SG, Ng D, Johnston JJ, et al. Using exome data to identify malignant hyperthermia susceptibility mutations. Anesthesiology 2013;119(5):1043–53.
65. Khalil H, Sereika SM, Dai F, et al. OPRM1 and COMT gene-gene interaction is associated with postoperative pain and opioid consumption after orthopedic trauma. Biol Res Nurs 2017;19(2):170–9.

66. Kim KM, Kim HS, Lim SH, et al. Effects of genetic polymorphisms of OPRM1, ABCB1, CYP3A4/5 on postoperative fentanyl consumption in Korean gynecologic patients. Int J Clin Pharmacol Ther 2013;51(5):383–92.

67. Landau R, Liu SK, Blouin JL, et al. The effect of OPRM1 and COMT genotypes on the analgesic response to intravenous fentanyl labor analgesia. Anesth Analg 2013;116(2):386–91.

68. Senagore AJ, Champagne BJ, Dosokey E, et al. Pharmacogenetics-guided analgesics in major abdominal surgery: further benefits within an enhanced recovery protocol. Am J Surg 2017;213(3):467–72.

69. De Gregori M, Diatchenko L, Ingelmo PM, et al. Human genetic variability contributes to postoperative morphine consumption. J Pain 2016;17(5):628–36.

70. Ren ZY, Xu XQ, Bao YP, et al. The impact of genetic variation on sensitivity to opioid analgesics in patients with postoperative pain: a systematic review and meta-analysis. Pain Physician 2015;18(2):131–52.

71. Henker RA, Lewis A, Dai F, et al. The associations between OPRM 1 and COMT genotypes and postoperative pain, opioid use, and opioid-induced sedation. Biol Res Nurs 2013;15(3):309–17.

72. Boswell MV, Stauble ME, Loyd GE, et al. The role of hydromorphone and OPRM1 in postoperative pain relief with hydrocodone. Pain Physician 2013;16(3): E227–35.

73. Ochroch EA, Vachani A, Gottschalk A, et al. Natural variation in the mu-opioid gene OPRM1 predicts increased pain on third day after thoracotomy. Clin J Pain 2012;28(9):747–54.

74. De Gregori M, Garbin G, De Gregori S, et al. Genetic variability at COMT but not at OPRM1 and UGT2B7 loci modulates morphine analgesic response in acute postoperative pain. Eur J Clin Pharmacol 2013;69(9):1651–8.

75. Bartosova O, Polanecky O, Perlik F, et al. OPRM1 and ABCB1 polymorphisms and their effect on postoperative pain relief with piritramide. Physiol Res 2015; 64(Suppl 4):S521–7.

76. Hayashida M, Nagashima M, Satoh Y, et al. Analgesic requirements after major abdominal surgery are associated with OPRM1 gene polymorphism genotype and haplotype. Pharmacogenomics 2008;9(11):1605–16.

77. Zwisler ST, Enggaard TP, Mikkelsen S, et al. Lack of association of OPRM1 and ABCB1 single-nucleotide polymorphisms to oxycodone response in postoperative pain. J Clin Pharmacol 2012;52(2):234–42.

Printed and bound by CPI Group (UK) Ltd, Croydon, CR0 4YY

03/10/2024

01040399-0006